The Effective Clinical Neurologist

סוֹמֵךְ נוֹפְלִ׳ם
וְרוֹפֵא חוֹלִ׳ם
וּמַתִּ׳ר אֲסוּרִ׳ם

Pick up the fallen
Heal the sick
Free chronic sufferers from their bonds
(From a daily Jewish liturgical prayer.)

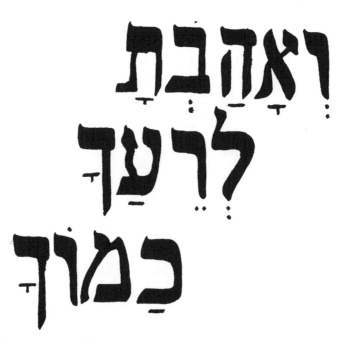

וְאָהַבְתָּ
לְרֵעֲךָ
כָּמוֹךָ

Do unto others as you would have them do unto you (literally, love thy neighbor as thyself).

The Effective Clinical Neurologist

Second Edition

Louis R. Caplan, M.D.
Professor of Neurology, Harvard Medical School, Boston;
Senior Neurologist and Director of Stroke Service,
Beth Israel Deaconess Medical Center, Boston

Joshua Hollander, M.D.
Associate Professor of Neurology, University of Rochester
School of Medicine and Dentistry, Rochester, New York;
Chief of Neurology and Chief of Physical Medicine and
Rehabilitation, Rochester General Hospital

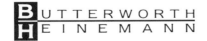

BUTTERWORTH
HEINEMANN

Boston   Oxford   Auckland   Johannesburg   Melbourne   New Delhi

Library of Congress Cataloging-in-Publication Data

Caplan, Louis R.
    The effective clinical neurologist / Louis R. Caplan, Joshua Hollander.—2nd ed.
      p. ; cm.
    Includes bibliographical references and index.
    ISBN 0-7506-7226-9 (pbk. : alk. paper)
    1. Neurology. 2. Physician and patient. 3. Neurologists. I. Hollander, Joshua. II. Title.
    [DNLM: 1. Neurology. WL 21 C244e 2001]
  RC346 C285 2001
  616.8—dc21

                                            2001025380

British Library Cataloguing-in-Publication Data
A catalogue record for this book is available from the British Library.

The publisher offers special discounts on bulk orders of this book.
For information, please contact:

Manager of Special Sales
Butterworth-Heinemann
225 Wildwood Avenue
Woburn, MA 01801-2041
Tel: 781-904-2500
Fax: 781-904-2620

For information on all Butterworth–Heinemann publications available, contact our World Wide Web home page at: http://www.bh.com

10 9 8 7 6 5 4 3 2 1

Printed in the United States of America

Contents

Preface

Joshua Hollander has joined Lou Caplan in writing this second edition of *The Effective Clinical Neurologist*. While we have pursued different paths in neurology, we both have been deeply involved as clinicians in caring for patients and in trying to teach the art and science of patient care to students and trainees. Since 1969, Joshua Hollander has directed a neurology unit at the Rochester General Hospital, an affiliate of the University of Rochester School of Medicine and Dentistry. Lou Caplan, after 14 years of serving as Chairman of Neurology at Tufts University and Neurologist-in-Chief at the New England Medical Center, returned in 1998 to the Beth Israel Deaconess Medical Center and Harvard Medical School—institutions where he began as a staff neurologist in 1970.

Much has happened since publication of the first edition more than a decade ago. Changes in health care have made the practice of medicine more difficult and reduced the ease of effective use of inpatients for training of residents and trainees. Hospital stays are shorter and much of the evaluation is performed outside of the hospital. Hospitals are financially stressed and patient care suffers. Managed care organizations have attempted to reduce specialist involvement as well as dictate protocols for patient evaluation and treatment. Despite these changes, medicine remains an encounter between two individuals—a patient seeking help and a physician rendering care. It is with this approach to this encounter that we attempt to guide our successors.

Careful rereading showed that much of the earlier edition remains timely. This book attempts to convey an approach to the care of neurologic patients, and this approach remains even more important today than it was a decade ago. The purpose stated in the first edition seems in fact more relevant now: "Present medical school and postgraduate education emphasize basic science and the clinical and pathologic features of disease. Often lost sight of in the morass of organs, symptoms, signs, tests, procedures, and drugs are the *patient* as a person dealing with illness, the *physician* struggling to apply science to the patient, and the *interaction* of the patient and the physician. Training programs and their faculty are often so focused on research that the training of medical students and house officers to effectively and humanely care for patients becomes a lesser priority far below research goals. No available books teach young physicians how to be effective clinicians-neurologists or, for that matter, clinicians in any field."

Changes in the text were needed to reflect the changes in patient care that have occurred since the first edition was written. The book is divided into three parts. The first part serves as an introduction to the role of the clinician-neurologist. The second part thoroughly discusses all aspects of the doctor-patient interaction beginning with the initial encounter and continuing with history taking, examination, selecting and interpreting investigations, selecting treatment, record keeping, and physician information-giving and interactions with the patient. Examples are used widely and new cases have been introduced. We have expanded the examination section but still emphasize a personalized approach. The section on neurologic investigations has been greatly expanded and updated to account for the dramatic changes in technology. The third part of the book discusses various types and sites of care, including hospitals, outpatient areas, and consultations. Academic considerations, house officer training, and medicolegal issues are also given attention. We have added material related to managed care but have tried to be concise in these discussions.

We hope that this edition will also prove of practical use for young physicians and students planning careers in clinical medicine, especially those who will care for patients with neurologic problems. Patient care remains an extremely worthy if demanding endeavor. This book should also interest physicians, educators, and senior neurologists who have responsibility for the teaching and training of clinicians and neurologists.

Louis R. Caplan
Joshua Hollander

Acknowledgments

I wish to thank my mentors and early role models in internal medicine training: Drs. Eph Lisansky, Ted Woodward, Maurice Pincoffs, T. Nelson Carey, and Phillip Tumulty; my successive chiefs of medicine, all remarkable scientists, teachers, and people: Drs. Howard Hiatt, Frank Epstein, Lou Sherwood, Jordan Cohen, and Shelly Wolfe; and my teachers in neurology: Drs. Charles Van Buskirk, Derek Denny-Brown, Miller Fisher, Raymond Adams, John Sullivan, Joe Foley, Rick Tyler, and Pierson Richardson. I thank my students, residents, and fellows at Harvard, the University of Chicago, and Tufts, and coworkers at the Beth Israel Deaconess Medical Center and the New England Medical Center in Boston as well as at the Michael Reese Hospital in Chicago for their stimulation, insights, help, and support over the years. Most of all, I thank my patients whose illnesses, personalities, strengths, and weaknesses have taught me so much about disease, caring, and life. My continuing debt to these patients can never be repaid. This book is dedicated to them. It will be successful if in any minute degree it helps in the care of future patients.

I thank Drs. Ron Cranford, Don Aaronson, Sara Charles, and Richard Beresford for reviewing and commenting on the medicolegal issues in Chapter 14. I am very grateful to Drs. Larry Levitt, Marty Samuels, Alex Reeves, and Matt Menken for reviewing the entire text of the first edition and making thoughtful suggestions.

Louis R. Caplan

It seems appropriate to acknowledge those physicians who were my teachers over many years. At Columbia, Robert Loeb and Kermit Pines taught me internal medicine, and exposure to H. Houston Merritt, Robert Fishman, and Lewis Rowland led me to pursue neurology. At Vanderbilt, David Rogers was my Chief of Medicine, and Bertram Sprofkin continued to keep me interested in neurology. C. Miller Fisher, Raymond Adams, and Pierson Richardson taught me neurology during my resident years. My colleagues have allowed me to share in the care of their patients. The patients are what the clinical endeavor is about and I owe them much. In Rochester, Robert Joynt has continued to be a source of fact and philosophy. Gerald Honch, a true clinician, and Sheila Hollander have recognized my failings and tolerated me nonetheless.

Thirty years of residents and students continue to ask questions, the answers to which I do not always know. While humbling, it keeps me young.

Joshua Hollander

Introduction

One of the essential qualities of the clinician is interest in humanity, for the secret of the care of the patient is in caring for the patient.[1]
—FRANCIS W. PEABODY, M.D.

The patient, like art, is bigger than we are. He will have the last word. He will outlast us. His pain will be ours, and his terror, and his hopes, and finally, perhaps, his illness. For what are we all, ultimately, but patients.[2]
—JOHN H. STONE, M.D.

This book is about the practice of clinical neurology and medicine. Though aimed primarily at the young neurologist, most of the principles apply equally to internal medicine and the other nonsurgical specialties. In this age of an ever-growing deluge of journals and books, why another book on doctoring? What made us write this book and why now?

THE PRESENT THREAT TO CLINICAL MEDICINE

First of all, we are very worried about the future of clinical medicine, as we now know it. The last decade has witnessed profound and rapid changes in the delivery of health care that in our minds threaten extinction of the clinical art of medicine. High costs have led to increased involvement in health care delivery by government, industry, and entrepreneurs who have created a potpourri of acronyms like HMOs and PPOs (health maintenance organizations and preferred provider organizations) and jingles like "docs in a box" (referring to commercial emergency stations). Patient care has become an economically oriented impersonal business. Congressional legislation in health care has recently been limited to large budget bills. Solo private practitioners are having more and more trouble competing financially and view themselves as a threatened species.

The revolution in technology has undoubtedly improved the physician's ability to diagnose illness but has also led to changes in economic incentives. Procedures and tests usually occupy little of the practicing physician's time but pay a lot more than time spent with the patient in traditional clinical tasks such as eliciting a detailed history, performing a careful physical examination, and discussing the findings and treatment plan leisurely and empathetically with the patient.

These factors threaten the art of medicine, but there are some forces on the horizon that could promote the quality of clinical encounters. The predicted surplus of physicians means fewer patients and patient encounters for many doctors but allows more time for each patient and for educational pursuits. Also, exploration of a change in physician payment mandated by Congress and called relative value scales (RVS) may lead to an upgrading in reimbursement for cognitive as opposed to procedural services. This change should have given more incentive for spending time with the patient. If a book needs to be written about the clinical art of medicine, now is the time to do it, before the chance is hopelessly lost.

THE FAILURE OF PRESENT TRAINING

The second impetus for a book on this subject is our perception and fear that somehow our medical schools and training programs (including those programs at Harvard, University of Chicago, and University of Rochester) do not prepare young physicians well for clinical practice. Most training in the "clinical" years of medical school and during internship and residency is on inpatient services (perhaps better termed in today's climate *impatient* services) in large teaching hospitals. The wards, intensive care units, and rooms of these institutions are now filled with very sick patients with serious cardiac, neurologic, and neoplastic diseases. Many diagnostic tests have been performed on these patients before admission so that patients come with attached diagnostic labels; and economic pressures have caused preprogrammed evaluation and treatment and a hurried, often not subtle, push out the door. There is little opportunity for the student or house officer to think out, plan, or review diagnostic evaluation or treatment. Moreover, the illnesses and patients seen in the hospital are by no means representative of those seen in doctors' offices and outpatient clinics, which means that doctors have little opportunity during training to become well-acquainted with the diseases they will probably encounter in practice.

As frequent examiners for the oral board examinations for certification in neurology, we are discouraged that fully trained neurologists often fail to acquire important clinical information and cannot assimilate clinical data to formulate differential diagnoses and cogent, practical evaluation and treatment plans. If they are not shown or told about the results of a computed tomography (CT) or magnetic resonance imaging (MRI) scan, many neurologists' chances of finding a diagnosis are sunk. As a member of the Patient Safety Committee of the Council of Medical Specialty Societies, one of us has had an opportunity to review data on malpractice claims and cases: a frighteningly increasing number of claims relate to the physician's failure to think of the diagnosis and to communicate meaningfully with the patient. How many medical schools or residency training programs instruct trainees in the art of delivering an effective summation interview to patients leaving the hospital or after an office evaluation or consultation?

As experienced attending physicians, we find that even very good, caring residents seem to know very little about the patients they care for—their occupations, accomplishments, families, hopes, problems, fears, and aspirations. The sick person in a hospital gown has been yanked from his or her customary environment and surrounded by a very complex array of potentially fearful machines and people. It is hard for anyone to catch a glimmer of the banker, teacher, lawyer, mother, or doctor in that person huddled in bed. Physicians need to be able to view and treat patients as whole people.

It has become fashionable now for neurology departments to change their title to Department of Neuroscience. No one would dispute the need for more scientists, especially neuroscientists, but we also badly need physicians. The training of scientists and physicians is not identical. This book is aimed at the medical student, the resident, and the beginning practitioner and clinician. For years, we have sought a book to give neurology residents about the art of caring for the patient. L.R.C. used to give Tumulty's book, *The Effective Clinician*,[3] to graduating residents. It is a fine book, but exclusively devoted to internal medicine with little neurology. This book is now out of print and is no longer available.

THE PATIENT

Finally, this book is written with the patient in mind. As Stone noted so aptly in the quotation at the beginning of this Introduction, ultimately we all are patients. Published letters from physicians about medical care delivered to themselves[4] or their families attest to increasing impersonalization and a failure of communication in our present system. Somehow in the race for success in science, we are leaving behind the patient. There is no inherent competitiveness or reciprocity between the science and art of medicine. Without a knowledge of science, a compassionate wish to improve the health of mankind is meaningless. But as Blumgart said, "Scientific knowledge without wisdom is a frozen storehouse."[5] The increased complexity of technology and diagnostic and treatment options makes even more critical the physician's skill in managing illness and the art of communicating with patients and their loved ones. There but for the grace of God go we all, for all of us and our families are or will eventually become patients. L.R.C. recently had to cross over the line to become a health care consumer, a patient—a state that he did not want or like, despite the ministrations of caring physicians. But the experience as a patient, we believe, helps us to be better doctors. Unfortunately, we cannot force all of our students and trainees to become patients during their apprenticeships (though perhaps we can and should do the next best thing: that is, ask them to work as nursing assistants ministering to the sick on an intimate level). If we had to transmit the art of medicine in a single sentence, the two best candidates in our opinion would be Peabody's famous dictum, "The secret of the care of the patient is in caring for the patient" and the Golden Rule, "Do unto others as you would have them do unto you."

ORGANIZATION AND STYLE

The text is divided into three main sections. The first is a short essay on the essence of being a clinician and the special aspects of being an effective clinical neurologist. The second part, the core of the book, focuses on the neurologist-patient interface. We have pointed a closeup camera lens at these two major dramatis personae of medical care, following them from their introduction, through the diagnostic process, treatment, and follow-up care. Communication is emphasized. Case examples are sprinkled liberally throughout to illustrate the method, lend a pragmatic tone, and clarify problems and suggestions. Though neurologic problems and patients with nervous system disease are emphasized, the concepts are applicable to all specialists and all patients.

The third part enlarges the scene to include different situations and settings of care and the other major actors in the drama. The hospital and ambulatory settings are explored, followed by an analysis of consultations, the main activity of many neurologists and other specialists. Neurologists have traditionally been academicians whose activities emanated from teaching hospitals and medical centers. Though many neurologists have spread out into the community, academic relationships and influences are still very strong. For this reason, and because we are lifelong academics who have thought long and hard about teaching and research, we could not omit this important sphere of influence. This section closes with a glance at the legal aspects of care, the neurologist-lawyer interface, and the neurologist in court.

Some of the chapters partially overlap, making some repetition unavoidable. Though we have tried to minimize replication, some degree of repetition is a very useful teaching device. We recall as medical students being convinced that something was important only when it was taught a second, third, or even fourth time. Consultations are discussed in the chapters on inpatient and ambulatory care and academic concerns, as well as receiving a more complete coverage in the chapter on consultations. Communications, a central theme of the book, are considered in many chapters as well as in the section devoted solely to this key topic. Though these and other general subjects are reintroduced often, we have attempted to consider various aspects from differing angles and have tried to avoid being redundant. We have also omitted consideration of pediatric neurology because of our meager experience.

REFERENCES

1. Peabody EW. The care of the patient. *JAMA* 1927;88:872–882.
2. Stone JH. The patient as art. *The Pharos of Alpha Omega Alpha* 1974;37:9–31.
3. Tumulty PA. *The Effective Clinician: His Methods and Approach to Diagnosis and Care*. Philadelphia: W.B. Saunders Co., 1973.
4. Rabin U, Rabin PL, Rabin R. Compounding the ordeal of ALS: Isolation from my fellow physicians. *N Engl J Med* 1982;307:5–9.
5. Blumgart HL. Caring for the patient. *N Engl J Med* 1964;270:449–456.

PART I

The Clinician-Neurologist

One of the essential qualities of the clinician is interest in humanity, for the secret of the care of the patient is in caring for the patient.

This book is about clinical neurologists, and we thought it best to begin by describing them and what they do. We first discuss the derivation of the term *clinical*, its modern usage, and the way we use the term *clinician* throughout the book. We next turn to the neurologist and describe and define the special approach recommended to effectively diagnose and manage patients with diseases of the nervous system.

1

The Clinician-Neurologist: Scope, Methods, and Uniqueness

A clinician is one whose prime function is to manage a sick person with the purpose of alleviating the total effect of his illness.[1,2]

—PHILLIP TUMULTY

The competent internist "understands the distinction between *disease*, as a set of biologic events, and *illness* as a complex human event, characterized by symptoms and other discomforts and representing the interaction of a person with his or her pre-existing physical and psychosocial characteristics, with a set of environmental events which often take the form of a disease. This orientation to the sick *person* as well as the sick *organ*, encourages restraint in the use of technology to resolve clinical problems.[3]

—JEREMIAH BARONDESS

Watson: You speak of danger. You have evidently seen more in these rooms than was visible to me.
Holmes: No, but I fancy that I may have deducted a little more. I imagine that you saw all that I did.[4]

—A. CONAN DOYLE

THE CLINICIAN

The word *clinic* is derived from the Greek term *klinicos*, pertaining to a bed. The adjective "clinical" came to mean activity centered about the bedside because in early times physicians were consulted as a last resort only when the sufferer was too sick to get out of bed. Later, when most patient-doctor encounters involved ambulatory people, the usage was broadened to include any activity that related directly to the patient. By definition, a clinician is someone who works with patients, but the adjective when applied to a physician usually implies praise. When we describe someone as a "clinician," we mean that he or she has particular skills in diagnosis and patient interactions.

3

Accurate diagnosis is central, but not absolutely essential, to a physician's success. Many clinicians, especially neurologists, are most stimulated by the intellectual challenge of deducing the cause of the patient's symptoms. Like Sherlock Holmes, himself modeled after a skilled physician, a clinician sleuth avidly hunts possible clues during the clinical encounter. The hunt begins with an analysis of the patient's dress, comportment, mood, style, and body signals. The physician listens carefully as the patient spontaneously describes his or her problems and self, and then interprets the patient's responses to the physician's pointed queries, comments, and pauses. Then the detective physician conducts a meticulous general and neurologic examination, testing clues, hunches, and theories generated by the history. Finally, the medical sleuth uses information from laboratory, imaging, and physiologic investigations to arrive at a complete differential diagnosis and a quantitative estimate of the probability of various pathologies. The clinician is versatile enough to use any and all available information as clues to the diagnosis. In some patients, the diagnosis comes mostly from the history, in another patient from an unexpected finding on examination, and in still others from careful analysis of a brain imaging abnormality.

The diagnosis should include not only the causes of present and past diseases but also an analysis of illness in its broadest sense as Barondess has described it. The clinician seeks information and clues from the patient, associates, and family (the patient's environment) as to how the symptoms and signs have affected the patient. How has the problem perturbed the patient's milieu? How have the patient's activities, attitudes, and feelings changed and how has the environment responded?

The complete clinician, as Tumulty suggests, is not just a superb diagnostician. Diagnosis is futile if it does not in some way help the patient and those in the patient's environment understand and deal with the illness. Optimally, accurate diagnosis will lead to curative treatment but everyone with experience in dealing with patients with medical and neurological diseases knows that true cures are few and far between. Doctors remember vividly with a smile and with pride the handful of patients who have dramatically and fully recovered because of their treatment. Patients with pernicious anemia, pneumococcal pneumonia, myxedema, colloid cysts of the third ventricle, and normal pressure hydrocephalus can often be cured if we are clever enough to make the correct diagnosis. Most diseases, however, are either chronic or less easily remediable. Loeb has been quoted as attributing human ailments to one or more of three basic faults: "Bad make, bad luck, and worn out." Doctors often feel like Hans Brinker temporarily plugging the floodgates with their fingers but knowing that they are just delaying the inevitable ravages of genetic programming, time, and disease.

The effective clinician plans specific treatment for the specific pathologies and pathophysiologies found in the individual patient. Most important is the doctor's ability to communicate skillfully and simply with the patient. It is important to explain to the patient the nature of the problem, the alternatives for treatment, and the reasons why particular advice has been given. The physician must also monitor the patient's understanding of explanations and advice. The true clinician helps the patient, family, friends, and caretakers understand what is wrong, what is likely to happen, how the problem will affect the patient and themselves, and how they might best respond. The clinician manages, advises, and befriends the patient in a time of need.

THE NEUROLOGIST AND NEUROLOGIC DIAGNOSIS[5]

"The proper study of mankind is man's brain; the ultimate purpose of the practice of medicine is to protect the brain."[6]

—FRED PLUM, M.D.

What Distinguishes Neurologists from Other Medical Specialists?

Neurology has been called by some the queen of clinical disciplines. Although the neurologist is really just a subspecialist in internal medicine with training, experience, and expertise in diseases of the nervous system, there are definite differences between neurology and other medical specialties. In our opinion, the three major distinctions are:

1. In neurology, *anatomy*, especially neuroanatomy, is of prime importance. Neurologists have a compulsive preoccupation with the anatomy of disease not shared by most general practitioners and internists. The nervous system is made of heterogeneous parts. Who could imagine body parts as different as the brain, spinal cord, peripheral nerves, and muscles? Each component of the nervous system is very distinct and made of diverse subunits with different appearances, functions, and susceptibilities to various diseases. In contrast, most other internal organs are more homogeneous. The parts of the lung, liver, pancreas, spleen, and bone marrow all look alike and have identical functions. In these organs, disease is determined by the amount of the organ rendered dysfunctional, not by the location or the anatomy of the illness.
2. The *neurological examination* when thoroughly and carefully performed is more complex and time consuming than the rest of the physical examination.
3. After the clinical encounter (the traditional history and physical examination), the skillful neurologist is able to arrive at a relatively *accurate differential diagnosis* more often than in other branches of clinical medicine.

In other medical specialties, for example, hematology, endocrinology, and gastroenterology, laboratory analyses of blood and body fluids and radiologic tests play a relatively more important role in suggesting the initial diagnostic considerations. How does a hematologist fare without a blood count or a glimpse at a blood smear? How well does a nephrologist do without knowledge of the blood urea nitrogen, creatinine, and electrolytes and without looking at the urine? How well does a gastroenterologist do without X-rays of the intestinal tract or the results of liver function tests? In neurology, imaging and other radiologic, physiologic, and laboratory procedures refine and elaborate on the diagnostic impression derived from the clinical encounter. Neurologists have the potential to learn more with their eyes, ears, hands, and minds without benefit of technology than most other medical specialists. The converse, of course, is also all too true: if neurologists have not hit on the correct differential diagnosis and disease anatomy after the clinical encounter with a patient, they are often hopelessly lost. It has been said that the true neurologist is one who can make a diagnosis when there has been a power failure. Put another way, in neurology, more rides on the clinical encounter and its interpretation than in any other specialty.

Is the Neurologist's Compulsion with Anatomy Reasonable and Justified?

The emphasis on anatomy, a fascination with the structure of the human brain and nervous system as the highest pinnacle of primate development, and the systematic logic of the neurologic clinical encounter are probably the major factors that attract physicians to neurology. Is the compulsion and concentration on anatomy justified? Is the desire to localize lesions precisely merely academic hair splitting (intellectual and pedagogical masturbation) or are there practical, pragmatic reasons for needing to know where the lesion is? Have newer imaging technologies such as computed tomography (CT) and magnetic resonance imaging (MRI) made clinical localization obsolete? We are firmly convinced that clinical localization is still of paramount importance in patient care and its importance has even increased in the CT/MRI era. There is some truth in the jest that only two indications for a neurologic consultation remain: (1) A positive imaging study and (2) a negative imaging study. Primary care physicians often do not try to localize the lesion and as a result may image the wrong part of the neuraxis or they may order tests not suitable for the most likely disease process.

Some Brain and Spinal Lesions Are Not Imaged Well by CT or MRI

A neurosurgeon asked one of us (L.R.C.) to consult on a patient who had recently noticed weakness of her right arm and leg. A CT scan had shown a single discrete, well-demarcated lesion that enhanced after intravenous contrast and was located in the region of the left precentral gyrus near the midline. Local mass effect was present, but the scan was otherwise normal. Clinical examination showed the expected right hemiparesis with moderate weakness of the right lower extremity and shoulder. The hand and leg were strong, and language function was normal. Unexpectedly, there was also a left upper quadrantanopia when visual fields were mapped by confrontation testing using a small white pin, and the patient had great difficulty in drawing a house, or copying a complex figure. There was clearly a lesion present at the right temporo-parietal junction detectable by bedside findings but not imaged by CT. L.R.C. urged the neurosurgeon to delay the planned surgical procedure that would remove the left cerebral hemisphere lesion. Subsequent investigation showed a renal cell carcinoma. Later CT also documented a deep right posterior temporal metastasis.

Transient ischemic attacks are usually not visualized by neuroimaging tests. Patients are commonly referred for seizure disorders with extensive imaging studies without electroencephalography. Lumbar spine imaging continues to be requested for possible spinal cord compression because the legs are weak without considering that the cord ends high in the lumbar area and an effort at establishing a sensory level might define the correct thoracic area to image. Of course, the most accurate cerebral imaging technology will not give useful information about a lesion in the spinal cord, peripheral nerves, or muscles.

Clinical Localization Allows Selection of the Best Imaging and Physiological Tests to Refine the Clinical Diagnosis

For cervical spinal cord disease, these tests might include plain X-rays of the cervical spine, neck CT or MRI, cervical myelography, or somatosensory evoked potentials. This evaluation schema would not only be inappropriate, but useless for lesions in the brainstem, cerebrum, or even the more caudal spinal cord. Consider a patient with a suspected vascular occlusive lesion affecting the left medulla that caused right limb weakness. The clinician will want to know the results of noninvasive ultrasound recordings from the left subclavian artery and the extracranial and intracranial left vertebral artery. Improved techniques in MR angiography and CT angiography may show the intraosseous segment of the vertebral arteries that was previously terra incognita for noninvasive studies. If angiography is needed, the left vertebral artery should be opacified first.[7] If in the same patient the right hemiparesis was due to left cerebral ischemia, the left common and internal carotid artery should be studied noninvasively and be opacified first at angiography.

Operations on the brain and spinal cord are quite different from abdominal or chest surgery. The presence of the bony skull and vertebral column dictate the need for precise preoperative localization rather than simply exploring the abdomen after a midline surgical incision.

The Location of a Lesion Often Tells What the Lesion Is Most Likely to Be

Let's consider a patient with weakness of all four limbs. If the weakness is due to a myopathy, the differential diagnosis would be completely different from that of a severe peripheral neuropathy causing weakness. Lesions of the brainstem, bilateral cerebral hemispheres, or spinal cord also can cause quadriparesis but the diagnostic considerations would be quite different for all of these three regions and completely different from diseases likely to cause myopathy or neuropathy. Occasionally, the clinical localization accurately predicts the probable pathology. A young woman with fatigue and frontal headache stops menstruating. You find a bitemporal hemianopia on examination, localizing the process to the optic chiasm. The probability is quite high that this patient has a pituitary tumor. Another patient, an elderly woman who cannot provide details of her illness had a left Horner's syndrome, loss of pain and temperature sensation on the left face and right body and limbs, left limb incoordination, hoarseness, and weakness of the left larynx and left pharynx. These findings clearly indicate a lesion in the left lateral medulla. The probability is very high that she has a lateral medullary infarct caused by occlusion of her left intracranial vertebral artery.

Knowing the Clinical Signs in Patients Whose Anatomy Has Been Defined by Brain Imaging Helps Localization in Patients with Similar Clinical Findings Even without Neuroimaging Tests

Localization also helps us learn how that part of the nervous system works. What could be more stimulating or challenging than understanding the human brain, for how can one understand human thought and behavior without coming to grips with the brain? Contrary to the beliefs of Galen and other ancients, the character, personality, intelligence, and actions of a person are surely more related to the function of the brain than to their lungs, liver, heart, pancreas, or humors.

WHAT ARE THE MAIN STRATEGIES AND RULES THE NEUROLOGIST USES?

Like any successful clinician, the neurologist must pay attention to the person and the environment to manage illness as Barondess has defined it. The major differences in strategy center around the diagnostic process. In our opinion, there are three basic rules of diagnosis essential for the neurologist (and also applicable for other clinicians):

1. The neurologist should always ask *what* is the disease mechanism and *where* is it located? These two queries should be pursued concurrently.
2. The neurologist generates and tests hypotheses, gradually refining them at each phase of the clinical encounter. During and after the history, during and after the general and neurological examination, and after each planned test or series of laboratory investigations, the skilled neurologist models and refines the anatomical and disease diagnoses much like a sculptor gradually chips away at the marble, slowly allowing a face to emerge.
3. The neurologist thinks in terms of probabilities, not absolutes. How likely is a particular diagnosis—80 percent, 50 percent? What are other possible diagnoses, and what is their probability of being correct?

What Data Help Answer the Question of What Disease Mechanism Is Operant in the Patient?

Disease mechanism simply refers to the pathologic entity or pathophysiology of the disease causing the patient's symptoms, signs, and laboratory abnormalities. The major clues as to what is wrong come from the history. See the following sections for what the data include.

The Demography of the Patient

Age, sex, and race affect the chances of a patient having a particular disease. A focal brain lesion in an elderly man has a different set of etiologic probabilities than a similar lesion in a young girl. Where the patient lives also affects probabilities. Multiple sclerosis is much more common in Minnesota and Great Britain than in Northern Africa or Central America. Cysticercosis is more common in Mexico and Los Angeles than in Wisconsin. Lyme disease is a leading possibility on Nantucket Island but deer ticks in Rochester, NY are not yet known to have acquired the causative organism.

The "Ecology" of the Patient's Illness

A patient's previous personal history and prior illnesses yield clues to the diagnosis. The presence of known lung cancer greatly increases the probability that neurological symptoms are due to direct spread or metastasis from the tumor or to an indirect effect of the cancer. An older man with a past history of coronary artery and peripheral vascular occlusive disease who develops a left hemiparesis has a high probability of having had a stroke due to either atherosclerotic disease of the right carotid artery or cardiogenic embolism. A patient with diagnosed systemic lupus erythematosus who becomes confused most likely has a steroid psychosis, a bleed into the brain caused by thrombocytopenia, or an infarct related to lupus anticoagulant or other coagulopathy, or an autoimmune encephalopathy.

The Family History, Occupation, and Exposures of the Patient to Various Risk Factors

These factors also affect disease probabilities. The data mentioned so far do not include the symptoms of the present illness; they include only demographic information about the patient and his or her past medical illnesses and environment. This information is often available even before the neurologist sees the patient and may have already been communicated by the physician or person arranging the visit or consultation. We call the accumulation of these data *a priori odds.*[8]

Suppose, as a neurologist, you are called by an internist from the emergency room who asks you to come down and consult for her patient, a 38-year-old woman with rheumatic mitral stenosis and atrial fibrillation who has developed weakness of the left arm. Without knowing any of the specifics of the recent symptoms, you mentally note the high probability that her nervous system lesion is due to a brain embolus from her known heart disease. Were the patient a 27-year-old homosexual playwright who had mental status changes, your a priori bet would be that his problem was related to AIDS. Of course, the a priori odds are just probability guesses that may have little relation to the present problem. The young woman with rheumatic heart disease could have slept on her arm, causing a radial nerve palsy, and the playwright could have been mugged, causing a head injury. Unfortunately, many nonneurologists rest their diagnoses entirely on these a priori odds—a kind of guilt by association. The neurologist just uses the a priori odds to suggest hypotheses worth pursuing during the clinical encounter. The hypotheses generated can be confirmed or rejected, depending on further information about the present problem.

The Onset of the Present Symptoms
Some diseases begin abruptly during activity (for example, cerebral hemorrhages or embolism), and others are more likely to be noticed during the night or on arising (such as cerebral thrombosis or carpal tunnel syndrome).

The Course of the Illness
In our opinion, this is the most essential item of historical data. A sudden onset brain lesion that is maximal at onset, improves, and clears quickly is most likely due to a brain embolus, whereas focal signs that develop and evolve during months and are gradually progressive are more likely due to tumor. Symptoms that progress gradually and inexorably during years are often due to degenerative disease. In multiple sclerosis, the neurologic deficit often advances during a period of days to a few weeks, stabilizes, then gradually remits, a time course unlike most other neurologic conditions. Because the establishment of the course of illness is so crucial to diagnosis, we will have much more to say about it in Chapter 3, which discusses history taking.

Accompanying General or Neurologic Symptoms
Symptoms such as fever, jaundice, malaise, headache, seizures, and loss of consciousness also contribute heavily to accurate diagnosis.

How Does the Neurologist Tell Where the Lesion Is?

The data that tell the doctor the location of the lesion (where?) are different than information that tells the nature of the lesion (what?). The most important information for localization of a lesion comes from the neurological examination and the results of imaging and physiological tests. The patient's account of the nature, as opposed to the timing, of the neurologic symptoms is also very helpful and may be the only available data in patients who have recovered from temporary symptoms. The patient may also perceive subtle deviations from normal before abnormalities are evident on examination. Tingling, altered somatic or visual perception, and unaccustomed imprecision in speech are often described by patients despite the fact that neurological examination is not sensitive enough to detect definite abnormalities in these spheres. Some general localization principles are as follows.

Some Symptoms or Signs Are Quite Specific for Certain Regions

Abnormal speech output characterized by the use of wrong words and poor comprehension and repetition of spoken language is diagnostic of a dominant hemisphere (usually left) temporal lobe lesion. Lights or unformed colored objects seen transiently but repeatedly in the left upper quadrant of vision with both eyes is diagnostic of a lesion in the lower bank of the right calcarine fissure.

The Distribution of the Particular Symptoms or Signs Helps Localize the Lesion

Weakness limited to the left abductor pollicis brevis, opponens pollicis, and first two lumbrical muscles is diagnostic of a left median nerve lesion. The patient who reports tingling in the little finger and the medial half of the fourth finger, which stops abruptly at the palmar crease nearly always has an ulnar neuropathy. Weakness of the left face and hand with increased left deep tendon reflexes and an extensor plantar reflex on the left means a lesion in or beneath the right precentral gyrus in the perisylvian area controlling the face and hand.

Combinations of Findings ("Fellow Travelers") Help Localize a Deficit

The strategy of trying to localize a lesion might be compared to trying to locate a car on a long road. Specific landmarks such as a restaurant, cross street, or traffic light are sought. Let us consider the example of a patient with loss of pin sensation in the left arm and leg. If she also had a left hemianopia, the localization would have to be in the posterior portion of the right cerebral hemisphere (or two separate unrelated lesions). If, however, she had also had loss of pin sensation in the right face, right palatal weakness, right arm and leg ataxia, and nystagmus, the lesion would have to be in the right lateral medulla. Each symptom or sign should not be considered merely as an individual complaint but instead the neurologist should try to define a locus or loci in the nervous system where these symptoms and signs may all localize.

The Topography of Local Symptoms Is Also Helpful in Localization

Headache in the forehead usually indicates a supratentorial lesion, but pain in the occiput or neck more often indicates an infratentorial posterior fossa localization. Pain and tenderness in the third thoracic vertebrae in a patient with paraparesis almost always suggests an extradural lesion at that location. Pain and tenderness in the left lower abdomen in a patient with left psoas and quadriceps muscle weakness makes it likely that the disease process affecting the left femoral nerve is located near the left psoas region.

The clinician generates and tests anatomical hypotheses during the history and examination much as he or she has tested disease mechanism hypotheses during the history. These anatomical hypotheses can usually be further refined or tested by neuroimaging or physiological tests.

Sequential Hypothesis Generation and Testing

Medical students may think of the clinical encounter as a passive, rote accumulation and recording of specific data items. They visualize a process much like filling out a checklist or completing a questionnaire. Then, after all the information is obtained, analysis and interpretation should lead to the correct answer. Medical students, to the surprise of many, seem to do as well as, in fact usually better than, seasoned clinicians in arriving at the correct diagnosis in the weekly clinicopathological conferences in the *New England Journal of Medicine*.[9] Given a written protocol containing the facts from the clinical encounter and laboratory tests and having readily available a library and able clinical teachers, intelligent students can deduce the diagnoses in this intellectual exercise.

Naiveté about the method of reaching a diagnosis is not limited to students. Some medical faculty members teach students to accumulate all data prior to systematic analysis. Weed described the major function of the ward attending physician as sitting in a conference room reviewing the problem lists generated by the students and house staff, using his or her own experience and savvy to teach interpretation of the data base.[10] We could not disagree more. The most difficult clinical task is generation of the relevant clinical data, not its interpretation.

We graybeards, and virtually every medical student and house officer, can vividly recall innumerable examples of "being taken to school" by an experienced clinician. The attending physician comes on the ward and in just a few minutes uncovers some new key information from the history, physical, or neurological examination that had been completely missed by the medical student and resident despite much longer previous exposure and interaction with the patient. These moments are indeed embarrassing, but instructive.

The secret is the method of approach. Generation of clinical data is not passive, but involves very active thought from the minute the physician meets the patient. The experienced physician thinking of a particular anatomical localization or a disease mechanism asks the patient questions that will test hypotheses he or she has in mind.

Patients are very naive about the workings of their own bodies, especially their nervous systems, and they are often just as naive about the behavior of disease. Most patients with weakness or numbness in the left arm attribute the problem to a local process within that limb. They would not ordinarily spontaneously volunteer the occurrence of a temporary buckling of the left leg a month before, thinking the two problems completely unrelated. Surely, the same patient would be unlikely to relate the occurrence of transient monocular blindness in the right eye unless specifically asked about visual loss in the eyes. Patients often mentally divide up their bodies into the domains of various different specialists. Eye symptoms are brought to their ophthalmologists and "female problems" to their gynecologists. Patients don't know what to tell the neurologist. By generating anatomical hypotheses, the clinician-neurologist asks the questions that will most likely lead to accurate localization. *It takes more experience to know which questions to ask than to provide answers.* Experience allows efficient interaction with the patient to ensure collection of all important relevant data. Data collection cannot be limited to a conference room.

The physician begins to generate hypotheses even before meeting the patient. These are based on information provided by the referring physician or layperson. We have already referred to probabilities suggested by this information as a priori odds. After the long initial statement of the problem by the patient, the physician begins to test these previous a priori hypotheses and new ones suggested by the patient's initial remarks. After asking a series of penetrating questions, by following and listening carefully and digesting the responses, the physician begins to organize and rate the hypotheses. When the history is completed, often while the patient is undressing, the physician should mentally list the active hypotheses about the disease mechanism and the clinical localization and be ready to test these during the examination.

As with the history, new, often unexpected findings are noted during the examination that alter previous hypotheses, change probabilities, or suggest new ideas. The findings can come from the general examination: A very high blood pressure, an unexpected black cutaneous lesion on the foot resembling a melanoma, clubbed fingers, or a loud carotid bruit or heart murmur will obviously be important. Unexpected neurologic findings such as papilledema, an extensor plantar response, or tongue fasciculations also will usually change the physician's thinking and somehow must be integrated into the working hypotheses. During the examination, the alert clinician often returns to points in the history for clarification, and new examination findings may suggest historical questions not already asked.

After the examination, the clinician should pause and again generate a modified list of diagnostic probabilities for both disease mechanism and localization. The physician is now ready to plan laboratory investigations to test these hypotheses. Again, sequential modification of the diagnostic lists should follow each important laboratory result.

In our opinion, this systematic, sequential process of deductive reasoning is crucial if the neurologist is to (1) make the correct diagnosis, and (2) avoid serious diagnostic omissions. Success in this method requires *thinking time.* After each part of the process, pause and think! We teach this method to internists and medical residents because we believe it is equally applicable to diagnostic problems presented to the internist. Unfortunately, the technique seems foreign to many of today's medical residents.

Probabilities and Other Diagnostic Concerns

We have already mentioned the importance of probabilities. Rarely is a given diagnosis absolutely certain. Failure to think of and consider other conditions or localizations is the commonest reason for failure to diagnose. We all know physicians who invariably diagnose "zebras" instead of "horses" when hoofbeats are heard on the street. The probability of the presence of a given diagnosis is an important factor in planning investigations and treatment.

Another important factor is treatability of a disease. Even though a particular condition may be less likely than another, if it is remediable by treatment, then it is very important to consider before excluding it. Hypothyroidism, pernicious anemia, and insulin-secreting adenomas are unusual but potentially reversible causes of confusion, dementia, and ataxia.

Another consideration is the cost of missing a given diagnosis. By cost, we do not mean economic or legal, though these issues are becoming much more prominent today. We refer to morbidity and mortality. Subdural hematoma is not a common cause of hemiparesis but failure to diagnose can, and has, led to the death of patients who would have survived if treated quickly and effectively. Subarachnoid hemorrhage causes only a very small fraction of headaches, but failure to recognize the unusual instances can be disastrous.

The function of this opening chapter has been to introduce the reader to the main attributes and methods of the clinician-neurologist. This outline will be elaborated on in the next sections that dissect the various parts of the clinical encounter.

REFERENCES

1. Tumulty PA. What is a clinician and what does he do? *N Engl J Med* 1970;283: 20–24.
2. Tumulty PA. *The Effective Clinician*. Philadelphia: W.B. Saunders Co., 1973.
3. Barondess JA. The training of the internist. With some messages from practice. *Ann Intern Med* 1979,90:412–417.
4. Doyle AC. The adventure of the speckled band. In WS Baring-Gould (ed), *The Annotated Sherlock Holmes*. New York: Clarkson N. Potter Inc., 1967;257.
5. Caplan LR. The method of neurologic diagnosis and treatment. In LR Caplan, JJ Kelly (eds), *Neurological Consultations*. Toronto: B.C. Decker and Co., 1988;1–6.
6. Plum E. From a speech given at the dedication of the Brown University Department of Neuroscience. Providence, RI, 1988.
7. Caplan LR, Wolpert SM. Angiography in patients with occlusive cerebrovascular disease: A stroke neurologist and neuroradiologist's views. *AJNR* 1991;12:593–601.
8. Caplan LR. Diagnosis and the clinical encounter. In LR Caplan (ed). *Caplan's Stroke: A Clinical Approach*. 3rd ed. Boston: Butterworth–Heinemann, 2000;51–71.
9. Frank AD. A review of the case records. *N Engl J Med* 1987;316:1219.
10. Weed LL. Medical records that guide and teach. *N Engl J Med* 1968;278:593–599, 652–657.

PART II

The Patient Encounter

The interactions of the person we have just described, the clinician-neurologist, and the patient are very complex and multifaceted. In this section, after first discussing general strategies and principles, we artificially and traditionally divide the physician-patient interface into its various components as follows: history taking, the examination, recording the data from the clinical encounter, test planning and interpretation, physician information transmittal, discussions with patients, and treatment. We try to tie the various components together by closing this section with patient examples that illustrate the clinician at work during the various phases of the doctor-patient interaction.

2

General Strategies

A sensible man confronted by a sick person would ask himself three simple questions. "What is wrong with him?" "How did he get this way?" "How can I help him?"[1]

—MACK LIPKIN

"Cheshire Puss," Alice began . . . , "Would you tell me, please, which way I ought to go from here?" "That depends a good deal on where you want to get to," said the Cat. "I don't much care where," said Alice. "Then it doesn't matter which way you go," said the Cat.[2]

—LEWIS CARROLL

The relationship between doctor and patient is extremely complex and multifaceted. We have introduced the technique of neurologic diagnosis first in the preceding chapter because of its central and critical role in the success of an effective neurological clinician. But even the most competent analysis and accurate diagnosis will be wasted if the physician cannot (1) gain the cooperation, respect, and confidence of the patient, (2) select, plan, and coordinate treatment, (3) communicate with the patient and others about the illness and its effects and management, and (4) help the patient battle and come to terms with the medical conditions and neurological problems. Table 2-1 outlines these various goals of the interview and of the clinician-patient interaction. Cohen-Cole emphasizes a three-function approach to the medical interview: (1) data gathering, (2) developing rapport with the patient, and (3) patient education and motivation.[3] Others have emphasized the importance of various techniques and strategies to obtain maximal data and to consider the patient's point of view and perspective.[4-7]

Before discussing various aspects of the physician-patient encounter in succeeding chapters, we thought it would be useful to map out general strategies. As the Cheshire Cat pointed out to Alice, it is always best to know where you are headed before starting on a complex journey.

17

Table 2-1 General Aims of the Clinician-Patient Encounter

1. Gaining rapport with the patient
2. Making a sound medical-neurological diagnosis
3. Considering the environment and full social-economic-psychologicsal context of the illness
4. Planning evaluation and treatment
5. Communicating with the patient
6. Clarifying the rules and pattern of the clinician-patient relationship

GAINING RAPPORT

Most patients come to a physician with positive feelings. The reasons for coming to that particular physician vary greatly. Patients may have investigated who would be best for them to see, just as they would choose a tutor, an electrician, or an accountant. More often, the patient's physician, family, friends, or a medical source has suggested your name as a specialist appropriate for them and their problem. In some instances, you may have been designated as the available caregiver by group practice or a managed care organization. In any event, there usually has been some type of preselection, and the patient is free to begin or end a doctor-patient relationship. The patient hopes for and wants the relationship to succeed.

During the initial interview, the physician has the difficult job of pursuing, collecting, and interpreting very complex data that will answer Lipkin's basic questions: What is wrong, how did it happen, and how can I help? At the same time, the patient is sizing up and evaluating the physician. Is the doctor competent? Does he or she seem to care? Will we be able to work together? While working very hard at making a complete diagnosis, the doctor must build on the patient's initial positive feelings. The physician must develop rapport with the patient. Without rapport, even the best intellectual analysis will not succeed. If the patient does not follow the physician's advice, or does not return for diagnostic testing and treatment, all of the physician's training and intellect will have been useless. The physician must, from the first moment of the encounter, work to build a relationship. There is no doubt that that relationship can be therapeutic. That relationship is indispensable.

MAKING A SOUND MEDICAL DIAGNOSIS

We have already commented on the central role of technical skill and accurate diagnosis. Centuries ago, barber-surgeons and other physicians were uneducated individuals who offered various remedies for specific types of symptoms.[8] Fortune tellers, medicine men, voodoo doctors, various soothsayers, and quacks continue this practice even today.[9,10] Herbal products and other nonstandardized supposedly medicinal substances are very widely used by patients, at least in part because of nontrust of the medical establishment and the failure of physicians to meet the needs of patients.[10–12] We call ourselves physicians primarily because of the vast advances in technical knowledge and the science of medicine.

A prominent newspaper columnist related his experiences with the diagnosis and treatment of his son's brain tumor. The columnist could not sufficiently praise his son's doctors for their caring, their humanity, and their skills in relating to his son and the family. They were fine human beings, but he said he would rather that they had been the worst possible bastards and had possessed the technical knowledge and skills to save his son. Of course, the two skills, technical and humane, are not mutually exclusive and should not even be competitive. The art and science of medicine are both critical, but the art is empty and impotent without the substance of science.

The physician must work very hard and be systematic, penetrating, and thorough at making an accurate, medically sound diagnosis. The process of meticulous pursuit of the diagnosis, more than any other physician behavior, makes patients respect and trust their physician.

Diagnoses are made mostly through three different but interrelated techniques: deductive reasoning, inductive analysis, and pattern matching.[13] Deductive analysis involves sequential hypothesis-making and testing to deduce diagnoses. Deductive exploration should be both positive (looking for features and information that suggest or confirm a diagnosis), and negative (queries that might elicit features that argue against diagnoses). Inductive analysis involves a thorough collection of data and then analyzing that data after it is collected for patterns and information that lead to the possibility of various diagnoses. Pattern-matching involves comparing features of the history and/or the examination that match conditions that the clinician knows well, has seen, or has read about in the medical literature.[13]

CONSIDERING THE ENVIRONMENT AND FULL SOCIAL-ECONOMIC-PSYCHOLOGICAL CONTEXT OF THE ILLNESS

No man is an island: the patient operates in a complex social, civic, cultural, economic, religious, and philosophic environment. It is not enough to understand and diagnose the illness; the physician must understand the person and the milieu. In addition to a medical diagnosis, there must be a comprehensive diagnosis that considers the totality of the illness. Many illnesses cannot be understood using only biomedical concepts. Physicians can divide up clinical data into three different types: (1) strictly medical—information relating to the pathology of the disease and its symptoms and signs, (2) social, in the broadest sense of the word—information about the patient's environment (where does the patient live, work, and play? Who are the significant others in the patient's life? What are the patient's cultural, religious, and economic background and resources?), and (3) intra- and interpersonal or psychological—more personal and potentially more charged information about the patient's feelings and stresses.

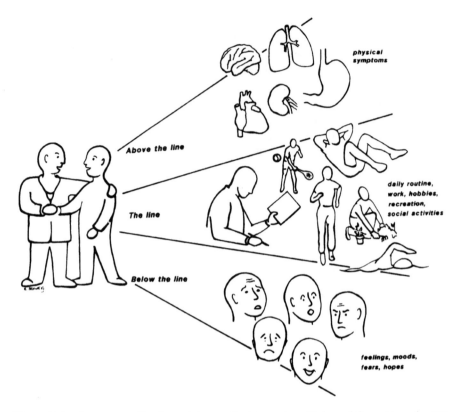

Figure 2-1 A conceptualization of the medical interview. (Adapted from Lisansky ET, Shochet BR. Comprehensive medical diagnosis for the internist. *Med Clin N Am* 1967; 51. Drawn by Evey Schweig.)

Lisansky and Shochet constructed a schema that we find very useful in conceptualizing the medical interview and data collection.[14,15] Modified after Felix Deutsch's "associative anamnesis," the construct (Figure 2-1) involves drawing lines to organize the clinical data. Above the line are written the physical symptoms and manifestations of the disease. Below the line are the personal relationships and feelings of the patient, and along the line in a "neutral" zone are the important social and environmental factors. The physician should arrive at a double diagnosis: (1) What medical disease does the patient have? and (2) What kind of a person is this and how do personality and life experiences relate to the illness, its etiology, recurrence, chronicity, and management?

PLANNING EVALUATION AND TREATMENT

While interviewing and examining the patient, the physician must not only make a comprehensive diagnosis but must begin to think about evaluation and treatment. After the examination, the physician will have to act. What will the next step be? How urgent is the situation? Should the patient return to the physician, to his or her own referring doctor, or to another physician? To whom should they report and when? Are further tests needed? Which ones and in what sequence? Should some medication or therapy be prescribed now, or should it wait for further clarification of the diagnosis?

These questions are all difficult and will be discussed in detail in subsequent chapters. Needless to say, the answers to these questions must be carefully considered, or the initial patient encounter may fail. When the patient finishes dressing after the examination, he or she wants and expects some words of explanation. Until then the physician has mostly collected information. The patient now sees the physician in action. How thorough and responsive are the plans? If they are constructed hastily and thoughtlessly, rapport may suffer greatly.

COMMUNICATING WITH THE PATIENT

Perhaps the single most common patient criticism of physicians is failure to communicate. Physician-patient communication begins with the initial introduction. Much of the communication in the early part of the interview is nonverbal. Facial expressions that show intent listening, concern, seriousness, and understanding give the patient assurance of the physician's full attention and empathy.[16] Touching and eye contact also convey feelings and have therapeutic value.

At the closing of the first encounter, the physician must communicate verbally with the patient about the session. At the minimum, this must include the relative gravity of the problem (is it relatively minor or potentially serious?), the initial diagnostic impression if one is possible, and a discussion of investigations, medicines, and other treatments, and suggestions about follow-up. The *patient should know what to do* and *what are the next steps*. The patient should also be able to tell whether the physician is worried about his or her illness, how certain or uncertain is the diagnosis, and whether extensive or invasive tests are likely to be needed. If the diagnosis is quite uncertain and data is so preliminary that the physician would rather not commit to an opinion, then a fuller discussion can be postponed until results of tests are evaluated or there have been further encounters.

At some point, the physician must conduct a so-called "dismissal" or summary discussion. We prefer to call this the *denouement* because it is the culmination or climax of the physician-patient encounter and tension builds up until it is accomplished. Delivering an optimal summary discussion is very difficult and requires experience and careful planning, yet students and residents are seldom taught or shown how it should be done. How many trainees have been present when a senior clinician conducts a summary discussion?

While conducting the history and examination, the physician must carefully consider what to tell the patient. How much and what should be said? Premature reassurance, a wrong diagnosis, or inadequate discussion can irreversibly damage the physician-patient relationship before it is solidified. The physician must work just as hard on communication skills as on diagnosis.

CLARIFYING THE "RULES" AND PATTERN OF THE RELATIONSHIP

Although most clinicians see lots of patients, the converse is often not true. Some patients have little experience with doctors. Others have much experience and know that there are vast differences among physicians. Few have seen neurologists before; the first encounter is a new experience for each of them. Patients have many questions about the "rules" or modus operandi of the relationship: Are they rigid, flexible, or negotiable? Will it be a single visit, a consultation, a potentially continuing and long-term relationship, or one that will be limited by the length of the particular incident of illness? What kind of material or symptoms or questions should be brought to the doctor? What will be the style: highly controlled by the doctor or interactive? Are questions welcomed or resented by the doctor? Or by the patient? Who will pay, when, and how much? How are appointments made and for how long and how often are they likely to be needed? How can the doctor be reached, and when is it appropriate to call? Ancillary office or hospital personnel can answer some of these questions. Some answers will come only after more encounters. Some answers are implicit from the doctor's behavioral reactions; others must be explicitly discussed. Again, experience and individual style must dictate how the doctor communicates the modus operandi that he or she is accustomed to and comfortable with. Patients also know their own preferences, and they should feel comfortable discussing them. The physician should be as flexible as possible without endangering his or her ability to diagnose, treat, and manage the illness. The physician must always integrate the patient's unique individual perspective into the process of care and communication.[6]

Always keep five things in mind:

1. The "game" is nearly always on a "home field" for the doctor and away on unfamiliar turf for the patient.
2. The encounter or experience and relationship involve not only the doctor and patient but also the total environment of the encounter. It is hard for the patient not to lump together the totality of the event. The doctor's furniture and layout, location, ease of parking or transportation, length of waiting time, attitude of the office staff, the cleanliness and efficiency of the operation, even whether urine sample bottles are left in the bathroom is all part of the experience. The person who answers the doctor's phone, for instance, is a very important person for the patient because he or she is the first contact.
3. Invariably, the patient is placed in a dependent or inferior position due to illness and neediness. The doctor is dominant from the first. Although this hierarchy has potential therapeutic value, it also conveys expectations that are sometimes appropriate to dispel.

4. The clinician must manage the illness, the disease that is causing the illness, the patient, and the socio-psychological-economic-interpersonal setting of the illness.[13]
5. Clinicians always must manage themselves as attentive concerned listeners and wise and thoughtful medical advisers.

REFERENCES

1. Lipkin M. *The Care of Patients.* New York: Oxford University Press, 1974;107.
2. Carroll L. *Alice's Adventures in Wonderland.* London: MacMillan, 1945;89.
3. Cohen-Cole SA. *The Medical Interview. The Three-function Approach.* St. Louis: Mosby, 1991.
4. Lipkin M Jr., Putnam SM, Lazare A (eds). *The Medical Interview: Clinical Care, Education, and Research.* New York: Springer-Verlag, 1995.
5. Billings JA, Stoeckle JD. *The Clinical Encounter: A Guide to the Medical Interview and Case Presentation.* Chicago: Year Book, 1989.
6. Delbanco TL. Enriching the doctor-patient relationship by inviting the patient's perspective. *Ann Intern Med* 1992;116:414–418.
7. Mathews DA, Suchman AL, Branch WT Jr. Making "connexions": Enhancing the therapeutic potential of patient-clinician relationships. *Ann Intern Med* 1993;118: 973–977.
8. Gordon, Noah. *The Physician.* New York: Simon & Schuster, 1986.
9. Snow LF. Folk medical beliefs and their implications for care of patients: A review based on studies among black Americans. *Ann Intern Med* 1974;81:82–96.
10. Eisenberg DM, Kessler RC, Foster C, Norlock FE, Calkins DR, Delbanco TL. Unconventional medicine in the United States: Prevalence, costs, and patterns of use. *N Engl J Med* 1993;328:246–252.
11. Brody JE. Alternative medicine makes inroads, but watch out for the curves. *New York Times* April 28,1998:89.
12. Planta M, Gunderson B, Petitt JC. Prevalence of the use of herbal products in a low-income population. *Fam Med* 2000;32:252–257.
13. Cox K. *Doctor and Patient: Exploring Clinical Thinking.* Sydney: University of New South Wales Press, 1999.
14. Lisansky ET, Shochet BR. Comprehensive medical diagnosis for the internist. *Med Clin N Am* 1967;51:1381–1397.
15. Lisansky ET, Shochet BR. History taking and interviewing. In J Noble (ed), *Textbook of General Medicine and Primary Care.* Boston: Little, Brown, 1987;13–25.
16. Waitzkin H. Doctors and patients—are they really communicating? *The Internist* August 1986:7–10.

3

History Taking

In taking the history follow each line of thought; ask no leading questions; never suggest. Give the patient's own words in the complaint.[1]
— William Osler

If you have thirty minutes to see a patient, spend twenty-eight minutes on the history, two minutes on the examination, and no time on the skull X-ray or EEG.[2]
— Adolph Sahs

Listen! Listen to your patient! He is giving you the diagnosis![3]
— Rene Laennec quoted by Eric Hodgins

If I listen sensitively, you may tell me what the illness "means" to you, how the illness is affecting your work or your social life, or what you fear about the possible disease, and what you really want from the consultation.[4]

— Ken Cox

Chapter 2 sketched the general outline and strategy of the physician-patient encounter. This chapter will discuss the content, style, and details of the history-taking interview.

RAPPORT—FIRST TRY TO MAKE THE PATIENT FEEL AT EASE

The first meeting with the neurologist is quite anxiety producing for the patient. The patient is worried about symptoms and what you will do, find, and say. Also the situation, the office or hospital, and the doctor are probably new experiences. Most patients are understandably nervous. After the introduction, take time to seat the patient near you and hang up hats, coats, and paraphernalia. Try to give the impression of being unhurried. Break the ice gently. An analogous situation might be the college admission interview. Applicants are nearly always jittery, and interviewers have learned to begin very slowly by introducing neutral, nonthreatening topics like the weather, sports, and so on.

One useful tactic is to begin the interview by asking patients to tell you a bit about themselves. This will provide some neutral background data about the patient, and what the patient chooses to tell you will provide insight into what the patient feels is important. Asking patients about themselves shows patients that you are interested in them as well as their illness, and helps them to relax.

The History Taking Session Should Be "Therapeutic" as Well as Informative

Continue to establish rapport as the interview proceeds. Don't miss the opportunity to be therapeutic while you are acquiring historical data. Whenever possible, show empathy. Spiro characterizes empathy as the capacity of the clinician to identify with the patient and to feel his or her pain.[5] Patients often resent sympathy but need empathy—a concerned listener. "Friendly professional interest" is another descriptor used to denote the key professional attitude that patients want and need.[6] A very common criticism of physicians is that they are too mechanical and too concerned with the disease and not sufficiently attuned to the patient. In a well-known painting, Picasso portrays the technocratic but emotionally uninvolved doctor (Figure 3-1). In this painting, the doctor is intently looking at his watch while feeling the pulse of a very ill woman. The doctor is paying no attention to the patient. In contrast, the nurse is showing support and is attending to the patient's needs. The attitude of friendly interest and feelings of empathy is conveyed by:

1. Appearing unhurried and patient.
2. Allowing the patient to present his or her problems. Patients should feel at the end of the initial interviews that they have been heard.
3. Listening intently.
4. Conveying concern and empathy when appropriate, for example, saying "that must have been very difficult for you" when the patient has told you of a serious injury or severe pain.
5. Supportive nonverbal behavior such as eye contact, a touch on the hand or shoulder, an understanding nod.
6. Allowing the patient to express emotions such as anger, anxiety, and sadness.
7. Showing emotion yourself, when appropriate, such as tension or anxiety when the diagnosis is difficult or the condition serious. This behavior convinces the patient that you are concerned.[7]
8. Thorough and meticulous pursuit of all relevant data.
9. Reviewing with the patient your understanding of some points in the history tells the patient that you have heard and digested the material and are reflecting on it.

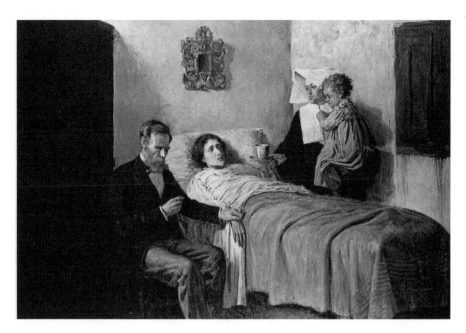

Figure 3-1 Pablo Picasso's *The Doctor's Visit*. (Displayed in the Museu Picasso, Barcelona, Spain.)

10. Spending a sufficient amount of time after the diagnostic information gathering to talk with the family and patient about their problem, your thoughts, and your proposed plan of management.

The interview with the patient takes time. Tumulty, in an article entitled *The Art of Healing*, stated, "Time personally spent with the patient is the most essential ingredient of excellence in clinical practice. . . . There must be time to assay the patient's intellectual and psychological elements; time to meticulously gather each piece of clinical evidence from the history and physical examination; time to analyze these data and to add to them helpful information from special studies and consultations; time to evolve a plan of management when diagnostic conclusions have been reached. And, above all, there must be time for the patient to communicate himself to you, and you to him. Without adequate time, you cannot possibly give sufficiently of yourself to your patients. Time is what they expect and what they need."[8] Unfortunately, time spent with the patient is a very expensive commodity and one targeted by managed care organizations that seek to severely limit the time of physician-patient encounters. Physicians must desperately resist this attempt to rob them and their patients of time.

INTERVIEW STYLES

Low and High Doctor Control

The verbal interchange between patient and physician can be thought of in terms of the degree of control the doctor exercises in the interview. Figure 3-2 graphically illustrates the extremes of the doctor control spectrum. The lowest doctor control style involves passive listening without influencing what the patient chooses to tell you. At the other end of the spectrum is very active inquisition by the physician, seeking specific answers to very direct questions. The low-control style has also been referred to as "patient-centered interviewing," while the high-control style is characterized as "physician-centered interviewing."[9] Both styles are important and useful, and ordinarily the interview should include shifts from one style to the other. The advantages and disadvantages of each style should be obvious. The high-control doctor style, when used prematurely, cuts off initiation of new material by the patient and risks omission of key aspects of the patient's problems. The main issue, the forest, may be lost by

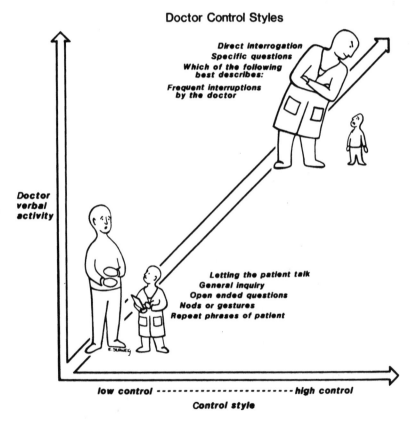

Figure 3-2 Doctor control styles. (Drawn by Evey Schweig.)

taking too much time to examine each tree with a magnifying glass. A good microscopist always first looks at tissue under a scanning low-power lens to identify major pathology or areas of interest before changing focus to high power for closer analysis of problem regions. The low-control doctor style risks excessive digressions by the patient, resulting in collection of a wealth of irrelevant material that does not contain specific answers to key questions.

We advise always starting with a low-control style. Begin by asking, "Tell me about your problem" or "What brings you here today?" Allow patients free rein until they seem to have completed their opening statement (usually three to ten minutes). What patients choose to tell you reveals a great deal about what is foremost in their thoughts. Even a seemingly insignificant aside may yield valuable insight into why the patient is there. One patient, who began by telling of four weeks of recent headaches, happened to mention that the headaches were not like those of her neighbor who died six months ago of a brain tumor. She had, of course, come to the physician out of concern that she had a brain tumor. The headaches were slight and infrequent and otherwise would not have been significant enough to warrant medical advice.

The doctor encourages the patient to continue by an expression of intent listening, a nod, or by saying "and" or "yes." Repetition of a patient's phrase signals the patient to elaborate further on that particular topic. If the patient said he had pain on the left side of the head, the doctor's echoing "left side of the head" encourages the patient to elaborate on the location and perhaps other characteristics of the pain but does not bias the answer with a leading question. If the doctor had asked, "Was the pain very severe?", some defensive patients, afraid that the doctor will minimize the significance of the symptom, might answer, "Of course it was severe. Would I bother a doctor with a trivial problem?" If the patient digresses prematurely, the doctor can gently lead him back to the prior subject ("Tell me more about your headache."). Switch topics by asking, "Was there anything else?" or "Were there other symptoms?"

Once the doctor is satisfied that the patient has sketched the outline of the material he or she feels is important, the doctor can switch to what has been called an "inquiry mode," asking more details about symptoms introduced by the patient ("How frequent were the headaches?", "Did they seem to occur more often at any particular time of the day?", "What were they like?", "Did anything seem to bring them on?"). The more general and less leading the question, the better the chance that the patient's reply will not be colored by his or her perception of what the doctor expects. Sometimes these general questions will not yield enough data. When asked about the characteristics of the headache, the patient may say she doesn't know what you mean. The doctor may have to offer choices ("Was it throbbing, steady, burning, or sharp?"). If none of those adjectives fits, the patient nevertheless might choose to elect a poorly fitting descriptor.

After eliciting specifics about the first symptom area, the doctor should switch again to a more low-control style. If the patient's initial statement was scanty or short, the doctor should make the invitation to continue as broad as possible ("Are there other things you feel are important?" or "Is there any-thing else?"). Be sure the patient has had a chance to relate all the symptoms, concerns, and relevant data. By echoing or focusing in on another area of symptoms, the doctor has changed focus to high power from a scanning lens. Switching back and forth from a cruising, low-control style to a higher-control inquiry mode maximizes the chances of hearing all that the patient feels is rel-evant but ensuring collection of sufficient details and specifics.

The inquiry mode has two major aspects or purposes: (1) elicitation of more detail about a symptom (for example, the character, location, duration, precipitants, and accompaniments of a headache) and (2) hypothesis testing. Knowing that many headaches in young patients are due to migraine, the physician will ask about accompanying visual symptoms such as bright lights, flashing objects, lines, and so forth and about sensitivity to light and sound, and the presence of nausea during and after the headache. Most medically unsophisticated patients would not have thought that nausea or visual abnor-malities were related to headaches unless specifically queried.

Defective interview style is an important reason for failure to diag-nose.[9–16] On average, doctors interrupt their patients 18 seconds into the clini-cal encounter.[14] Well intentioned, most doctors do this in the interest of efficiency and time saving since most physicians believe that the first symp-toms mentioned are the most significant ones. Frequent interruptions lead to an inadequate historical database. In a recent study, among 264 taped physi-cian encounters, only 28 percent of patients completed their opening statement of concerns before being interupted.[15] Patients have on average one to five symptoms to relate. Because of frequent interruptions, fewer than a quarter of patients can complete their opening statement, and only half are allowed to explain all of their symptoms. In one study, only 1 of 52 patients interviewed went on to complete their concerns after the initial interruption.[14] The most common concern expressed by the public and an important cause of medical malpractice suits is about whether the patient's problems are heard and under-stood.[16] Failure to "hear" the patient begins reactions of disaffection and frus-tration that lead to poor doctor-patient communication, and sometimes ultimately to legal action on the part of the patient or family.[16] The patients' concerns are often practical. More important to them than naming the disease are the implications, for example, how long might they have to stay in the hos-pital, how much will it cost, how will it affect work and family and recre-ational activities.

Seeking Primary Data—Don't Accept Secondary or Tertiary Data

Patients and, unfortunately, many doctors have a reverent belief (or hope) that doctors' diagnoses are always correct. Like the *deus ex machina* direction of classic plays when a god descends from a prop, the doctor deity waves a hand or reflex hammer and proclaims or ordains a fact or diagnosis.

Patients also seem to think that doctors want to hear "doctor information" that somehow must be superior to what they, who are only unsophisticated lay persons, can relate. A recent patient began his statement by saying: "A month ago I went to Dr. X who gave me a penicillin shot for infectious mono; then Dr. Y, the best doctor in town, treated me for an ear infection and a heart attack, and now he wants me to see you because of a stroke." So far you have heard nothing about the symptoms and have no way to evaluate, verify, or disagree with any of the four diagnoses mentioned. All or none might be accurate.

Some past diagnoses given the patient may be quite relevant; some may be remote and unimportant. In a patient suspected of having a stroke, past diagnoses of angina pectoris or myocardial infarction are obviously very important. Don't be content with the patient telling you that he or she has angina or that the doctor is treating him or her for angina. Inquire more about the symptoms: Was there pain? If so, what was its duration, characteristics, precipitants. Does the medicine help? The doctor is less likely to be interested in this stroke patient's amplification of childhood measles or appendicitis surgery. In a different patient who reports weakness of the left leg since youth, amplification of the childhood measles, its primary symptoms, and their evaluation may be quite relevant. In a patient who might have porphyria, the symptoms that precipitated past operations on the appendix and gall bladder may be well worth inquiry, but the details of the same surgical procedures, if remote, may be unimportant in the patient with a recent stroke.

House officers in their case presentations and write-ups often record past diagnoses without being inquisitive or critical. For example, a patient admitted to the hospital with a sudden onset of paralysis of the left arm and leg is reported to have had a "lacunar infarct with left hemiparesis" nine months before, but the young physician has not recorded the primary data from the chart or asked the patient about the symptoms and signs that occurred. The patient was able to give an excellent account of the event nine months ago and mentioned she also had had transient loss of vision in the right eye just before that event. Clearly, the initial diagnosis of a lacuna was incorrect, and both episodes of left hemiparesis were due to severe carotid artery disease. Unfortunately, even doctors' letters or summaries sometimes do not include the details of patients' symptoms and the findings from the general and neurological examinations but always seem to include the results of laboratory tests.

Patients hear what they want to hear. They may have heard that they had "infectious mono" when in actuality the doctor said, "you could have a number of different kinds of infection such as flu or infectious mono." They relate their own translations of the diagnosis.

We have two basic rules about information concerning care by other doctors and hospitals. (1) *Doctor or hospital information is best obtained from that doctor or the hospital chart.* If the information is important and relevant, be sure to obtain the original data. (2) *Don't read or study the hospital chart or doctor's notes before starting the patient interview.* Reading what someone else has said biases your observations and lessens your chances of finding something new or different. The patient may be seeing you because the preceding opinion or care did not fully solve the problem; for whatever reason, they want your help and advice. It is, however, very important to read the notes and available data before the interview is complete or at least before the summary discussion with the patient. You don't want to miss key points of information that the patient has omitted, and you will need to know the refer-ring physician's questions.

The same approach, in our opinion, is applicable to the review of X-rays and images. Look at CT and MRI scans first without clinical data; see what hits you as you systematically examine the images. Then look at the clinical data and the radiologist's report if available. This information will tell you which region to examine more closely and for what findings. Premature concentration on the left cerebral hemisphere in a patient with aphasia might cause you to overlook an unsuspected posterior fossa meningioma. On the other hand, not knowing the area to focus on could allow you to miss a subtle abnormality in the region of clinical interest.

Similarly, take the history from the patient yourself, then read the case notes or doctor's report, then return to parts of the history for clarification or amplification. Just as the patient's spontaneous statements are more likely to be unbiased than if they are responsive to deep probing, so are you more likely to be an objective observer and diagnostician if you are not biased by prior opinions and information that are more than occasionally erroneous. The patients are often the experts on their own diseases. No other individual has as much inside information on the causes, precursors, precipitants, and potential implications and meaning of the illness to them.[16]

Ask for Examples

We all use words differently. One patient may say "dizzy" and mean faint, another might mean vertiginous, and a third will mean mixed up, confused. One patient may describe "weakness," "numbness," or "discomfort" and have in mind something quite different from other patients who use the same words. Always ask for clarification and examples.

A woman complained of memory lapses. When asked for an example, she described unexpectedly meeting an old friend on the street and being unable to recall his name. She said that she could vividly recall where and when they had been friendly and could even picture his wife but could not recall his name. On another occasion, she said she wanted to sweeten her coffee and could not recall the word "sugar." The abnormality was clearly a naming problem, not amnesia. Another patient who complained of memory lapses gave an example of suddenly "coming to," sitting in a department store, not being able to recall what had transpired during the last few minutes. On another occasion, she real-ized her friend was berating her because she had missed several moments of a conversation. The friend said that the patient had "stared blankly." This patient was having partial complex seizures. A third patient with "memory lapses" gave two examples of typical incidents. One day he went into a store and could not recall what his wife had told him to buy. He would have to stop and ponder in the morning when he left his house, momentarily not being able to recall where he had parked his car the preceding night. He did not forget important engagements, events, phone numbers or complex details of client files at work. This patient suffered from "absent mindedness"; his preoccupation with other matters made it difficult for him to record and retain relatively unessential data. The examples given by these patients clarified their problems, each different, but all described by them as memory loss.

"Walk Through" Parts of the History, Especially the Present Illness

We have already commented on people's naiveté about the anatomy and functions of the nervous system. Many cannot report the distribution and severity of their weakness or numbness. This might be because they did not know what to look for, were too anxious or frightened, ignored or denied symptoms, or had an organic right cerebral hemisphere syndrome with impaired recognition of their deficit. We find a technique that we call "walking through the events" very helpful for clarifying the nature and development of symptoms.

Two examples of the technique will illustrate its utility. A 50-year-old, previously hypertensive woman said she fell out of bed and couldn't get up. She was not able to tell why it happened or what was wrong with her. I asked her to describe for me the events beginning with the preceding night. She had prepared dinner the night before and had washed the dishes with her husband, watched TV, and retired uneventfully. During the night, she awakened and went to the bathroom, which was about 50 feet away. She recalled reaching for and using the toilet paper with her left hand because the dispenser was located to the left of the toilet. She walked back to bed and fell asleep. The next morning she awakened late, after her husband had left for work, reached up to switch on the light and turn off the radio-alarm on the night table to her right. She usually exited the bed on her left but somehow could not turn in that direction. She swung her right leg over the right side of the bed and then fell to the ground. She inched toward the phone on her right but could not reach the rug, which was on her left, or stand up. In this patient, this detailed account showed that she had developed a left hemiparesis with anosognosia sometime between her nighttime trip to the bathroom and arising in the morning.

Another patient said that she had suddenly developed weakness of the right arm and leg that morning. When asked to describe the events of the morning, she gave the following account. She had been fine until, during breakfast, the coffee cup slipped from her right hand and she could not move her right fingers. She was not burned. Worried, she went upstairs to her room to lie down. As she went up the stairs, she noted a slight limp and had to make a conscious effort to lift her right leg up to the next step. She could hold the rail with her right hand. She called her daughter on the phone and spoke normally and understood what was said to her. She fell asleep. When she awakened an hour later, she could easily descend the stairs and was surprised and greatly relieved to find that her right hand, arm, and leg worked normally. After cleaning the kitchen and putting the dishes away using both hands, she suddenly felt weak and her right leg buckled. She tried to return to her bed but now could not navigate the stairs because she could not lift her right leg at all. She could not move her right hand or arm but could stand holding on to a chair with her left hand. When her daughter arrived 30 minutes later, she was able to walk to the car with a definite limp but without support. She could open the door with her right hand though it was still a bit weak and clumsy. She had described a fluctuating course quite typical for an evolving ischemic lesion.

From a patient's detailed description of events, a clinician is better able to localize and quantitate the deficits and their clinical course of evolution.

Repeat to Patients What You Think They Have Told You

We are all able to improve a paper, letter, or oral presentation when given an opportunity to review and edit. The patient's history has been elicited with interruptions and complex interactions and may not accurately represent what happened. We find it useful, at times, to recount for the patient the major features as derived from his or her account. Most patients are encouraged and pleased that the physician has retained and can recall the details. This means that the physician has been listening carefully. When the patient has heard the physician's recounting, he or she may want to add, edit, or elaborate on some aspects. The physician may have gotten an erroneous impression that the patient can correct, if given an opportunity. When the account of the woman who had fallen from bed was repeated, the patient now "remembered" that, after she had returned from the bathroom the night before, she and her husband had had rather rigorous intercourse that left her exhausted. The diagnosis of paradoxical embolism through a patent foramen ovale was later confirmed.

History Taking Does Not End with the Initial Interview

There are many reasons why patients are "poor historians" during the initial interview. They may be anxious, worried, ill, or in pain. Some questions may be new and unexpected. Repeating key questions sometimes uncovers important material missed the first time. A patient with a left hemiparesis was asked five times in several different ways about visual symptoms in the right eye. He denied their occurrence. On the sixth day of hospitalization, he called his doctor to his bedside and volunteered, "You know, doc, on the day before my stroke I was checking out food at the supermarket when a black curtain slowly descended over my right eye. After about 30 seconds, the shade lifted and I could see normally. The store clerk said I must have gotten some dirt in my eye. I don't know why I hadn't thought of that till now. Do you think it had anything to do with my stroke?"

We find it useful after the history portion of the encounter seems to be over to ask, "Is there anything else that you feel is important, or that we have not already discussed?" Most experienced doctors have often been the victims of the "hand on the door" syndrome[16] in which as the patient grasps the door to leave, he or she mentions the real reason for the visit or another important symptom not touched on during the encounter.

When evaluation seems to be drawing a blank and the diagnosis is unknown, we sometimes find it useful to start over, especially in hospitalized patients, and retake the history. The same maneuver is often useful after a series of unproductive outpatient visits. The clinical history is the foundation of the diagnostic edifice the doctor is building. Be sure that you have obtained all relevant data.

MEDICAL DATA

Present Illness Diagnosis

Diagnosis of the cause of the present illness is the critical part of nearly all neurological initial encounters. We always accumulate information first about the recent symptoms. Information about past illnesses and events is more easily assimilated and digested with a reference frame—the present illness. The technique or style of making the diagnosis has already been discussed: (1) Switching back and forth from low to high doctor control styles after the opening statement by the patient, (2) "walking through" events, and (3) hypothesis testing. The neurologist must make two medical diagnoses: an anatomical location diagnosis and a diagnosis of the mechanism of the illness. The diagnosis will usually consist of the probabilities of various differential diagnoses, not a single answer.

Let us illustrate the method first with an anatomical diagnosis. The patient describes numbness of the left hand. The neurologist first considers a local process in the hand or arm, such as a median or ulnar neuropathy. He or she asks about the distribution of the numbness. Was it primarily the thumb and adjacent two fingers (median) or the little finger and adjacent half of the fourth finger (ulnar) or both? Was there pain in the wrist or arm? Knowing that carpal tunnel syndrome is the commonest cause of neuropathy in the hand, the physician asks about precipitation or relief of numbness by various positions or activities and about past wrist trauma. The patient responds that the distribution is in the entire hand and the numbness is constant and not altered by position or activity. The doctor should now explore an alternate hypothesis, having not confirmed the original ideas. Could the lesion be at the neck, affecting the left cervical roots or the spinal cord? Questions now relate to the presence of neck or shoulder pain, past cervical arthritis, past neck injury or wearing of a collar. Is there weakness or numbness of the legs or feet, difficulty walking or a change in gait, urinary dysfunction, decreased potentia? Any of these symptoms suggests a myelopathy. If the patient responds negatively, the neurologist pursues another anatomical hypothesis: the brainstem. The clinician asks about dizziness, double vision, staggering, and other brainstem symptoms. Pursuing a cerebral localization, the neurologist asks about headache and numbness or weakness of the left face or lower extremity. Now, when asked specifically, the patient recalls minor tingling of his left cheek and left tongue. Knowing now that the lesion is most likely right cerebral, the medical sleuth focuses in on anatomical subdivisions of the cerebral hemisphere. Numbness suggests a post-Rolandic localization. The presence of symptoms of a hemianopia would localize the process far posteriorly in the occipital lobe or occipito-parietal junction or in the deeper temporal lobe structures adjacent to the geniculo-calcarine tract. Did the patient have difficulty seeing to the left? Did he bump into things? Was there difficulty reading? The neurologist recalls that right parietal lesions often cause visual spatial problems. Did the patient have difficulty finding his way, did he get lost? The neurologist does not simply wait and listen, using a low-control style, but switches to an inquiry mode, pursuing the localization just as a detective would pursue clues to the solution of a crime. In this case, the neurologist has localized the process to probably involve the right cerebral hemisphere, but the right brainstem is still possible. The neurologist makes a mental note to pursue the functions of these areas in the examination and subsequently in imaging and physiological investigations.

Let's use another example of a localization problem. A middle-aged woman reports severe spinning rotational dizziness after arising the previous morning. The neurologist first thinks of a lesion of the labyrinth on either side and inquires about ear pain, hearing loss, tinnitus. Knowing that labyrinthine origin dizziness is quite sensitive to changes in position and movement, the neurologist asks if the dizziness worsened when the patient turned her head or rolled over in bed. Also knowing that labyrinthine disorders such as Meniere's syndrome are often recurrent, the clinician probes for prior attacks. Because labyrinthine disease can be caused by infection, medicines, head trauma, and migraine, the neurologist might now choose to pursue those possibilities. The clinician has now mixed disease pathology with localization but primarily to influence the probability of an anatomical labyrinthine localization. Suppose all questions are answered in the negative. Knowing that the afferent pathway of the labyrinth through the vestibular nerve goes to the brainstem, the neurologist mentally pictures the brainstem, visualizing the location of the vestibular nuclei in the lateral medullary and pontine tegmental regions. Now the clinician proceeds, asking about symptoms that could indicate dysfunction of structures adjacent to the vestibular nuclei. Was there sharp pain, burning, or numbness of the face (nucleus and spinal tract of V)? Was there loss of ability to appreciate pain or water temperature on one side of the body (spino-thalamic tract)? Was there difficulty swallowing or hoarseness (nucleus ambiguous); was there diplopia (VI nerve nucleus, vestibular nucleus, or medial longitudinal fasciculus)? Was the face weak (VII nucleus or nerve)? Knowing that the most frequent cause of lateral tegmental disease is lateral medullary infarction, the clinician may now decide to probe for evidence of vascular risk factors such as hypertension, diabetes, high cholesterol, and coronary artery disease. The patient may be questioned about mastoid or occipital pain that might suggest occlusion or dissection of a vertebral artery or about prior transient ischemic attacks. The neurologist pursues the anatomical hypotheses as far as possible from the history. The neurological examination will later be planned to attempt to separate the still viable possible anatomical loci.

Let's now turn to a problem illustrating diagnosis of disease mechanism. A 27-year-old man has an epileptic seizure during the night, witnessed by his wife. Mentally, the neurologist reviews the most likely pathology of lesions causing seizures after inquiries lead to conviction that the incident was a true seizure. In a young person, congenital lesions and perinatal injury lead the list of possibilities. The doctor explores the history of the mother's pregnancy if known to the patient. Was the patient born prematurely? What was the birth weight? Did the patient have to stay in the hospital after the mother went home? Next, the doctor asks about developmental milestones or evidence of early life signs of cerebral dysfunction. When did the patient walk, talk? Was his development different from siblings? Did the patient learn to ride a bicycle? Was he agile and athletic as a child or clumsy and poorly coordinated? Was there a learning or reading problem? Was the patient a good student? Did he have to repeat one or more grades? If the patient cannot answer the questions, this is the appropriate time for the doctor to encourage him to ask his parents for details not known to him. Since the probability of various etiologies depends on the chronicity of the seizures, the clinician may next hunt for evidence of prior attacks. Did the patient ever have a febrile convulsion in childhood? Did he ever pass out and under what circumstances? Has he had transient olfactory, auditory, visual, or somatosensory phenomena? Has he ever had a lapse of memory, realizing suddenly that he could not account for the past few minutes? After being toilet trained, did he ever awaken with the bed wet or find that he had bitten his tongue during the night? Has he ever awakened with unusual exhaustion or diffuse unexplained muscle pains? Suppose that the history fails to elicit suggestions of past seizures or early life abnormalities. Infection is now pursued. Has there been recent fever, headache, ear pain, cough, sore throat? Does the patient belong to a group with a high risk of AIDS? If so, the seizure could reflect infection with toxoplasmosis, cytomegalovirus, or other opportunistic infectious agents. Has the patient traveled recently to Mexico (cysticercosis) or to the San Joaquin Valley (coccidioidomycosis)? Alcohol withdrawal is another very common cause of seizures. Is the patient a heavy or binge drinker, and what was his alcohol consumption during the days preceding the seizure? Could the etiology be a tumor? Are there any headache, sleepiness, focal neurologic symptoms, or behavioral changes? Arteriovenous malformations (AVM) are also a common cause of seizures in young people. Have there been recurrent migraine-like headaches? Is there a family history of seizures, a fact that would suggest an inherited or metabolic disease? Drug abuse is another frequent cause of seizures these days, so both the patient and spouse should be sensitively questioned about drug use. As the reader can see, the neurologist's process of inquiry has been very active, always thinking and exploring, probing and listening for any clues that direct the next line of attack. Diagnostic hypothesis testing is hard work!

Try to Disprove the Diagnosis

A tactic frequently taught in high school geometry is called reductio ad absurdum, literally reducing a hypothesis to an absurdity. The technique involves attempting to knock down or disprove the thesis. The same tactic is useful in medical diagnoses. Seek alternate hypotheses and try to substantiate or negate them.

Suppose that a 19-year-old college student comes to your office because of a very severe right throbbing headache the day before. The headache was preceded by shimmering white spots in her left visual field that lasted 15 minutes. She had no prior similar attacks. As she relates the history, the diagnosis of migraine with aura immediately comes to mind. Certainly this diagnosis is by far the commonest condition causing headache and visual obscurations in youth. Is there anything atypical for migraine? Ask for more details about the visual symptoms and the headache. What are possible, even if remote, alternative diagnoses? A vascular malformation? Seizures? Pseudotumor cerebri? Think of features that might be important in discriminating between these alternative differential diagnoses; for example, prior seizures and past attacks all referable to the right occipital region would favor an AVM. Make the differential diagnosis as wide as possible at the beginning. Don't prematurely eliminate an alternative diagnosis without convincing evidence.

Course of Illness Graphs and Creating a Mental Reference Library

The key historical feature predictive of disease mechanism is the course of the development of symptoms and signs, the pace of the illness. In neurology, assessment of the pace of illness is more feasible than in most general medical illnesses because of the anatomy and physiology of the nervous system.

Most other organs have relatively homogeneous compositions and functions. A patient might lose over 50 percent of his or her liver and have no clinical effect since the remainder of the liver can adequately manage the metabolic functions. There is much built-in reserve. Not until 80 percent or more of the liver is destroyed would symptoms appear, so that the gradual loss of the first three quarters of the liver would not be easily detected. Similarly, dyspnea, adrenal insufficiency, and renal failure develop when a sufficient amount of lung, adrenal gland, and kidney tissue become dysfunctional. Patients are usually unaware of early loss of function of these organs.

The brain and nervous system are quite different from other organs, being composed of very heterogeneous disparate parts. Also, normal nervous

Table 3-1   Patterns of Localization, Disease Onset, and Course

Location	Onset	Course	Disease
Focal	Acute	Remitting or fluctuating	Ischemic stroke
		Progressive (minutes to hours)	Intracerebral hemorrhage
	Gradual	Progressive (days)	Subdural hematoma Ischemic stroke
		Progressive (weeks to months)	Abscess, tumor
		Remitting	Demyelinative Focal infection
Diffuse	Acute	Stable or remitting	Metabolic Toxic Self-limited infection Subarachnoid hemorrhage
	Gradual	Progressive (months to years)	Degenerative diseases

system function is important for all of the routine functions of daily living—seeing, hearing, talking, walking, thinking. Observant patients are often acutely aware of any slight loss of agility, strength, speed, and mental facility and can report and describe the changes if carefully questioned. The neurologist can sketch at least a rough graph of the course of the development of the deficit from the patient's account, augmented by information from other observers (family and friends), and the neurologist's own observations.[17] Constructing course-of-illness curves is a useful exercise. We tell students and residents that, after they have finished their initial assessment, they should be able to draw such a graph. Simply knowing two pieces of data—whether the neurologic process is focal or diffuse and the course of the illness—predicts the disease type. A focal lesion that develops acutely and that improves gradually is most often a stroke. A focal lesion that has a gradual onset and then progressively worsens is most often neoplastic. Table 3-1 lists the possible combinations and the disease mechanisms they suggest.

What is the best way to construct a course-of-illness graph? Some patients can directly tell the physician the course of some signs. Good examples are monocular visual loss and weakness of one limb. A recent patient with optic neuritis described the onset of visual symptoms as gradual, with grayness and loss of focus in the left eye in the first few days, gradually progressing to near-blindness, with retained perception of the faint outlines of objects during a period of two weeks. After remaining stable for three weeks, vision gradually improved, leaving a central scotoma. This pattern (Figure 3-3) is quite characteristic of demyelinating disease.

Another patient with sudden weakness in the right arm and leg was fully aware of the deficit and could quantitate the severity of the weakness during a period (Figure 3-4) of 24 hours. The weakness first appeared when he was sitting

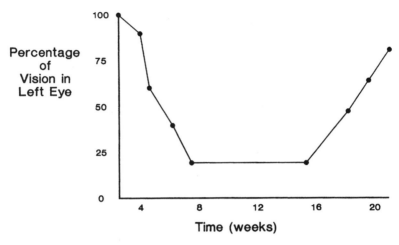

Figure 3-3   Monocular visual loss in a patient with demyelinative disease.

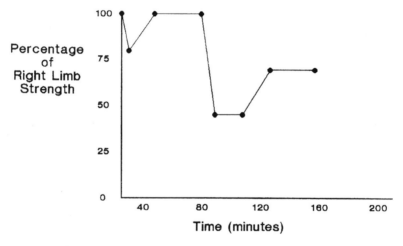

Figure 3-4   Right hemiparesis due to an ischemic stroke.

in a chair reading a book. The book dropped from his right hand, and he tested the limb and found that he could not move the fingers but could flex the elbow and lift the arm above his head. Ten minutes later, the hand and arm regained strength, and by twenty minutes, the coordination and the strength had returned to normal. One hour later, weakness returned, but this time he could not move his shoulder, elbow, or hand and had some difficulty lifting his right leg. He went to the hospital and thirty minutes later had improved to the point where he could move his arm, but it was still quite weak. By the time he was examined thirty minutes later, he believed there had been no additional improvement. This fluctuating deficit (see Figure 3-4) is quite typical of a thrombotic stroke.

Other patients, because of anxiety, naiveté, or cognitive deficits, cannot describe the development of even rudimentary deficits. Some other difficulties, for example, an attentional hemianopia or aphasia, are much more difficult to quantitate, and the patient may not be fully aware of the deficit. The doctor then uses the technique of "walking through the events." An example of this has been given previously in the patient who had a left hemiparesis and anosognosia from a right hemisphere stroke. Another patient was brought to the hospital stuporous by ambulance, with a note that he had developed a right hemiplegia at a store. The alert physician called the store and spoke to the salesperson who had waited on the patient. After trying on a sweater, the patient had become quite upset with the clerk and had begun to berate her. The clerk noted that during the tirade the patient's speech became slightly garbled and his mouth and face looked twisted. She asked the man to sit down and recalled that he had gestured appropriately with his right hand and walked naturally to a chair thirty feet away. The clerk called an emergency police ambulance and returned to the patient who now could not speak or move his right hand. When the ambulance came, the patient was able with support to walk a few steps and was assisted onto a stretcher. He was still awake and gestured goodbye and thanks with his left hand. When he arrived at the hospital ten minutes later, he had a severe right hemiplegia, his eyes were now deviated conjugately to the left, and he was very sleepy and barely arousable. This gradually progressive course of the acquisition of the clinical deficit with mounting intracranial pressure during a period of thirty minutes was typical of an intracerebral putaminal hemorrhage and is shown in Figure 3-5. In

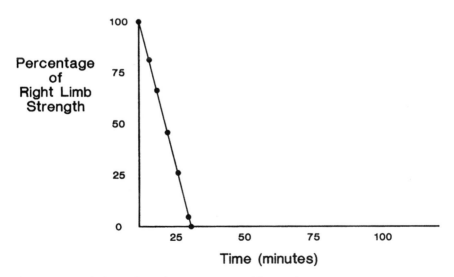

Figure 3-5 Right hemiplegia due to a putaminal hemorrhage.

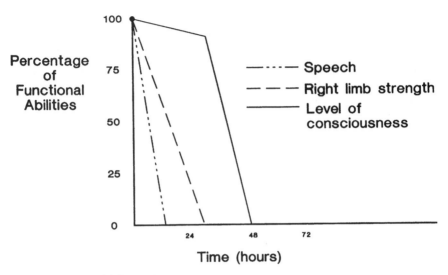

Figure 3-6 Loss of different functions in a patient with a left frontal lobar intracerebral hemorrhage.

order to construct this graph the physician had to walk through the events and use information from observers.

Sometimes there is more than one type of clinical deficit and different deficits evolve at slightly different paces. These also can be depicted on course-of-illness graphs. An example is shown in Figure 3-6, which graphs the deficits of another patient with a progressive intracerebral hemorrhage.

The course of some illnesses evolves over months or years and can still be graphed diagrammatically on a course-of-illness graph. Figure 3-7 is a graph of the course of illness of a patient with multiple brain emboli. This graph is more schematic. Because of the multiple types of deficits and varying time intervals, the nature of the deficits and time intervals are written in the graph, which is not drawn to scale as were the other graphs.

The patient's description not only makes the diagnosis, it educates the doctor for the next patient. In many patients, the diagnosis will be readily apparent during the early part of the interview. A young patient with repeated episodes during five years of scintillating scotomas that last twenty minutes and are followed by severe unilateral throbbing headaches with nausea has migraine. An obese young woman with severe headaches for months and transient visual obscurations lasting seconds probably has pseudotumor cerebri. A young man with four separate remitting attacks during a period of three years characterized successively by gradual loss of vision in the left eye, numbness of the left face, arm, and leg, dizziness with dysarthria and ataxia, and paraparesis has multiple sclerosis. Because the diagnosis in these cases is so obvious, many physicians are tempted to think "next case" and stop accumulating the details of the current problem. In these patients, it is espe-

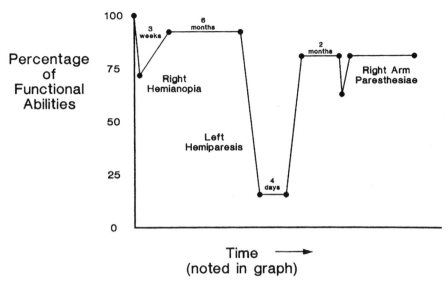

Figure 3-7 Multiple brain emboli from an atrial myxoma.

cially important for the physician to spend extra time in listening to the details of the symptoms.[18] Hearing exactly what the visual abnormality in migraine is like will help the physician decide if the next visual deficit he or she hears about from a different patient is migrainous. Hearing the details of the description of an optic neuritic visual loss and transient obscurations caused by increased intracranial pressure give the doctor vivid detailed patterns for a mental reference library.

Doctors often diagnose by pattern recognition. That fellow walking down the hall is John because he looks like John. We do not add up the features—long hair, glasses, mustache—to come to the answer John; we simply match the pattern of the face we see with an internal recalled image percept of John. Similarly, physicians make diagnoses by matching the pattern of visual loss their patient describes with patterns reported by past patients with known diagnoses. The more detailed your own mental library, the better a diagnostician you will be in the problem case. The wise physician is an eternal student who takes every opportunity to learn. Each patient can teach the doctor something—some about an illness or a symptom, some about human nature and coping with disease or disability. Some, during the examination, can serve as normal controls, giving the physician normative data about a special area of interest—picture looking, sensory functions, reading, and so on.

Past History

We find it much better to review important past history after taking the history of the present illness. After the present problem is clarified, the doctor can sense whether past events are irrelevant or might provide clues. At times, a past illness will yield unexpected data and engender new hypotheses about the present illness that will then require reexploration. A recent middle-aged patient had gradual onset of weakness of the legs, with impotence. In surveying the past history, the patient mentioned an old injury to the left eye. When asked to elaborate, he described being scratched on his left eye by another child; then, beginning ten days later, he noted gradual loss of vision in the same eye, with difficulty seeing the center of objects. No eye pain accompanied the visual loss. The eye returned to "nearly normal" after four months. The episode was diagnosed as a corneal injury by his eye doctor but, in retrospect, sounds more compatible with an optic neuritis. This raised the question that both the eye symptoms and the paraparesis were caused by multiple sclerosis. The doctor asked about other common symptoms of multiple sclerosis attacks, for example, paresthesiae, odd sunburnt feelings, and tingling in the limbs with neck flexion. The doctor also made a mental note to examine carefully the pupillary reaction and optic fundus for signs of a partially healed optic neuritis. Past hospitalizations, operations, injuries, and prolonged medical treatment should be systematically, but briefly, explored.

System Review

We find it most convenient to pursue the review of systems while performing the general and neurological examinations except when the system is directly relevant to the present illness. Before examining the heart, we ask about chest pain and palpitations; while palpating the abdomen, we ask about appetite, abdominal pain, and bowel habits. We also use the same strategy of neurologic system review while performing the neurologic exam. While examining the cranial nerves, we ask about visual loss, diplopia, dysarthia, hearing loss, and dysphagia. While examining each limb, we ask about loss of strength, numbness, and paresthesiae.

Family History

In some neurologic problems, the family history is the most critical part of the history. A 40-year-old patient with chorea, a 29-year-old person with progressive gait and limb ataxia beginning in youth, and a 9-year-old boy with proximal pelvic girdle weakness and a waddling gait are all highly suspect for familial degenerative diseases—Huntington's chorea, spinocerebellar degeneration, and Duchenne's muscular dystrophy. The diagnosis will rest on a parent, sibling, or other relative having similar problems. Yet few patients can give a detailed family history. Relatives may have died, moved, or become estranged. Forms fruste (minor forms) may have gone unrecognized.

One of us (L.R.C.) remembers vividly a service station attendant named Pettiput who had developed a gradually progressive, severe, paralyzing neuropathy during a period of twenty years. He had marked distal atrophy, loss of deep tendon reflexes, very slight loss of vibration sense, and thick peripheral nerves. He and the family were repeatedly queried about other members with trouble walking, thin legs, and neuropathy, with consistently negative answers. At the time of hospital discharge, when the diagnosis was still in doubt, he spoke to all the family members about the prognosis and treatment and again inquired about other family members with similar problems. A sister who had not visited before said, "Well, you know, doctor, our family name comes from the French word for small feet, and all of us in the family have odd-shaped feet." Examination of the feet of those present showed that most individuals had pes cavus deformities. Some had stork-like distal atrophy and absent ankle reflexes. This was a family with a hereditary neuropathy of the Charcot-Marie-Tooth type.

Patients often erroneously assume that their parents and siblings did not have a symptom or problem if that relative did not discuss it with the patient. The patient reasons that relatives know about their problems and would have shared similar symptoms. We can recall eliciting a history of classic migraines (migraine with aura) from a number of patients, in the presence of one or both of their parents. The patients all denied any family history of migraine. We asked if they had directly questioned their parents and siblings about past or present headaches, and they all said no ("Knowing about my bad headaches, they would have told me."). Even when we talked to the parents, most parents denied a similar problem. Some said they had "normal headaches." Two mentioned throbbing unilateral headaches diagnosed as eye strain. Several mentioned only "premenstrual syndrome," characterized by very severe pounding headaches and nausea during the first trimester of pregnancy and puerperium and during the early part of most menstrual cycles, symptoms probably indicative of migraine.

Whenever possible, if familial disease is seriously suspected, it is wise to question and examine available family members personally. Examination of family members proved to be one of the most important single diagnostic procedures in a large series of patients with neuropathy seen at the Mayo Clinic.[19] A next-best technique is instructing the patient to ask relatives specific questions such as, "Did you ever have headaches?"

OTHER CONCERNS IN THE INTERVIEW

Questioning of Others

When one or more intimates accompany the patient to the office or hospital, we prefer to interview the patient with the intimate present unless the patient objects or asks to be seen alone. It is not necessary that the intimates be close family. They might be roommates, lovers, caregivers, or very concerned friends. We have several reasons for this preference. The intimate can often provide crucial information that the patient is unaware of or has minimized or denied. Often the intimate wants to be sure that the patient has told everything to the doctor. Intimates may have their own agenda and questions that may be very important for the patient's well-being and treatment. Often the problems of the patient originate in the milieu in which they live. Meeting and understanding a young patient's wife or husband may yield valuable insights into the patient's illness and behavior. Also, intimates can give the patient a feeling of security and support in a difficult setting.

Unfortunately, especially with hospitalized patients whom a neurologist is asked to see in consultation, the observers' history is too often neglected. We have interrupted office visits to call a spouse who had witnessed an episode of loss of consciousness that the patient could not describe. In many patients, description of the problem event is so central to diagnosis and analysis that all possible steps should be taken to find observers. Their testimony may be worth much more than all the intricate and expensive investigation tools at your disposal. Yet too often the consultant is content to copy the description of the illness taken third hand that has been scribbled in a hospital chart.

Just as it is important to obtain all relevant information, it is equally essential to respect the patient's privacy and wishes. Patients should always be asked initially if they would like their intimates to be present during the interview. Even when they choose to be accompanied, we always seize an opportunity to be alone with the patient to ask for any information that they might not share with their relatives or intimates present. An excellent opportunity for this is during gait testing. We always ask ambulatory patients to walk along a hall or corridor outside the office, examining room, or hospital room. Out of vision and hearing of the intimate, some patients will reveal important data previously concealed. A young woman may tell you about use of oral contraceptives or cocaine, facts that she would never relate in her mother's presence.

Caution should be exercised when contacting people at the patient's work site. Although it may be important to obtain information from witnesses to an event that took place at work or from employers and employees of the patient, the information revealed to these individuals by your questioning could affect the patient's return to work and ability to earn a livelihood. It is always best when possible to obtain the patient's permission before you contact others. Needless to say, information about the patient's diagnosis and prognosis should never be revealed to strangers without the patient's permission.

What Does the Patient Think Is Wrong? Is He or She Worried about any Specific Disorder?

Patients are usually laypersons, often with serious misconceptions and misinformation about disease. They harbor impressions, fears, and concerns that are totally unexpected and would not have occurred to you.

A young man with intermittent tingling of his left foot revealed that he was "deathly afraid" of muscular dystrophy. He had seen a childhood chum become progressively disabled by that disease and had watched the Jerry Lewis Muscular Dystrophy Telethon two weeks before. Of course, muscular dystrophy would not have been remotely entertained in a doctor's differential diagnosis for this patient because it does not cause numbness. Simply reassuring him about the absence of this dreaded disease was extremely therapeutic. The actual cause of the trivial symptom was not very important to the patient who didn't wish to pursue expensive and time-consuming tests and investigations such as electrodiagnostic testing or imaging.

We usually ask the patient about any insights into the cause of the problem and any specific worries or concerns. If the patient mentions a particular disease or cause of illness, we make certain that we pursue further his or her reasons and concerns. The patient's ideas and reasoning are often very helpful in understanding their motivation to consult a neurologist, and will be very important to deal with in the summary discussion. Understanding the patient's perspective of the encounter is a most important key to establishing effective doctor-patient communication.[20] Sometimes during the discussion of the patient's ideas about the symptoms or disease, the patient will reveal new data not previously forthcoming during the interview.

Patients' Reasons for and Expectations of Consulting a Doctor

Patients come to doctors for different reasons. Some seek a cure of their disease, others simply want relief from or amelioration of their symptoms. Some want a clarification and explanation of their problem in terms that they can understand; they have not received this from previous caregivers. Some seek a more sensitive, caring, concerned approach; they may not be dissatisfied or critical of the competence of their prior care, only unhappy with the "bedside manner" and style of delivery. Some patients come to satisfy their spouses, lovers, bosses, or parents whom they feel are needlessly concerned and who will be "on their back" until they do get medical attention. Some come to legitimize the fact that they are infirm or disabled, not to ameliorate their symptoms, which serve an important function in their equilibrium with their environment. Some want confirmation of a diagnosis of serious disease or, more hopefully, a different, more favorable opinion. Some seek guidelines in choice of physicians. Some have simply come because their doctors told them to, or because that is what people do when they are sick.

The answer to the question of why the patient has come is difficult and more complex than what the patient thinks is the cause of the symptoms. Many patients have not thought of their motives and cannot analyze or describe them. Answers will come from observation and discussion. Some articulate and direct patients will tell you, "I want your advice about the surgery that Dr. X has prescribed" or "Doctor, I am not so much bothered by the tingling in my leg—I wouldn't take any pill for it. I just want to know what is causing it." We sometimes ask patients which is more important to them: learning the cause of the symptoms or obtaining relief from the symptoms, or are both of equal importance?

One patient seen years ago provides an excellent example of the importance of learning the patient's expectations. She was a 39-year-old, upwardly mobile African American woman who had very severe headaches. After the initial visit, L.R.C. explained to her that she had migraine and shared with her treatment alternatives. The first medicine did no good, and she returned in three weeks, emphasizing the terrible pain she suffered and how it was ruining her life. L.R.C. gave her another pill to prophylactically prevent headaches, and again there was no effect. The third prescription was a different matter: She entered the office crying and said that the pill had such bad side effects that she had to stop it. The calendar on which she had been asked to record the frequency, duration, and severity of her headaches showed that during the first two weeks after beginning the new pill, she had had no headaches. When this was pointed out, she said, "Yes, but the side effects were very bad. It changed my whole personality." L.R.C. asked her to explain. She then described her activities. A divorcee, she rose early to get her children off to school, then worked until dinner. She rushed home and prepared dinner; afterwards, her two teenage girls went upstairs to do homework, watch TV, and talk on the telephone. She explained that when she had a headache (two or three times a week), her girls came to her room, brought her warm milk, rubbed her neck, and consoled her. They also talked to her about their problems, triumphs, and activities. During the two weeks that she was headache-free, they spent very little time with her. She erupted and was very critical of the children and berated them. "You see," she said, "the pills made me lose control and yell at my children." She was telling me that her headaches served a very important function in her relationship with her children and she did not really want the headaches to go away, only to be relieved a bit. She wanted me to be sympathetic. She wanted some easing of her headache surely, but not a cure. From that time on, she was given advice and a mild analgesic. She returned periodically for three years, always bitterly complaining of the headaches. She used the visits to seek advice (from an experienced father and a man) about raising her children. The tacit "contract" between her and L.R.C. became clear only during a period of time. It may not be possible during the initial interview to elicit the nature of the doctor-patient "contract" desired by a particular patient, but the physician should at least begin to seek insight into this issue early.

The timing of the office visit or hospitalization is also important. Why is this patient here now? Why today? Did the symptoms change abruptly or worsen? Did new symptoms occur? Did someone else press them to come now? Is the other physician that he or she has customarily seen away, ill, or unreachable? We always ask about the timing of the visit. This also gives important insights into the patient's history, the pace of the illness, and motives for seeking consultation.

Exploring the Social and Environmental Aspects of the Illness

Patients are seldom completely isolated. Many have very complex social, family, moral, religious, professional, and economic environments. The nature of their environments sometimes explains the symptoms. Often, doctors must know about the environments to help patients respond to their illness. To treat disease, physicians must know about patients as well as their diseases.

A detailed study performed in the 1950s provides important insight into the importance of the social context of illness.[21] The authors studied over 3,000 patients, divided into five different social groups (two American working groups, one group of Chinese origin, one of American college graduates, and one of Hungarian refugees). Illness episodes were not randomly distributed among members of any of these groups. In each group, during two decades of adult life, a quarter of the individuals had about one-half of all the episodes of illness of their group. These were not single diseases and their sequelae; the susceptibility to illness involved unrelated diseases of different organ systems. Moreover, these episodes of illness clustered during periods of one to two years, with intervals of relatively good health between. Physicians took historical accounts of illness while, concurrently and separately, social scientists questioned the individuals about their life histories and experiences. A remarkable number of illness clusters surrounded important life events—college, marriage, divorce, moving, a new job, death or illness of family or friends, an affair, or economic difficulties. The great majority of illness clusters in the lives of members of each group occurred at times when individuals perceived their situations to be threatening, unsatisfying, overdemanding, and in conflict. They often could not make satisfactory adaptations to their situations.

Obviously, during the initial visit, the physician cannot learn all the details of the patient's life. The patient's family and work situation and any presently perceived important stresses are significant. One useful technique is to ask about activities during a single typical day. As a patient describes her day from awakening to retiring, a great deal is revealed about her and individuals with whom she shares her life. This technique also gives insight into whether or how the symptoms affect the patient's daily routines.

Below the Line: The More Personal and Intimate Milieu

We have already introduced the concept popularized by Lisansky and Shochet of the comprehensive medical diagnosis—disease and personality, the double diagnosis.[22] In this schema, the more intimate personality features are drawn below the line, physical symptoms go above the line, and environmental factors are recorded along the line in a neutral zone. Personal intimate data are the most difficult to elicit. This type of data are usually best elicited by a low-control, patient-centered approach of interviewing.[9] Usually multiple visits are needed for the doctor to fully gain the confidence of patients, enabling them to share their innermost fears, guilt, and anxieties. The physician must ask what sort of person the patient is. How will the patient respond to treatment suggestions? Will he be compliant? Is he reliable? Is he likely to return for needed tests and treatment? Is he likely to decompensate psychologically? How? With depression? Manic behavior? Psychosis? Denial?

Be sensitive both to patients' words and nonverbal behavior. Dress, facial expressions, voice intonation and inflection, gestures, and body movements can be very revealing. Note cues that show that the material being discussed is sensitive. Some patients will "go below the line," introducing sensitive subjects such as problems at work or marital discord. You can follow the lead gingerly, watching for indications that the patient is uncomfortable and wants to switch the topic. If the patient resists further discussion, make a mental note to explore the issues later at a more appropriate time.

Let's consider a middle-aged lawyer who consults you about a seizure and mentions excessive use of alcohol. You might ask, "How long have you been drinking? Do you drink alone or with others? Does your drinking affect your work or your family life?" Be sensitive to the patient's changing the subject or evasive replies. Avoid focusing prematurely or too aggressively on sensitive issues.

Some patients show emotion during the interview. Sighing, a catch in the throat, and crying are often spontaneous during the interview. Let patients express their feelings. Be empathetic. Don't act indifferent or unconcerned, and don't switch topics until the patient has had a chance to express feelings. The patient's perception as to your concern and caring or lack thereof may derive from your handling of the patient's emotional displays.

After completing the formal history taking, while the patient is undressing, the physician should mentally list the major differential diagnoses in order of likely probability. This is the time to plan the physical examination.

We have tried to emphasize in this chapter the importance of style and the methods of the history-taking process. Doctors should become more self-conscious and aware of the techniques they use and the potential gains and shortcomings of these stylistic choices. The essence of effective history taking is the use of hypotheses that are sequentially tested. The data elicited must be very detailed and exacting. Especially important is the pace of the illness. Attention must also be devoted to the environment in which the patient lives, works, and became ill.

REFERENCES

1. Bean RB, Osler Sir William. *Aphorisms from His Bedside Teaching and Writings.* Springfield, IL: Charles C Thomas, 1961;41.
2. Sahs A (quoted by Robert Joynt, M.D.). A eulogy delivered to the American Neurological Association, October 20, 1987.
3. Hodgins E. Listen: The patient. *N Engl J Med* 1966;274:657–661.
4. Cox K. *Doctor and Patient: Exploring Clinical Thinking.* Sydney: University of New South Wales Press, 1999;ix.
5. Spiro H. What is empathy and can it be taught? *Ann Intern Med* 1992;116:843–846.
6. Brewin TB. Not TLC but FPI. *J Roy Soc Med* 1990;83:172–175.
7. Carter WB, Inui TS, Kukull WA, et al. Outline based doctor-patient interaction, analysis II, identifying effective provider and patient behavior. *Med Care* 1982; 20:550–556.
8. Tumulty PA. The art of healing. *Johns Hopkins Med J* 1978;143:140–143.

9. Smith RC, Hoppe RB. The patient's story: Integrating the patient- and physician-centered approaches to interviewing. *Ann Intern Med* 1991;115:470–477.
10. Barrows H, Bennett K. The diagnostic (problem solving) skill of the neurologist. *Arch Neurol* 1972;26:273–277.
11. Platt EW, McMath JC. Clinical hypocompetence: The interview. *Ann Int Med* 1979,91:898–902.
12. Waitzkin H. Doctor-patient communication: Clinical implications of social scientific research. *JAMA* 1984;252:2441–2446.
13. Waitzkin H. Doctors and patients—are they really communicating? *The Internist* August 1986:7–10.
14. Beckman HB, Frankel RM. The effect of physician behavior on the collection of data. *Ann Intern Med* 1984;101:692–696.
15. Marvel MK, Epstein RM, Flowers K, Beckman HB. Soliciting the patient's agenda. Have we improved? *JAMA* 1999;281:283–287.
16. Cox K. *Doctor and Patient: Exploring Clinical Thinking*. Sydney: University of New South Wales Press, 1999.
17. Caplan LR. Course-of-illness graphs. *Hospital Practice* 1985;20:125–136.
18. Caplan LR. Fisher's rules. *Arch Neurol* 1982;39:389–390.
19. Dyck PJ, Oviatt K, Lambert EH. Intensive evaluation of referred unclassified neuropathies yields improved diagnosis. *Ann Neurol* 1981;10:222–226.
20. Delbanco TL. Enriching the doctor-patient relationship by inviting the patient's perspective. *Ann Intern Med* 1992;116:414–418.
21. Hinkle LE, Wolff HG. Ecologic investigations of the relationship between illness, life experiences, and the social environment. *Ann Intern Med* 1958;49:1373–1388.
22. Lisansky ET, Shochet BR. Comprehensive medical diagnosis for the internist. *Med Clin N Am* 1967;51:1381–1397.

4

The General Systemic and Neurologic Examinations

Was man weiss, man sieht.[1] (What one knows, one sees.)

—Goethe

Let someone say of a doctor that he really knows his physiology or anatomy. . . . These are not real compliments; but if you say he is an observer, a man who knows how to see, this is perhaps the greatest compliment one can make.[2]

—J.M. Charcot

Here is a gentleman of a medical type, but with the air of a military man. Clearly an army doctor, then. He has just come from the tropics, for his face is dark, and that is not the natural tint of his skin, for his wrists are fair. He has undergone hardship and sickness as his haggard face says clearly. His left arm has been injured. He holds it in a stiff and unnatural manner. Where in the tropics could an English Army doctor have seen much hardship and got his arm wounded? Clearly in Afghanistan.[3]

—Sherlock Holmes speaking, Arthur Conan Doyle

As the direct clinical observation may be a very lengthy procedure it is understandable that many an unripe youngster in this machine-ridden era of hustle and bustle finds some difficulty in settling down to patient observation and clinical examination of the living individual, hoping that the modern technical methods will offer short cuts to diagnosis. In the face of this tendency it cannot be emphasized strongly enough that the direct clinical observation and meticulous clinical examination of the patient still constitute the main pillars of neurological clinical science, representing, as they do, "the sacred facts."[4]

—G. Monrad-Krohn

What is the most unique and specific feature that separates doctor-patient interactions from those in other professions, businesses, and endeavors? The examination of the human body. The examination is often sensitive, occasionally uncomfortable, and nearly always accompanied by anxiety as to what the doctor might find. The visit to a neurologist may add an element of additional concern about the nature of the interaction with this new type of physician. Patients often visualize physicians as individuals in white coats, listening, looking, and feeling with various commonly recognized instruments such as stethoscopes, tongue blades, and reflex hammers. The doctor's handling of the examination is very important to the patient and is one of the major factors a patient uses to rate the doctor's abilities and sensitivity. A careful neurologic examination is especially important when the patient has a grave diagnosis. A hurried, cursory, or insensitive examination is not easily forgotten. Some physical examination should take place during every encounter. Touching (physical contact during the examination) is usually therapeutic and reminds patients of the doctor's special relation to them. The policy of most psychiatrists to eschew physical examinations remains an extremely unwise and counterproductive rule that needlessly separates psychiatry from the rest of medicine.

Clinicians should generate a list of diagnostic possibilities after the initial history. The physical examination allows the clinician to validate these hypotheses. There is a tendency to see what we expect to see and care must be taken to observe what is there rather than what we have decided should be present. Generating hypothetical diagnoses after the history adds some challenge and fun to the diagnostic chase. We must be sure to objectively reevaluate the hypotheses during the physical examination as abnormalities are found.

The physical examination is a mixture of routine procedures and hypothesis-driven testing. We find what we look for! Unfortunately, all too often believing is seeing. It is important to observe and record what is really there rather than that which our preliminary hypotheses would lead us to expect. If the examination is perfunctory, the yield will be small. A truly complete examination is too long and tiring for both patient and physician. Effective clinicians tailor the examination to the problems presented and to the hypotheses generated from the history, while at the same time they remain alert for unexpected findings.

The doctor must decide whether to allow a relative or intimate, who was present during the history, to stay during the examination or to ask them to step outside. Sometimes it is advantageous to have them stay. Spouses serve a chaperone function when the doctor examines a patient of the opposite sex who is even partially disrobed. Some patients feel more secure and relaxed when an intimate remains with them, especially if the patient is a child or a frail elderly person. Other patients are embarrassed or very sensitive about undressing before their children, parents, or friends. Especially during mental state testing, some elderly people do not want intimates present to witness their deficiencies and failings. I usually ask the patient and the intimate if they would feel more comfortable waiting outside or would prefer to stay during the examination. Both may say yes but embarrassment may develop during the examination. If there is any doubt at any time, it is best to ask them to leave.

GENERAL EXAMINATION

The extent of the general examination depends on a number of factors. Was the patient referred by a competent family practitioner or internist? Was the patient recently examined? How complete was the recent examination? Are there systemic symptoms? How much can the neurologist narrow the differential diagnostic probabilities from the history? Do not be trapped into merely uncritically accepting prior medical diagnoses. Often a finding on general examination will clarify the neurologic diagnosis. Finding the typical rash of Lyme disease or secondary syphilis, the adenopathy of infectious mononucleosis or AIDS, enlarged lacrimal and parotid glands of sarcoidosis, or palpating a prostatic or rectal tumor often explains previously obscure neurologic symptoms.

We always check and record the blood pressure in one arm. Even when there is no history of hypertension and the blood pressure is normal, the baseline values will be helpful to the neurologist and the referring generalist for future reference. For efficiency and to save time in dressing and undressing, the general examination is integrated into the neurologic exam. Mental state testing blends naturally with the completion of the history, before any disrobing. Then the head, neck, facial structures, eyes, ears, nose, and throat are examined while testing cranial nerve function. The pulses and skin and joints of the extremities are examined when limb, motor, sensory, and deep tendon reflexes are tested. We usually test first the arms, then the legs. When dizziness is a concern, we often evaluate the Barany maneuver before having the patient lie down. If needed, the chest, heart, abdomen, and back are examined next. Gait is checked either before the general and neurologic examination or just before patients reseat themselves for the discussion. We prefer to watch patients as they are ushered into the examination room and seat themselves. This gives considerable insight into their motor performance at a time when they are not aware that they are being assessed. When appropriate, we take them out into the corridor for gait testing before they disrobe rather than have them walk the few feet most examination rooms allow.

Let's take several examples of eclectic general examinations tailored to hypotheses generated by the history. A 56-year-old man has had two attacks of spinning dizziness lasting thirty seconds and two minutes, respectively. One was accompanied by visual blurring. Neither left any residual deficits. He has a past history of hypertension and is being treated for angina pectoris. This patient has described transient spells of dysfunction of the vestibular system either peripherally or in the brainstem. The most important cause by far is attacks of transient ischemia due to disease of the subclavian-vertebral-basilar arteries of the posterior circulation. The past hypertension and cardiac disease support the fact that the patient is an arteriopath prone to arteriosclerosis of the extracranial and intracranial large arteries and also suggest the possibility of cardiogenic embolism. In this patient, the heart and vascular system should be carefully examined. The most common site for arteriosclerosis causing the symptoms is the proximal subclavian and proximal vertebral arteries. The upper limbs should be carefully examined for ischemia. Feel the radial pulses simultaneously. Is one smaller, delayed, or less forceful than the other? Is one arm or hand cooler than the other? If the pulses are different, check the blood pressures in both arms. Next feel the innominate and subclavian arteries in the supraclavicular notch and listen for bruits in this region and along the mastoid areas where the vertebral arteries course. Is there asymmetry of the supraclavicular area? A cervical rib? In this patient with probable cardiovascular disease, it will also be important to listen over the carotid arteries and feel the facial pulses for asymmetries or augmented flow.[5,6] The pulse and heart should be carefully examined for arrhythmia, heart size, and murmurs. Palpation of the pedal and femoral pulses will also give an indication of atherosclerosis in these or tributary arteries. In this patient, special attention should also be directed to the eyes. The retina will give good information about the severity of hypertension and the presence of degenerative or arteriosclerotic changes. While the patient's complaint of visual blurring in one attack may merely reflect oscillopsia from transient vestibular nystagmus, one needs to be alert to a possible subtle abnormality of eye movement or visual field testing that may give a clue as to the location of the process. The ears will also require special attention because of the nature of the main symptom, spinning dizziness.

The second patient is a 75-year-old widow who described unpleasant tingling, prickly feelings in her fingers. She reported some change in her balance and gait. Her feet feel odd—sometimes cold, and at other times there are sharp almost stabbing pains in her legs and thighs and a strange feeling of ants crawling on the skin of her lower extremities. The symptoms were compatible with a peripheral polyneuropathy or a myelopathy. The doctor should think of metabolic diseases that might be potentially remediable or important to detect. Leading the list are pernicious anemia, hypothyroidism, and diabetes mellitus. Search for clues of the presence of pernicious anemia; by checking the conjunctiva and color of the skin creases in the hand, the hemoglobin can be estimated. Look for splenomegaly, blue eyes, and an atrophic tongue. Look for signs of hypothyroidism. What is the skin and hair texture? Is the thyroid enlarged or nodular? Is axillary and pubic hair distribution normal? Is the voice hoarse? Check the ocular fundus particularly for signs of diabetic retinopathy.

The third patient is a 34-year-old woman referred from another city because of multiple strokes. Exhaustive laboratory testing during three hospital admissions and innumerable outpatient visits including multiple MRI scans, several catheter digital subtraction angiograms, and extensive blood tests for coagulopathy had proven negative. She sought another opinion. L.R.C. asked her to undress. As soon as he entered the room, he was stunned to see very extensive livedo reticularis involving her trunk and limbs. She said that this finding had been present since youth. She also said that he was the first person to completely undress her for examination. The diagnosis of Sneddon's syndrome was apparent even without laboratory tests. We have had similar experiences with other patients with Sneddon's syndrome. The angiokeratomas of

Fabry's disease, and the cutaneous findings in patients with pseudoxanthoma elasticum and tuberous sclerosis have also provided valuable clues to the diagnosis of patients with complex neurologic symptoms.[7] Disrobing patients (leaving underwear and bras on) can be a very helpful diagnostic procedure. In any case, be sure to examine the skin carefully. Many other systemic and neurologic disorders have prominent dermatological manifestations. Anemia, jaundice, hypothyroidism, neurofibromatosis, scleroderma, purpura, melanoma, and lupus erythematosus are just a few examples.

The final example patient is a 47-year-old house painter. He reported gradually progressing weakness of the legs, stiffening of his gait, impotence, urinary frequency, and tingling of the feet during the past two weeks. He also had some pain in the upper back. He had no important past illnesses but had felt poorly for the past three months. He smoked two packs of cigarettes a day and drank to excess when no painting jobs were available. In this patient, the motor, sensory, and autonomic symptoms are most likely due to disease of the spinal cord. What might cause spinal cord disease in this setting, and where is the lesion? The slowly progressive nature of the symptoms and back pain suggest cancer. It will be important to look for signs of lung or other cancers. Are the fingers clubbed? Are there supraclavicular or axillary nodes? Is the liver enlarged or nodular? Is percussion and auscultation of the chest normal? Does the prostate gland feel normal or hard and nodular? The back should also be carefully examined for any unusual deformities (kyphosis, a gibbus, or scoliosis). Look for tenderness by fist percussion of the thoracic vertebrae. Is the neck tender? Is there normal mobility of the neck? The emphasis of the general examination of this patient has been quite different from that of the other patients.

At times, diagnoses of systemic diseases will be suggested after the neurologic examination is completed. As mentioned, we usually examine the heart, chest, abdomen, and skin after the extremities and after the neurologic examination. This allows testing of hypotheses of systemic disease generated from the neurologic findings. The neurologic findings might suggest the possibility of conditions such as sarcoidosis, Whipple's disease, systemic lupus erythematosus, acromegaly, hepatic encephalopathy, or arsenic or lead toxicity that would then lead the alert clinician to look for findings in the general examination that would give evidence for or against these conditions.

Some systemic findings will be unexpected from the history. A strikingly high blood pressure, fever, cardiac murmur, enlarged spleen, rheumatoid nodules, impressive lymphadenopathy, a cutaneous melanoma, or jaundice should stimulate rethinking of the original hypotheses concerning the neurologic symptoms generated from the patient's history. Some findings, of course, will be unrelated to the neurologic diagnosis, while others may be critical.

THE NEUROLOGIC EXAMINATION

The neurologic examination is also discussed elsewhere in more detail.[8] In our experience, the two aspects of the neurologic examination that are seldom if ever tested adequately by nonneurologists are the mental state and neuro-ophthalmologic functions. Cognitive and behavioral abnormalities related to cerebral hemisphere dysfunction, and perceptual and oculomotor abnormalities related to dysfunction of the eyes, afferent visual pathways, and oculomotor systems are extremely common and important in patients with neurologic diseases. Neurologists must master testing of the mental state, vision, the visual fields, and oculomotor function. Neurologists should be able to make an initial assessment of cognitive functions to determine when formal neuropsychological testing is indicated and allow adequate imaging and other testing to proceed without excessive delay. When formal intellectual testing is indicated, neuropsychologists can be much more helpful than psychologists or psychiatrists who perform psychometric testing. Mental state and neuropsychological testing is described elsewhere in detail.[9,10] All too many ophthalmologists and optometrists are relatively weak in or inattentive to neuroophthalmology. It is essential that neurologists be capable of evaluating the visual fields and eye movements. In patients with neuromuscular disease, testing of muscle power is most important since this is seldom done adequately by nonneurologists.

Mental State

We divide mental state evaluation schematically into two broad types of observations:

1. Observation of the patient's intellect and behavior during the interview and examination. We call this *gestalt* observation since it is general, unfocused, and informally assessed.
2. *Formal* testing of intellect and behavior. Formal testing should routinely consist of assessment of:
   a. Memory
   b. Language functions
   c. Visual-spatial abilities
   d. Tests of orientation, attention, and concentration

We emphasize these four functions, because focal brain lesions can cause isolated dysfunction of one or more of these capabilities and because these functions are difficult to assess and quantitate without formal testing. Neurologists should assess the mental state in each patient they see. When the symptoms suggest possible disease of the central nervous system, formal testing should be done. In some patients with symptoms that indicate disease of muscle or the peripheral nervous system, testing can often be informal gestalt-type evaluation.

Before elaborating on suggestions for mental state testing, we need to explain the reasons for emphasizing these specific functions and omitting some standard tests contained in medical, psychiatric, and neurologic manuals describing examination of the mental state. We believe that the purpose of examining the mental state is to detect focal brain disease, not to quantitate the patient's intelligence or degree of impairment. Although lack of intelligence is quite common in the general population, most have no important neurologic disease. Moreover, the brief time usually spent on mental state testing does not allow adequate quantification of intellectual ability. In practice, physicians who test general knowledge and try to quantify intelligence make a quick, biased judgment of whether a patient is up to his or her usual par. They then gauge the questions by a rough estimate of the patient's education and possible intelligence quotient (IQ). If the patient is dressed humbly and works as a cleaning lady, very simple questions are asked. If the patient is a bright-looking college student, quite different questions are used. In either case, the examiner can find the patient's intelligence wanting by making the questions too difficult, or can overlook loss of intelligence by aiming the questions too low.

Let's look at the usual general intelligence questions asked: Who's the president? Who are your senators, congressmen, and the mayor? Name in reverse the last six presidents. What are the capitals of Colorado, Vermont, and the Netherlands? Who won the Super Bowl and the World Series last year? Who pitches for the Boston Red Sox? Who won last year's world cup in soccer? Tell me about Kosovo, the impeachment of President Clinton, the Hillary Clinton New York state Senate race (or whatever current events are in the news). What were the dates of the Civil War and World War II? Response to these questions is quite variable in "normal" people encountered on the street or in the doctor's office. People's interests, experiences, and backgrounds are quite different. Also, many patients are offended or put off by this type of questioning. I believe that when the neurologist needs to measure and quantify the patient's IQ, it should be done by formal full-length evaluation using standardized tests such as the Wechsler Adult Intelligence Scale (WAIS) test-revised.[11] General gestalt estimates based on dress, hairstyle, manners, interpersonal behavior, hygiene, mannerisms, gestures, and vocabulary are probably as useful as biased, nonstandard brief questioning.

Much can be learned in each patient by close scrutiny during the history-taking interview. Ask the patient for specific data—names, address, dates, times. When the patient gives a general answer, try to pin him down for more specific information. When did that happen? What was the doctor's name? Do you recall the address, phone number, date of your visit? How is the history organized? What vocabulary does he use? Are his reports consistent? If the patient's history is totally disorganized and inconsistent, the physician should not get upset but instead realize that important diagnostic information has been obtained.

A brief diversion during the history to a description by the patient of an aspect of his work or hobby with detail may contribute not only occupational history but also tell much about mental status. It also establishes rapport with the patient and educates the physician. Most people are willing to discuss their children or grandchildren: How many? Ages? Schooling? Work? The confident description of ten great-grandchildren is a reassuring sign of preserved mental function.

Let us now turn to the content of formal testing. We illustrate by sharing the usual routine of one of us (L.R.C.) and the rationale for the method. He usually begins by asking the patient to write a paragraph. Evaluating the patient's use of written language is an excellent way of screening language capability. No aphasic patient writes and reads normally. The paragraph can be about a general topic of the patient's choosing or a specific topic that you dictate. Sample topics include: Write a letter to a relative describing your symptoms. Write a paragraph about your hometown. Tell a young person why he or she should or should not practice your profession. Evaluate for me the present president. Alternatively, a busy practitioner could ask the patient, while waiting to be called into the office, to write unassisted a long paragraph describing her medical symptoms and why she has come to see the physician. All patients are asked to identify the paragraph by writing their name, address, and the date at the top of the paper. This tests their orientation without calling attention to it. Note the vocabulary, grammar, syntax, and organization of the paragraph and the patient's use of space. If the clinician is suspicious of a language problem, he or she then asks the patient to write lists of objects, for example, ten animals that might be found in the zoo, the ten largest cities in the United States, ten articles of clothing, five means of transportation, ten common hobbies or avocations. This tests naming, spelling, and ability to persevere with a task. Some patients lack English language skills, which can be overcome if they are literate in their native language and a knowledgeable person accompanies the patient. Functionally illiterate patients may be able to write a short sentence only with great effort. It is best to minimize this part of the examination in these individuals.

While the patient still has pencil and paper in hand, L.R.C. next tests *visual-spatial* capabilities by asking the patient to spontaneously draw an object. He chooses a common object with some symmetrical features such as a clock, house, daisy, or bicycle. A clock face requires little artistic skill but can be most informative in patients with what might otherwise be subtle problems. Next he draws an abstract figure (Figure 4-1) and asks the patient to copy it as exactly as possible.

Disorders of drawing or copying can be caused by either left or right cerebral lesions, usually located posteriorly in the hemispheres. Patients with right parietal damage usually copy very poorly. In their spontaneous figures, they often omit objects on the left; size, angles, and proportions are often misjudged. Copying does not improve performance.[12-14] In contrast, patients with left parietal damage often draw very simple rudimentary figures but do not omit one side of the drawing and generally estimate size, angles, and proportions well. They are able to copy well, greatly improving their spontaneous performance. Their problem is conceptualization of the abstract idea of the object, while patients with right parietal lobe damage have a normal concept of the object, but they cannot construct the visual-spatial components of that concept.[15]

It is just as important to test constructual abilities in patients with right cerebral lesions as it is to test speech function in patients with left cerebral pathology. Speech abnormalities usually predict dominant hemisphere perisylvian disease, while constructual dyspraxia with poor copying ability suggests an abnormality of the right inferior parietal lobe. While paper and pencil are still

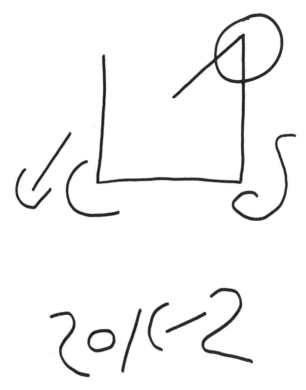

Figure 4-1 Two examples of abstract drawings to be copied.

in hand, in some instances give the patient arithmetical computations to perform. Arithmetic tasks are important in patients in whom the history suggests difficulty with numbers and their manipulation and in patients suspected of having intellectual loss who use mathematics in their jobs or pay the bills at home.

He then asks patients to put the pencil and paper aside and gives them a paragraph to read. He chooses a suitable paragraph from a packet of materials collected for higher cortical function testing kept in his doctor's bag. He most often uses an Aesop's fable of about one hundred words in length, which is copied in large print on a 5 × 8-inch white index card. He asks patients to read the paragraph aloud. He especially notices the articulation of the words, listening for the rhythm and ease of speech production and for dysarthria and dysphonia. He listens for omissions, word errors, pauses, and paralexic errors. Does the patient become distracted from the task? Does the loudness or force of speech diminish as the patient reads? Does tone become more nasal, as in some myasthenics? He then asks patients to describe the point of the story. If they were reading the story to a child, how would they explain the message that the author is trying to transmit? Have patients understood what they read? Can they explain the message in abstract terms? An example of a typical paragraph

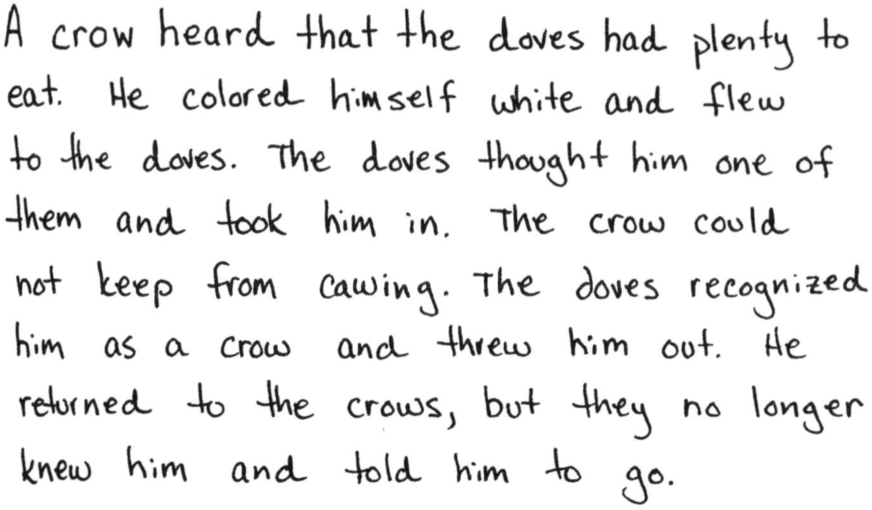

A crow heard that the doves had plenty to eat. He colored himself white and flew to the doves. The doves thought him one of them and took him in. The crow could not keep from cawing. The doves recognized him as a crow and threw him out. He returned to the crows, but they no longer knew him and told him to go.

Figure 4-2 Paragraph to be read aloud by the patient.

is shown in Figure 4-2. He later uses the paragraph as one memory item to test the patient's recall ability. If the examiner has no packet of test materials handy, an appropriate paragraph for reading can be chosen from a nearby newspaper, magazine, or book—ubiquitous objects in doctors' offices and in the wards and patient rooms of hospitals. Alternatively Gray's standardized reading paragraphs are useful for quantifying reading abnormalities.[16]

He next shows patients a series of pictures. Dr. Caplan is particularly interested in how normal patients and those with brain lesions handle visual information. While some patients seem to resent "school tests" of general information, objecting that the doctor is checking to see if they have "lost their marbles," they usually do not object to looking at pictures. He usually prefaces the testing by saying that he is interested in their vision. He chooses pictures or scenes that have been cut out from magazines such as the *National Geographic*. The pictures usually have multiple people or objects scattered on the left and right sides. He holds the picture in front of patients for about ten seconds. If the patient has poor visual acuity, he gives the picture to the patient to examine. After withdrawing the picture, he asks patients what they saw. After their general description, he asks for specific details. When and where did the scene take place? How old are the individuals? How are they dressed? (Figures 4-3, 4-4, and 4-5 are sample pictures used.) Much can be learned from the patient's performance. Watch the patients' eyes as they scan the picture. Do they search symmetrically? Have they seen the whole picture? What vocabulary do they use to describe the contents? Have they grasped the general gestalt of the picture or gotten lost in a minor peripheral aspect? An alternative useful picture is the Cookie Theft Picture that is used in the NIH Stroke Scale (Figure 4-6).[17] Patients with right cerebral hemisphere lesions often neglect the left details of

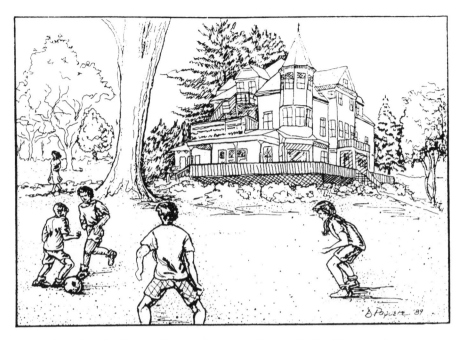

Figure 4-3 Sample picture of a complex scene. (Drawn by Dari Paquette.)

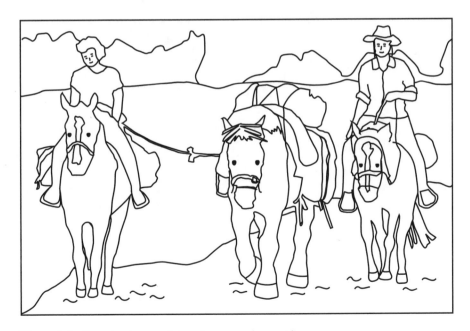

Figure 4-4 Sample picture of three horses and two riders.

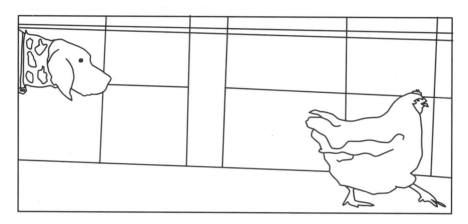

Figure 4-5 Sample picture showing a dog chasing a hen.

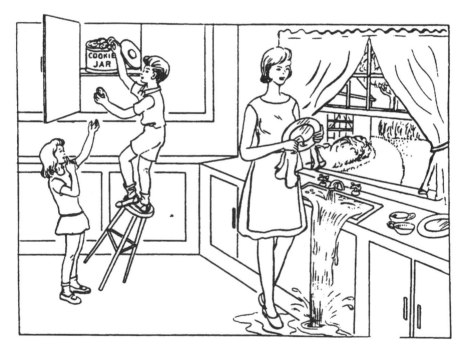

Figure 4-6 The cookie theft picture. (Reprinted with permission from Lyden P, Brott T, Tilley B, Welch KMA, Maacha EJ. NINDS TPA Stroke Study Group. Improved reliability of the NIH Stroke Scale using video training. *Stroke* 1994; 25.)

the picture.[14,18] Figure 4-5 or a similar picture is especially useful in patients with right hemisphere disease who might have neglect of the left side of visual space. These individuals will fail to see the dog on the left of the picture. Patients with frontal lobe disease often scan poorly and are satisfied with describing the first feature that catches their eye. They do not extract further information from the scene. He usually shows two or three pictures and uses them for memory items later. Pictures from magazines, especially advertisements, can substitute for your own pictures.

He next shows patients pictures of well-known individuals pasted on index cards to test *memory*. He carries in the testing packet pictures of a variety of different individuals—prominent men and women in the fields of politics, entertainment, sports, and comic characters. He selects from these five or ten individuals, chosen with the age, sex, and background of the patient in mind. He asks patients to name the individuals as they are shown. If they cannot name the character shown in the picture, he asks them to describe the individual if they can. After patients are finished naming all of the individuals, he reviews with them the pictures while they are still laid out on the desk. He encourages grouping, for example, pictures showing two individuals together and pictures of men or women, and figures from different occupations. For example, he might say, "I have shown you four single pictures, all women (Jacqueline Onassis, Julia Roberts, Hillary Clinton, and Oprah Winfrey); five men, all political figures—two pairs (Franklin Delano Roosevelt and Winston Churchill, and Bill Clinton and Al Gore), one single picture of Ronald Reagan; and one comic character, Mickey Mouse. As he names the individuals, he points to the pictures grouped together to facilitate recall. He always warns patients that he will later ask them to remember what pictures they were shown. A patient's ability to name and describe the individuals tells something about naming and language functions and recall of past information. Formal facial recognition testing can utilize the Benton Photographs.[19]

When the rest of the neurologic examination has been completed and the patient has dressed and reseated himself, L.R.C. asks the patient to recall (1) the paragraph that was read, (2) what scenes were shown, and (3) the names of the people in the pictures. This usually includes fourteen data items from memory—one paragraph, three scenes, and ten individuals. Amnesia, the inability to make new memories and to recall recent events and recently learned data, can be caused by focal lesions of the brain. Lesions causing memory loss usually affect structures within Papez circuit—mammillary bodies, mammillothalamic tract, medial thalamic nuclei, fornices, and medial temporal lobes including the hippocampi and amygdala. Bilateral lesions of these structures are usually required to produce permanent amnesia, but unilateral left-sided lesions can cause amnesia lasting as long as six months.[20,21] Lesions of the septal nuclei and basal frontal lobes involving the basal nuclei of Meynert, often due to rupture of an anterior communicating artery aneurysm, can also cause abnormalities of memory function. It is always important to test memory actively by giving patients material and later checking their recall ability. Passive memory testing, that is, asking patients what they had for breakfast or what they did yesterday, is unsatisfactory since answers can be made up or confabulated and the doctor usually cannot check the accuracy of the answers.

We sometimes use other active tests to check memory. We give patients three items to recall: for example, a horse, Santa Claus, and 125 Park Avenue. Patients should be told that their recall of the items will be tested later. We ask patients to repeat the objects to be sure that they have heard and registered them. Alternatively, the doctor can tell patients a story with a number of data items. We often use the following story: "Tom, Bill, and Harry went fishing in the Adirondack Mountains on July 4. They caught three mackerel and two bass, and then each had a roast beef sandwich and a bottle of Budweiser beer." This story contains ten key facts. At the end of the examination, the number of items recalled can be assessed. Patients with aphasia may be unable to reliably recite items; in patients with important language dysfunction, it is usually best to hide objects in the room. The patient later is asked to point to the objects. Money is especially effective. For example, hide a five dollar bill under the phone, one dollar in the desk drawer, and fifty cents under a piece of paper.

We have now screened the patient for language, visual-spatial, and memory dysfunction, and orientation. If abnormalities are found on the screening tests, the evaluation of these functions should be pursued further. If an abnormality of speech is present, more extensive testing of spoken language production, naming, repetition of spoken language, and comprehension of spoken and written language is necessary. A set of simple pictures for naming can be assembled from magazines, or the booklet from the Boston Naming Test may be used.[22] A particularly useful test easily administered at the bedside is the token test of DeRenzi and Vignolo.[23] Tokens of different sizes (small and large), shapes (triangles and rectangles), and colors (red, yellow, blue, green) are used (Figure 4-7). These can be easily made from wood, cardboard, or plastic and colored with a child's painting set. The patient is first given directions using a single descriptor: ("pick up a small one, red one, or triangle"), then two adjectives ("small red, large triangle, yellow rectangle"), then three descriptors ("the large red triangle"). If the patient performs correctly, six descriptors are used ("put the small blue square alongside the large red triangle"). Relation words, especially difficult for aphasics, can be checked ("hold the blue one above, below, over, instead of, with the red one").

Visual-spatial abnormalities can be further checked by having the patient copy the Rey-Osterrieth figure[24-26] (Figure 4-8) or constructing mosaic patterns using Koh's blocks[27] (Figure 4-9). Koh's blocks are small cubes that have surfaces that are red, blue, and white; red and white; blue and white; and red and blue. Diagrams of models of mosaics to be copied are available in WAIS-R testing kits since testing with red and white Koh's blocks is a standard part of this IQ test.[11] This subtest of the WAIS is easily administered in the office or at the bedside and is very useful in quantifying the severity of constructional, visual-spatial deficits.

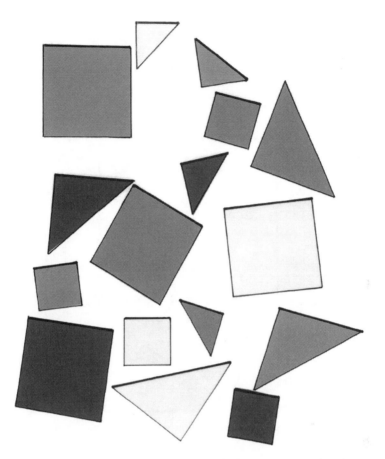

Figure 4-7 Different shapes, sizes, and colors of tokens. (Reprinted with permission from DeRenzi E, Vignolo L. The token test: A sensitive test to detect receptive disturbances in aphasics. *Brain* 1962;85.)

More detailed tests of memory using various items from different sensory modalities for presentation (visual, auditory, tactile) can be given. Usually patients with left thalamic-temporal lobe disease find it difficult to remember verbal language material, while right thalamic-temporal pathology causes more visual memory difficulty.

The other types of screening procedures used as part of the mental state evaluation are aimed at testing the patient's ability to concentrate on and handle tasks that require persistent effort. Lack of concentrating ability is a common, but nonspecific problem; it can be caused by psychological factors, depression, head injuries such as concussion, sedative drugs and alcohol, or any toxic or metabolic encephalopathy. A standard test for concentration is repetition of series of numbers forward and backward. The numbers are given slowly ("1...7...9...5"), and

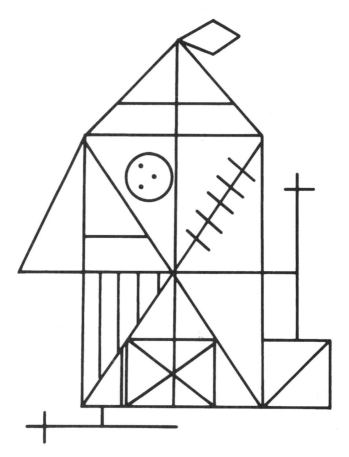

Figure 4-8   The Rey-Osterrieth figure for copying.

then the patient reports them as given or transposes them (5, 9, 7, 1). Most patients should be able to retain at least six numbers forward and five in reverse. Some patients perform this task inconsistently, transposing six numbers correctly and then failing to transpose five in the next attempt. Spelling the word "worlds" backwards is a similar task. Addition or subtraction of serial 2s or 3s is a similar type of concentration task (not of calculation) since the patient must concentrate on and recall the previous number before each addition and subtraction.

Patients with a variety of different lesions have difficulty performing long tasks. Patients with large frontal lobe lesions or extensive bilateral cerebral disease often show abulia.[28] Abulia can be defined as (1) lack of spontaneity in speech and activity, (2) long latency in initiating a task or in responding to queries or directions, (3) short, terse replies, and (4) difficulty persevering with tasks. Some tests that are useful in screening for abulia are counting backwards as quickly as possible from 20 to 0, crossing off all the As in a long paragraph, instructing the patient to say "up" or "down" each time you move

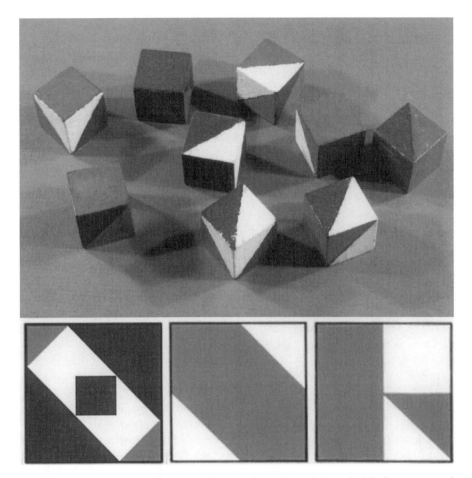

Figure 4-9   Koh's blocks. Mosaics to be copied are shown below the blocks. (Reprinted with permission from Wechsler D. WAIS—R. Wechsler Adult Intelligence Scale—Revised. New York: Psychological Corporation, 1981.)

his finger. Abulic patients will often wait to begin the task, sometimes requiring repetition of the directions and exhortation. Shortly after starting, they will often slow down, become distracted, or stop. For example, counting backward, they will say "20...19...18...17...16." They will require stimulation from the doctor to continue ("come along," "what's next?"). Some, after beginning to count backward correctly, will start to count forward ("20...19...18...17...16...15...16...17...18"). When asked to cross off all the As on a page, they will correctly identity the first few As and then become sloppy or simply stop the task. When testing position sense, abulic patients may respond correctly after the first few finger displacements, then will stop responding. The examiner will have to prompt them ("what direction was that?" or "now") each time the finger is moved to elicit a verbal response.

Luria[29] and others[30,31] have outlined a number of tests for perseveration and other abnormalities often present in patients with disorders that affect the frontal lobes. Patients with frontal lobe lesions often have difficulty switching from one subject or task to another. The patient is asked to write repeatedly a series of two squares, one circle, two squares, one circle, two squares, and one circle; patients with frontal lobe disease may have difficulty in switching from square to circle and will write more than two squares. A similar task involves tapping with palm down twice alternating with palm up once. The patient can be asked to alternate positions using one hand. The patient is told to hit the top of the desk, first with a fisted hand, then with the palm, then with the side of the hand. These alternate hand postures are continued for 20 seconds or more. Patiuents who perseverate will have difficulty inhibiting repetition of postures. Another test involves alternating actions of the two hands such as palm down with the left hand followed by palm up with the right hand then palm up with the left hand and palm down with the right hand.

Frontal lobe pathology can also affect the patient's planning of a task. Ask the patient to make a floor plan of a one-story house that they would like to live in. This task requires preliminary thinking to decide on the number of bedrooms and baths and their relation to the rest of the house. Patients with frontal lobe dysfunction will often begin impulsively with little forethought, and the relations, sizes, and proportions will be poorly considered.

Another common paradigm used in patients suspected of having frontal lobe lesions involves go/no-go responses.[31,32] These test the patient's ability to follow stimulus-response behavior rules and to be able to change the behavior when the rules change. The patient is asked to hold the hand in one position in response to the examiner holding his or her hand in one position and to hold the hand in a different position when the examiner holds his or her hand in a second position. Then the rule is switched so that the first examiner's hand position requires the patient to respond as they did to the second hand position in the first test. Another way of performing the test is to ask the patient to hold the hand in one posture when the examiner holds his or her hand in a certain position but not to act if the examiner holds his or her hand in a different posture.

We have now finished the routine screening for mental status abnormalities. The entire testing should take no longer than seven to ten minutes (less if patients write their paragraph while waiting to be seen). We have omitted a number of standard tests suggested by others, for example, tests of general information, proverb interpretation, subtraction of serial 7s from 100, and so-called tests of judgment. We have already given the opinion that general information tests are biased and not diagnostic. Most individuals have heard proverbs since they were children and associate them with didactic sermons about proper behavior. By adulthood, they are sick of hearing proverbs and cannot interpret them as fresh problems. Orally presented computations are quite variably handled by normal people, and difficulty performing sequential arithmetic manipulations is a very nonspecific finding. Putative tests of judgment usually involve asking the patient how they would behave under certain hypothetical conditions (What would you do if someone in a movie theatre yelled fire? What would you do if you found stamped, addressed letters on the street?). These are intellectual tests of gamesmanship, not tests of judgment.

Throughout this chapter, we have mentioned paraphernalia that are useful during cortical function testing. We believe it is very important for neurologists to keep a small test kit in their bags or offices for ease of testing. This kit is probably more practically useful than a reflex hammer or sharp disposable pin—objects that most neurologists find indispensable. We list here suggested components of such a kit. These materials are easily collected and should be maintained and refurbished as times change.

1. A series of paragraphs, for example, Aesop's fables.
2. Gray's reading paragraphs.[16]
3. Scenes from magazines such as *National Geographic*.
4. Pictures of well-known individuals.
5. Small pictures of common objects, for example, telephone, window shade, lamp, chimney, etc.
6. Common objects, for example, comb, spoon, paper clip, or safety pin.
7. Koh's blocks and mosaic patterns.[11,27]
8. Tokens.[23]
9. Identical photographs of faces for matching.
10. Colored plastic or fabric swatches for color matching and naming.
11. Rey's figure.[24–26]
12. The cookie theft picture.[17]
13. Short written directions and queries (stick out your tongue, close your eyes, touch your left thumb to your right ear, how old are you?, are you wearing a hat?).

Cranial Nerves

I. Olfactory Nerve

Smell need not be routinely tested, but neurologists should have olfactory stimuli readily available. We use the following indications for testing the sense of smell:

1. *Head injury.* The olfactory nerves or tracts can be torn or contused. When the olfactory nerves are injured, sometimes cerebrospinal fluid rhinorrhea is also present.
2. *Dementia.* Basal frontal lobe tumors such as olfactory groove meningiomas are important diagnostic considerations. Decreased sense of smell may also occur in Alzheimer's disease.
3. *Meningoencephalitis.* Unilateral or bilateral anosmia may be a clue to the presence of herpes simplex virus encephalitis.
4. *Unilateral gradual loss of vision in one eye.* Some processes that involve the optic nerves also affect the more medially placed olfactory nerve.

When smell is checked, be sure not to use caustic volatile substances (such as ammonia), which can irritate fifth nerve endings in the nose, giving the patient a false sense of smell. We keep five vials or test tubes handy for testing smell and taste. We fill them with coffee, cloves, water, salt, and sugar. For smell, we use the water, salt, or sugar as controls. Have the patient occlude one nostril by putting a finger against it and, with eyes closed, smell one of the vials with the open nostril. The patient should be able to differentiate no odor (control vials) from an odor and should be able to tell that the two odors, coffee and cloves, are different. It is not necessary that the odor be recognized or named. Identification of odors requires experience, intelligence, memory, and speech, functions that involve a large portion of the brain. We are now testing just the olfactory nerves.

At times, medicolegal and other considerations may require more elaborate testing and the use of multiple scratch test odors may be helpful. Identification of these batteries is subject to all the concerns previously addressed.[33]

II. Optic Nerve

Visual Acuity   Even if there are no visual complaints, so many neurologic disorders affect vision and the eyes that a baseline visual acuity measurement may be useful later. We use a handheld card calibrated for visual acuity; others might prefer an acuity chart affixed to a wall in the office. If a chart is not handy, acuity can be estimated by whether the patient can see the head of a small pin or read newspaper print. If visual loss is severe, can the patient count fingers, see your hand, or detect gross movement or light? If patients wear glasses, it is best to check corrected vision. If they do not have their glasses, a pinhole can be used. When visual loss can be corrected by glasses or a pinhole, it is due to ocular refractive problems and is not of neurologic importance.

We are reminded of renting a car in France. The packet in the glove compartment asks if the driver can see the print in which the directions are written. If not, the driver is told to look at the print through a pinhole provided with the kit. If the pinhole doesn't work and the driver still cannot read the print, he or she is instructed to return the car and not to drive it.

Visual Fields   Nonneurologists seldom check the visual fields. We have even seen patients who came for consultation with several pairs of glasses prescribed by ophthalmologists, whose hemianopia was not detected because visual fields were not tested. We generally test the visual fields by confrontation, testing each eye individually while the patient holds one hand over the other eye. We watch the patient's eyes to ensure they are fixating on the examiner's nose or eye, whichever direction we have given them. We generally begin with finger movements in the periphery of each field; we then use a white- or red-topped pin. The key to interpretation of the patient's response is the question asked ("Say when you see something move to the side of your vision. Say when you know it is a pin. Say when you know the color of the pin."). The field for movement is much larger than the field for color. Although central vision can be tested with red

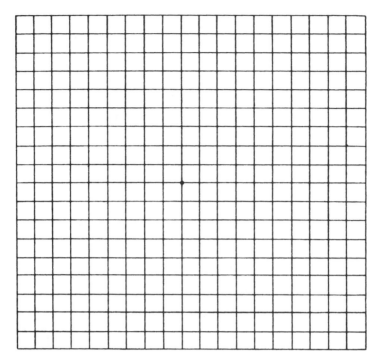

Figure 4-10 Amsler grid. (Reprinted with permission from Amsler Charts Manual. Keeler Limited, 456 Parkway, Lawrence Park Industrial Estate, Broomhall, PA 19008.)

matchheads or pins, we find the examiner's face a more useful test object. The patient covers one eye and is asked to look at the examiner's nose. "Are all the parts there?" If there is only one eye or no mouth, a central field defect is likely. Somewhat more precise estimation can be obtained by using the Amsler grid[34] (Figure 4-10). The patient fixes on the center of a red quadrille lined box containing grids that look like a checkerboard and is asked to point to the area that is poorly seen or in which the grids are absent or distorted. This allows the patient or physician to plot the defect on a quadrille pad.

In patients with cerebral lesions, we also test functional use of their visual fields. We often walk patients over to a window and ask them what they see outside. What do they see in the pictures on the wall, or in an advertisement or picture in a magazine, or a picture in the cortical function testing kit? Neglect may be much more apparent during functional testing than in formal testing of the visual fields. Patients with neglect may not see the head of the dog that is chasing the hen in Figure 4-5 or the children on the left of the "cookie theft" picture (see Figure 4-6).

Ophthalmoscopic Examination Careful observation of the ocular fundus is one of the most important parts of the physical and neurologic examination.

Be sure to take time to view the disc, vessels, and peripheral fundus oculi adequately. While you are fixing on the optic disc, the patient may show rhythmic small eye movements (nystagmus). Nystagmus is sometimes easier to detect and quantify during opthalmoscopy than when directly watching eye movements. The disc will be seen to move rhythmically. House officers are reluctant to take adequate time to study the fundus of sick patients and patients are quickly dismissed as having cataracts obscuring the fundus. If the patient can see out, you can probably see in. The more practice one has the easier and the more helpful the examination becomes. Remember to keep your head out of the way of the fixing eye, if you wish the patient to hold his eyes still.

Recently, one of us (L.R.C.) went onto a large medical floor to see a consultation without his doctor's bag. He tried to borrow an ophthalmoscope from one of the interns and residents (6 physicians) on the floor. None had an ophthalmoscope with them and the ward nurse had no ophthalmoscope available to borrow. No one had looked into the eyes of this patient (who had papilledema). Unfortunately ophthalmoscopy is becoming a lost art among many nonneurologists and nonophthalmologists. All the more reason for the neurologist to become proficient at this very valuable part of the examination.

III. Oculomotor, IV. Trochlear, and VI. Abducens Nerves

Be sure to check the pupillary reaction to light carefully. The miosis of Horner's syndrome is quite subtle because the eyes are usually viewed with the lights on and both pupils are then constricted. Dim light with side illumination of the pupils is needed. Look at the position of the eyelids in reference to the corneas and pupils, noting ptosis or asymmetries. We always test eye movement in the left and right eyes individually, before checking conjugate horizontal and vertical gaze. Both saccades and pursuit can be tested quickly if normal. Note any nystagmus and whether it is horizontal, rotatory, or vertical and whether it is present on primary gaze or on gaze to one side or only on up or down gaze. Red glass testing is not used unless the patient complains of diplopia. If the ocular axes are not conjugate, use the cover/uncover test to see if the patient fixates alternately with each eye. This indicates strabismus as opposed to an acquired oculomotor disorder. Diplopia not readily attributed to myasthenia, third nerve palsy, sixth nerve palsy, or internuclear ophthalmoplegia, is likely a fourth nerve palsy.

V. Trigeminal Nerve

We check the corneal reflex using a wisp of cotton on the lateral cornea when symptoms suggest a possible middle or posterior fossa lesion such as an acoustic neuroma. It is important to approach the eye from the side to eliminate visual threat and to be sure the cornea has been touched. In some patients, excessive blinking makes testing of corneal sensation difficult. Touching the eyelash in these patients elicits a blink response that is also a V–VII reflex. Nasal tickle is also V mediated. We check appreciation of touch and pin or cold sensation on the face when (1) the patient complains of face pain, numbness, or paresthesiae; (2) a middle or posterior fossa lesion is suspected; and (3) a hemispherical process involving the parasylvian sensory cortex might be present. Especially on the face, we find warm and cold stimuli preferable to a sharp pin. Patients, especially the very young or very old and those with trigeminal neuralgia, do not like to be jabbed with a pin on their faces and cannot maintain objectivity in reporting their pin perception. A cold object (we use a tuning fork) is usually tolerated well, and patients can report if one area is cooler than another.

In patients with cerebral hemispherical lesions, it is very useful to test localization of touch stimuli on the face and extinction of bilateral stimuli. In patients suspected of having a peripheral lesion involving the Vth nerve, the sensory loss may be limited to the ophthalmic, maxillary, or mandibular divisions. In patients suspected of having peripheral nerve or upper cervical spine lesions, checking carefully the distribution of the sensory loss may be very helpful in localization. The sensory innervation of the face and occiput and neck is shown in Figure 4-11.[35] In patients with brainstem lesions, both sides

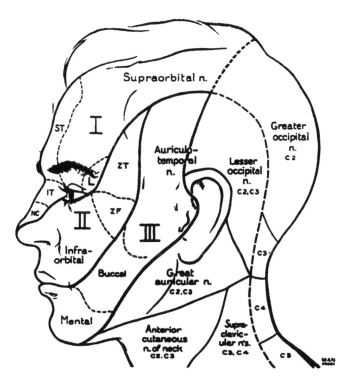

Figure 4-11   Diagram of the cutaneous fields of the head and upper neck. The three divisions of the trigeminal nerve (I ophthalmic, II maxillary, III mandibular) are indicated by heavy black lines. The boundaries of cutaneous nerve distribution are shown by light broken lines: B = buccal, IT = infratrochlear, L = lacrimal, NC = external nasal branch of nasociliary, ST = supratrochlear, ZF = zygomaticofacial, ZT = zygomaticotemporal. Cervical roots are noted as C2-C5. (Reprinted with permission from Haymaker W, Woodhall B. *Peripheral Nerve Injuries.* 2nd ed. Philadelphia: W.B. Saunders Co., 1953.)

of the face may lose sensibility but in a different way—the ipsilateral loss due to involvement of the spinal tract of V and its nucleus, and the contralateral loss due to a lesion affecting the nearby quinto-thalamic tract.[21,36] In that cicumstance it is important to compare pain or temperature sensation on the face with that on the trunk as well as comparing the two sides of the face.

VII. Facial Nerve

Carefully observe the patient's face during the interview not only for asymmetries, but for blinking and facial expression. Are there Parkinsonian features? Facial weakness can be elicited by asking patients to show their teeth, close their eyes, wrinkle their forehead, or grimace. Asymmetries are sometimes more noticeable when the patient smiles. A nonsensical query (for example, "What would you do if you found a hyena in your bathtub?") will usually elicit a grin. We find the platysma an especially useful muscle to test since asymmetry of its function is common in patients with upper motor neuron facial paresis. Ask the patient to jut out her chin and grunt; this maneuver shows the platysma muscles bilaterally. The platysma contraction will be less present on the side opposite the upper motor neuron facial weakness.

We do not routinely test taste. It should be checked if the patient has a lower motor neuron facial paralysis to differentiate a brainstem lesion from a lesion within the fallopian canal and when the patient complains of abnormal smell or taste function. When taste is tested, use salt and sugar. Hold the tongue out with a pad, moisten a swab, and apply salt or sugar water to the side of the anterior part of the tongue where the taste buds are located. Ask the patient to raise one hand if he tastes something, while the tongue is still protruded. The patient should be able to tell water from salt, and salt from sugar.

VIII. Auditory Nerve Portion

The Weber and Rinne tuning fork tests take time and are unrevealing if the patient has no hearing problem. We only perform these tests when there is a hearing problem. It is easy to perform a simple audiogram at the bedside by using stimuli of different frequency. Going from highest to lowest frequency, a watch tick, fingers rubbing, whispered number, and 256- and 128-hertz tuning forks provide a wide spectrum of sound frequencies. Patients with neurologically important hearing loss usually have difficulty with voice ranges. Inability to hear a watch tick is frequently caused by presbycusis or noise trauma, and patients are usually quite deaf before they lose ability to hear the tuning forks (low ranges). Test each ear separately, masking the other ear by finger rubbing or other noise. The Weber and Rinne tests are helpful when there is a unilateral hearing loss. Performing these tests with a 128-hertz fork gives spurious answers because of vibratory sensation. Whispering in one ear (like, link, look, lake) while masking the other gives a quick test of speech discrimination more useful early in neural lesions.

VIII. Vestibular Nerve Portion

Vestibular testing is not done routinely and residents seem to have considerable difficulty when confronted with a dizzy patient. Nystagmus is sought in the primary position (head upright). Check for past pointing. This term does not mean cerebellar-type overshooting of the target. The patient, with eyes open, lifts the outstretched arm and reaches out to touch the examiner's finger. After several efforts with the eyes open, this is then repeated with eyes closed. Patients with vestibular lesions will often misjudge the direction, pointing past the finger to the same side no matter which arm is used. The patient can be asked to march in place with eyes closed and may slowly rotate to one side. When gait testing is performed with eyes closed, they may drift to one side. The Romberg test elicits a fall to one side. The direction of the slow phase of vestibular nystagmus, the Romberg fall, the compass turn, or the gait drift all point to the bad side. Obviously the Romberg, compass turn, and gait drift are all performed when gait and station are tested.

When the patient reports episodic or persistent dizziness or light-headed feelings, we perform positional maneuvers and simple caloric testing in the office or at the bedside. Most important, if the patient says he becomes dizzy in certain positions or circumstances, watch him as he performs these maneuvers (for example, stooping, turning, lying with head to the right, bending to look under a table).

Watch for nystagmus. We find examining for positional nystagmus very useful. In the office, L.R.C. uses two adjoining chairs. He asks the patient to sit sideways on one chair with his back not restricted by a chair arm or back. Holding the patient's chin in one hand, the head and trunk are gently eased backward, holding a knee under the patient's back for support. The head is turned to one side. He looks carefully for nystagmus as the patient is brought into the head-to-the-side position. Then the patient is quickly brought to the upright position, again watching for nystagmus and asking about subjective sensations of dizziness. The maneuvers are then repeated with the head turned to the other side. These maneuvers are depicted diagrammatically in Figure 4-12. Alternatively the test can be performed by having the patient sit on the side of the bed or near the head end of the examining table, as in the original Hallpike maneuver[37] (Figure 4-13). The examiner propels the head and trunk backward, turning the head to the side. The patient should finish flat with the head extended slightly and turned 45 degrees to one side. The patient should not have been flat prior to testing and should not fixate visually on an object. With benign positional vertigo, the commonest cause of positional dizziness, after a brief delay, subjective vertigo with brisk nystagmus will appear and fatigue after about one minute. The patient is then brought back upright to the primary position and the symptoms recur with the nystagmus in the opposite direction after a similar latency.

The minicaloric test of Nelson can also be administered at the bedside.[38] A small quantity of ice water is introduced into the external ear canal using a tuberculin-sized syringe. The duration of the nystagmus on the two sides is com-

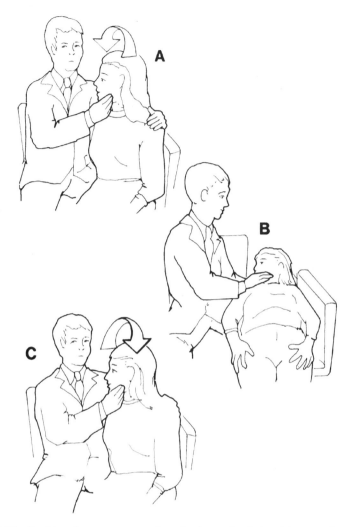

Figure 4-12 Positional nystagmus testing: **A,** the patient's head is turned to one side and brought down; **B,** the patient's head is kept in the position until the response fatigues and then brought up to the primary position; **C,** and observed. Please see text for more detailed description. (Drawn by Harriet Greenfield.)

pared. J.H. omits the minicaloric test because some patients tolerate it poorly and prefers to perform electronystagmography (ENG) when this is needed. ENG offers little over the conventional bedside examination but allows (1) recording of nystagmus in the dark to avoid visual fixation suppression of nystagmus and (2) allows quantitation of the velocity of the slow phase nystagmus during caloric testing, which is more reliable than the duration of the nystagmus.

The positional maneuvers and the caloric tests frequently reproduce the patient's sensation of vertigo. When we reproduce the sensation that patients

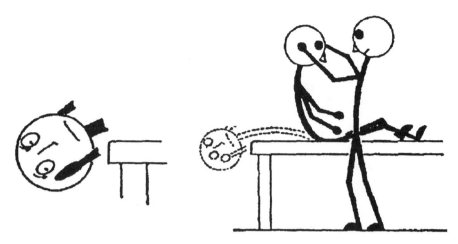

Figure 4-13 Original Hallpike diagram of testing for positional nystagmus. (Reprinted with permission from Matsumoto S, Okuda B, Imai T, Kameyama M. A sensory level on the trunk in lower lateral brainstem lesions. *Neurology* 1988;38.)

experience spontaneously in their attacks, they gain confidence that we understand their symptoms and will be able to help. Other dizziness simulation maneuvers could include hyperventilation, a potentiated Valsalva maneuver (have patient do deep knee bend and then hold breath and stand), and Barany rotation. This can be done by utilizing a secretarial chair and slowly rotating the patient. The chair is then abruptly stopped, causing some patients to develop vertigo. All of these maneuvers can elicit dizziness. What is critical is whether the dizziness elicited is the same as the dizziness that the patient spontaneously experienced. These patients should also have orthostatic blood pressure determinations.

IX. Glossopharyngeal and X. Vagus Nerves

Testing of the gag reflex is unpleasant for the patient and is seldom revealing. We do not check the gag reflex routinely. For some reason that is difficult to understand, many physicians and nurses believe that patients with neurologic lesions should not be fed until they have a gag reflex. The relationship of the gag reflex to swallowing is the same as the relation of the biceps reflex to arm flexion. Patients with an absent biceps reflex still may have normal biceps muscle strength. Similarly, some patients with absent gag reflexes swallow normally; other patients with active and hyperactive gag reflexes swallow poorly and repeatedly aspirate. Many residents seem to believe that the important part of the gag reflex is retching and miss the fact that the palate has elevated and deny the patient food. We don't usually retch with swallowing. The only way to judge the patient's swallowing ability is to watch the patient swallow water. The patient is given 90 ml of water in a cup to drink. Coughing or spluttering is a failed test as is a gurgling sound during postswallow speech.[39] It is also important to watch the uvula and pharyngeal pillars as the patient says "ah."

When the patient complains of numbness inside the mouth or a posterior fossa lesion is suspected, sensation in the mouth and soft and hard palate can be checked with a swab or tongue blade.

XI. Spinal Accessory Nerve

Neck flexor weakness is a prominent finding in patients with myopathy and motor neuron disease. Neck muscle strength should be tested in any patient with prominent widespread or diffuse muscle weakness and in patients with abnormalities of adjacent cranial nerves (X and XII). Local lesions in or near the jugular foramen can affect cranial nerves IX, X, and XI together; sometimes the process spreads to the more medially placed hypoglossal foramen, causing tongue weakness.

XII. Hypoglossal Nerve

Ask the patient to stick out her tongue. When protruded, the tongue will often deviate to the weak side. Tongue strength is best tested by having the patient push the tongue forcefully into the cheek while the doctor tries to resist the force of the movement. Can the patient protrude the tongue fully and in the midline? Is there tongue atrophy or fasciculations? Remember that fasciculations are seen at rest and the tongue should be examined in place in the mouth.

Motor System

Although we routinely watch for drift of one arm when the patient's arms are outstretched, there are a number of other things to look for with this maneuver. In some patients, the wrist or hand on the weak side will flex, showing asymmetric weakness. Extension of the metacarpalphalangeal joints and flexion of the proximal and distal interphalangeal joints are early signs of hand weakness. In some patients, when the hands are held outstretched, the little finger on the weak side will become hyperabducted (digiti-minimi sign). When the limbs are extended palms up, pronation is an early sign of central weakness.

Muscle Strength

It is important to check proximal, middle, and distal muscles in each limb, and muscles in each nerve root and nerve distribution. These are listed in tabular form in Table 4-1. Check deltoid (C5, axillary nerve), supra and infraspinati (C5, nerve to the spinati), biceps (C5–C6, musculocutaneous nerve), triceps (C7, radial nerve), wrist flexors (C6–C7, median nerve), wrist extensors (C6–C8, radial nerve), abductor pollicis brevis (C8, median nerve), and abductor digiti minimi (T1, ulnar nerve) routinely in the upper extremities. Testing internal (medial) and external (lateral) rotation of the arm at the shoulder (Figure 4-14) is especially useful. External rotation (Figure 4-14A) depends mostly on the infraspinatus while internal rotation (Figure 4-14B) depends on the pectoralis major, teres major, and the lattissimus dorsi.[35] When there is a myopathic disorder affecting proximal muscles both movements are weak.

External rotation is primarily C5 (suprascapular nerve) while internal rotation involves C5–C8 and different nerves. In lesions of C5, the deltoid and supraspinatus as well as lateral rotation of the shoulder are weak but internal rotation of the shoulder is preserved. In the lower limbs, check psoas (L2–L4, femoral nerve), thigh adduction (L2–L4, obturator nerve), thigh abductors (L4–S1, superior gluteal nerve), thigh extensors-glutei (L5–S2, superior and inferior gluteal nerves), quadriceps (L3–L4, femoral nerve), hamstrings (L4–S1, sciatic nerve), tibialis anterior (L4–L5, peroneal nerve), foot flexors (L5–S1 posterior tibial nerve), foot invertor-tibialis posterior (L5–S2, posterial tibial nerve), and foot abductors (L5–S1, peroneal nerve). The simple MRC muscle, peripheral nerve outline is inexpensive and quite helpful as one is learning muscle testing.[40]

Grade the degree of muscle weakness so that later you can determine whether the weakness is the same, worse, or improved. L.R.C. uses and teaches

Table 4-1 Muscle Strengths to Test Routinely

Muscles	*Nerve Roots*	*Peripheral Nerves*
Upper limbs		
Deltoid	C5	axillary
Supra and Infraspinati	C5	nerve to the spinati
Biceps	C5–C6	musculocutaneous
Triceps	C7	radial
Wrist flexors	C6–C7	median
Wrist extensors	C6–C8	radial
Abductor pollicis brevis	C8	median
Abductor digiti minimi	T1	ulnar
Lower limbs		
Psoas	L2–L4	femoral
Thigh adduction	L2–L4	obturator
Thigh abductors	L4–S1	superior gluteal
Thigh extensors-glutei	L5–S2	superior and inferior gluteal
Quadriceps	L3–L4	femoral
Hamstrings	L4–S1	sciatic
Tibialis anterior	L4–L5	peroneal
Foot flexors	L5–S1	posterior tibial
Foot invertor	L5–S2	posterior tibial
Foot abductors	L5–S1	peroneal

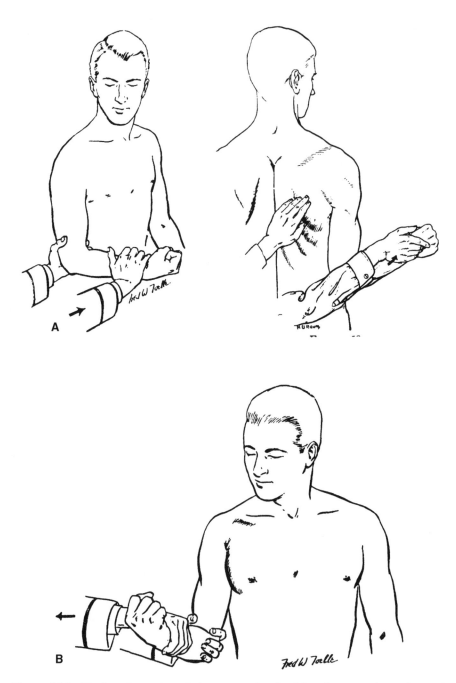

Figure 4-14 Testing of rotation of the arm at the shoulder: **A**, external rotation and assessing infraspinatus muscle contraction; **B**, internal rotation. (Reprinted with permission from Haymaker W, Woodhall B. *Peripheral Nerve Injuries*. 2nd ed. Philadelphia: W.B. Saunders Co., 1953.)

Table 4-2   Muscle Strength Grading Scale

1. No contraction.
2. Minimal muscle contraction, no movement.
3. Stronger muscle contraction, no movement.
4. Slight movement of part with gravity eliminated.
5. Moves limb well with gravity eliminated. Can resist gravity feebly and temporarily.
6. Can lift limb well against gravity but not against resistance.
7. Limb easily overcome by resistance.
8. Moderate resistance needed to overcome limb.
9. Slight but definite weakness.
10. Normal.

a 10-point scale that is simply a doubling of the standard 5-point system. In the 5-point system, nearly all patients can exert force against resistance and so fall between 4 and 5; 4 represents loss of 80 percent of muscle power. Decimal differentiators, for example, 4.2 or 4.4, are awkward. In the 10-point system, 6 is resistance against gravity and is equivalent to a 3 in the 5-point scale. We have outlined the grading system in Table 4-2. Whether one uses a 10-point, 5-point, or the Mayo 0- to 4-point scale, when communicating with others it is essential that the scale used be spelled out.

Muscle Tone

Muscle tone should be commented on as normal, spastic, rigid, paratonic, or flaccid. Bulk should also be noted. Observation for fasciculations requires that the patient be disrobed. Myoclonus, asterixis, chorea, athetosis, dystonia, and tremor require clear descriptions to enhance clarity.

Coordination

Coordination in the limbs should be routinely checked. We use finger-to-nose and toe-to-object testing routinely. Rapid alternating movements of the hand, hand patting, quickly touching each finger with the thumb, tapping quickly the end of the bent index finger on the distal interphalangeal joint of the thumb, drawing a small circle or square with the toe, tapping the foot in rhythm, and rebound are other cerebellar tests.

Gait

Gait is the single most important motor function to test. Some physicians like to watch the patient walk before they begin formal neurologic testing. Others watch gait after the rest of the examination. Be sure to notice the posture and movements of the upper limbs, in addition to the legs.

Station

Station is important for assessing trunkal stability. When this is done, it is a convenient time in patients with suspected spine problems to observe the spinal curvature, mobility, and tenderness.

Reflexes

In our experience, the usefulness of testing of muscle stretch reflexes is exaggerated. Very seldom is one or more abnormal reflexes the only abnormality. More often abnormal reflexes corroborate other symptoms or signs. When looking for a subtle reflex asymmetry, we find it useful to check reflexes that are often hard to elicit—pectoral, trapezius, wrist extensor, finger flexor, adductor, hamstring, and posterior tibial reflexes. On the side opposite an upper motor neuron lesion, it is often possible to elicit these reflexes while they are absent in the contralateral limbs. It is easier to differentiate a positive reflex from a negative than a 2+ from 3+ reflex. It is important to have the limb in an appropriate position to put the muscle at the correct length when testing reflexes. The sitting position may be the easiest for most. The presence and grade of reflexes can be recorded on a stick figure (Figure 4-15) or recorded on a simple reflex chart (Table 4-3).

Abdominal reflexes are cutaneous responses. They are often lost on the side opposite an upper motor neuron lesion. The upper and lower abdominal reflexes (above and below the umbilicus [T10]) are also useful to test in cases of suspected thoracic spinal cord lesions. The lower abdominal reflexes may be lost in lesions of the lower thoracic spinal cord (T11–T12) while the upper, and also often the lower abdominal reflexes are lost in lesions between T5 and T9.

For a variety of different reasons, the plantar response may be difficult to interpret. Ticklishness, hypersensitivity, toe grasp, and withdrawal are commonly observed when the Babinski response is elicited in the usual way with a

Table 4-3   Simple Reflex Chart

Reflex	Right	Left
Pectoral	+1	+1
Biceps	+3	+3
Triceps	+2	+2
Brachoradial	+2	+2
Abdominal (upper)	+	+
Abdominal (lower)	+	+
Knee	+3	+3
Ankle	+2	+2
Plantar	Flexor	Flexor

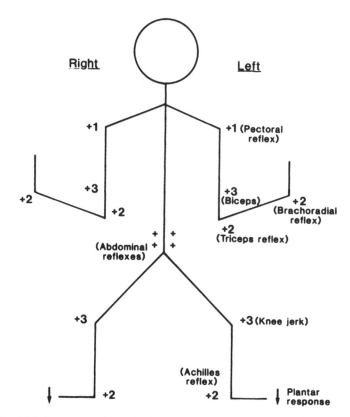

Figure 4-15 Stick figure recording of reflexes.

key or sharp object. In these patients, either gentle stimulation with your own thumb, or using the patient's thumb to elicit the plantar response avoids withdrawal. Testing the jaw, facial, and glabella reflexes is important in patients with upper motor neuron brainstem and cerebral lesions.

A number of "abnormal" reflexes such as the grasp, groping, sucking, snout, rooting, and palmo-mental reflexes are often elicited.[30,41] The presence of these reflexes is considered by some to represent loss of cortical inhibitory influence on the brainstem and more specifically to indicate frontal lobe dysfunction. The *grasp reflex* is elicited by the examiner touching or stroking the skin especially between the thumb and index finger of the patient's hand and eliciting forced grasping. The maneuver can also be performed on the foot. In the *groping reflex* the patient's hand as well as the eyes tend to follow an object or the finger of the examiner. The *sucking reflex* is elicited by touching the lip of the patient with a cotton swab and seeing if the patient will suck on the swab. The *snout reflex* is elicited by tapping the skin of the perioral region above the lip with a finger or a reflex hammer or simply pressing firmly on this region using a finger looking for a pursing-pouting reaction of the lips. The *rooting reflex* is elicited by stroking the corner of the mouth with a finger or tongue blade, watching for movement of the mouth toward the object. The *palmo-mental reflex* is elicited by vigorously stroking the thenar eminence in the palm of the patient's hand. A positive response is contraction of the mentalis muscle of the chin. We do not put much emphasis on these signs; they are present in some otherwise normal elderly patients and they are rarely if ever present in isolation. Their utility is very limited and their presence is a nonspecific sign of brain atrophy and ventricular enlargement. These signs do not correlate well with dementia.[41]

Sensation

Patients often report subtle sensory symptoms—numbness and paresthesiae—before the doctor can elicit any objective sensory abnormality. The sensory examination can be the longest, most frustrating, and least informative portion of the neurologic examination. Extensive routine sensory testing is seldom very helpful when there are no sensory symptoms. We generally carefully check regions with sensory symptoms; we also check the distal limbs for touch (cotton), cold (cool tuning fork), and vibration sense. A few suggestions:

1. When objectively testing sensation, ask patients to close their eyes and see if they can distinguish one object from another. We usually use cotton, finger touch, sharp end of the pin, and blunt end of the pin. This type of testing is more useful than comparing the degree of normality (for example, if a dollar represents normal sensitivity, does this patient's reaction rate 75?, 50?, 25?, etc.).
2. Check vibration sense carefully with a 128-hertz tuning fork. See how long the patient can continue to feel the vibration; compare with your own ability to continue to feel the vibration.
3. In patients with reduced alertness or those who might not be reliable observers, intersperse controls (such as no vibration, dull finger instead of sharp pin) amidst the test stimuli to be sure that the patient is paying attention and the responses are accurate. Holding the point of the pin against the tip of the finger and using a minor change in position of the finger allows presentation of either a touch or pin stimulus without the patient being able to see the different stimuli.
4. When evaluating sensation, it is much easier for the patient to recognize the transition from dull to sharp than the other way. When a preliminary survey suggests a spinal cord, nerve root, or peripheral nerve lesion, the boundary can be more readily defined by moving from abnormal to normal.
5. The best tests of cortical sensation are point localization, ability to recognize objects in the hands, and extinction of bilateral tactile stimuli. Some normal patients have poor graphesthesia, making this test less useful than stereognosis. Two-point discrimination is a tedious test that requires extensive patient attention and cooperation. Findings differ in the proximal, middle, and distal limbs and vary with the

stimuli—a compass point, pin, or the sharpened end of the pencil. Abnormalities of two-point discrimination are not reproducible. For these reasons, we no longer use two-point discrimination. It is useful to start with one or two tests on all patients until one is comfortable with what to expect from normals.

6. Thermal testing is preferred over the use of a pin. We find cool objects such as a spoon, tuning fork, or metal portion of the reflex hammer to be good stimuli. Some patients, especially youngsters, lose their objectivity when approached with a sharp object.

7. Record the findings on a sensory chart when there are abnormalities of sensation. Charts or sketches are much more revealing than verbal descriptions for depicting the distribution of sensory changes on a limb or the trunk. On the chart, you can also record the results of vibration sense and position sense testing and severity and gradations of sensory loss. A sample sensory chart is shown as Figure 4-16. On such a chart the relative severity of sensory loss can be shown. For example in Figure 4-16, which was elicited in a patient with a peripheral polyneuropathy, the sensory loss to all modalities is most severe in the very distal foot and lessens more rostrally.

Figure 4-17 from Haymaker and Woodhall[35] are dermatome charts modelled after Foerster.[42] Foerster's maps are derived by cutting a number of posterior roots above and below a root left intact and then determining the region of preserved sensibility in the zone of the intact root. This information was supplemented by studies of patients in whom contiguous roots were cut and Foerster then mapped out the upper and lower borders of sensory loss.[35,42] The maps of Foerster have proven generally more useful than the other often used maps of Keagan and Garrett (Figure 4-18),[35,43] which were based on the distribution of decreased sensitivity to pin scratch in patients with herniated intervertebral discs.[43]

The diagrams of the brachial and lumbar plexi and the distribution of the motor and sensory nerves and their cutaneous skin innervation in Haymaker and Woodhall[35] and the diagrams of the peripheral nerves and their innervations in two books on entrapment neuropathies (Dawson, Hallett, and Millender[44] and Kopell and Thompson[45]) have proven virtually indispensable in the diagnosis of patients with peripheral nervous system lesions. We urge having these books handy for reference.

The most important aspect of the examination is that it be directed toward the testing of hypotheses generated from the history. We see what we look for, to paraphrase Goethe's words quoted at the outset of the chapter. When the physician does not know what to look for, the odds are high that little of importance will be found. Even during the examination, positive findings should generate new hypotheses that are then tested as the examination proceeds. An example is a recent patient seen by one of us (J.H.). A 76-year-old retired merchant had an

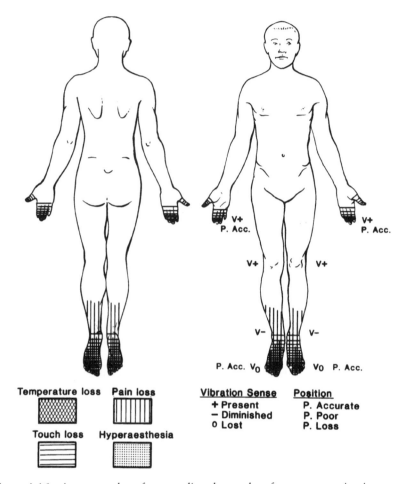

Figure 4-16 A sensory chart for recording the results of sensory examinations.

extensive decompressive laminectomy of C3–C6 for bilateral lower limb weakness and difficulty walking. Spinal stenosis with cord impingement was evident on MRI. He tolerated the surgery well and was sent home with home care services. One month later he was admitted because of significant progressive deterioration in his gait and bilateral increasing numbness and tingling. The neurosurgeon repeated the MRI, which showed a kinking of the spinal cord at C2–C3. Because spinal fluid was seen surrounding the cord, the neurosurgeon was concerned that the MRI failed to explain the progression of his symptoms and neurologic consultation was requested. Past medical history included nontophaceous gout, hypothyroidism on replacement, cardiogenic syncope due to complete A-V block with pacemaker, and osteoarthritis. On examination a cervical gibbus was noted. Mild decline in calculation and recall was noted in an otherwise normal mental status. Cranial nerves were normal. A somewhat

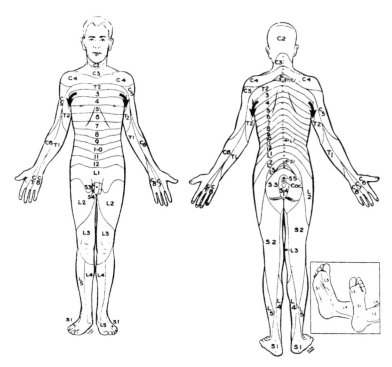

Figure 4-17 Segmental innervation of the skin after Foerster. The left diagram shows the segmental innervation of the skin from the anterior aspect. The curved arrows indicate the lateral extensions of the T3 dermatome. The diagram on the right shows the segmental innervation of the skin from the posterior view. The curved arrows in the axillary regions show the lateral extent of the T3 dermatome. The straight short arrows next to the vertebrae point to the T1, L1, and S1 spinous processes. (Reprinted with permission from Haymaker W, Woodhall B. *Peripheral Nerve Injuries*. 2nd ed. Philadelphia: W.B. Saunders Co., 1953.)

asymmetric tetraparesis was noted. Lower limbs were hypertonic. Striking loss of light touch and position sense was noted in the lower limbs, despite near normal temperature and pinprick sensation. Reflexes were slightly hypoactive in the lower limbs but the plantars responses were extensor. One might have assumed a progressive cervical myelopathy due to the postoperative gibbus and the damage induced by the spinal stenosis. The disparity between the findings in the sensory modalities and the absence of hyperreflexia did not fit well with the diagnosis of compressive cervical spinal cord myelopathy. Since subacute combined degeneration fit better with the neurologic findings, J.H. looked more carefully for the presence of splenic enlargement, tongue abnormalities, and skin coloration. His tongue was unusually smooth. Laboratory findings included a hematocrit of 40 but his MCV was 105. B_{12} level was unusually low at 75. Despite therapy with injectable cobalamin his improvement was incomplete.

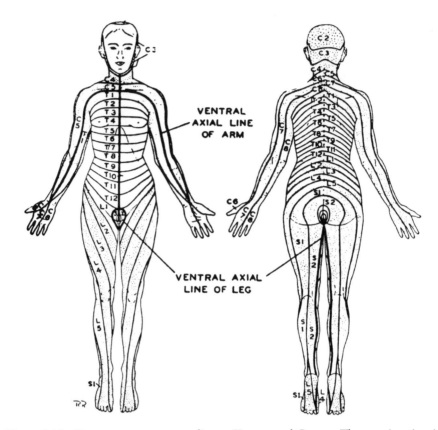

Figure 4-18 Dermatome maps according to Keegan and Garrett. The anterior view is shown on the left diagram and the posterior view is shown on the right diagram. (Reprinted with permission from Haymaker W, Woodhall B. *Peripheral Nerve Injuries.* 2nd ed. Philadelphia: W.B. Saunders Co., 1953.)

Combined system disease may occur with relative sparing of the blood. One should be alerted when findings do not fall into an expected pattern.

The neurologic examination should be thorough and complete. The information gleaned cannot be duplicated by any present or future technology. Unquestionably, the neurologist should be far more proficient in performing the neurologic examination and interpreting the abnormalities found, than any of his nonneurologic colleagues.

REFERENCES

1. Goethe JW. *Einleitung in die Propylaen,* 1798.
2. Goetz CG, Charcot JM. *The Clinician: The Tuesday Lessons.* New York: Raven Press, 1987;175. (Translation and comments from Bun, Charcot, Cohn, *Leçons du Mardi a ha Salpetiere Policlinique 1887–1888.* Paris: Progres Medical, 1892.)

3. Doyle AC. *The Complete Sherlock Holmes: A Study in Scarlet.* Garden City, NY: Garden City Books, 1971;14.
4. Monard-Krohn GH, Refsum S. *The Clinical Examination of the Nervous System.* 12th ed. New York: Harper and Row, 1964;8.
5. Caplan LR. Diagnosis and the clinical encounter. In LR Caplan (ed), *Caplan's Stroke: A Clinical Approach.* 3rd ed. Boston: Butterworth–Heinemann, 2000;51–71.
6. Fisher CM. Facial pulses in internal carotid artery occlusion. *Neurology* 1970;20: 476–478.
7. Caplan LR. Nonatherosclerotic vasculopathies. In LR Caplan (ed), *Caplan's Stroke: A Clinical Approach.* 3rd ed. Boston: Butterworth–Heinemann, 2000;295–342.
8. Caplan LR. The neurologic examination. In J Bogousslavsky, M Fisher (eds), *Textbook of Neurology.* Boston: Butterworth–Heinemann, 1998;3–18.
9. Cronin-Golomb A, Corkin S, Rosen TJ. Neuropsychological assessment of dementia. In PJ Whitehouse (ed), *Dementia.* Philadelphia: F.A. Davis, 1993;130–164.
10. Strub RL, Black FW. *The Mental State Examination in Neurology.* Philadelphia: F.A. Davis, 1977.
11. Wechsler D. WAIS—R. Wechsler Adult Intelligence Scale—Revised. New York: Psychological Corporation, 1981.
12. Hecaen H, Assal G. A comparison of construction deficits following right and left hemisphere lesions. *Neuropsychologia* 1970;8:289–304.
13. Gainotti G. Constructional apraxia. In P Vinken, G Bruyn, H Klawans (eds), *Handbook of Clinical Neurology,* Vol. 45, *Clinical Neuropsychology.* Amsterdam: Elsevier Science, 1985;491–506.
14. Caplan LR, Bogousslavsky J. Abnormalities of the right cerebral hemisphere. In J Bogousslavsky, LR Caplan (eds), *Stroke Syndromes.* Cambridge: Cambridge University Press, 1995;162–168.
15. DeRenzi E, Scotti C, Spinnler H. Perceptual and associated disorders of visual recognition. Relationship to the side of the cerebral lesion. *Neurology* 1969;19:634 –642.
16. Gray's Standardized Oral Reading paragraphs, Revised 1975. Old Tappan, NJ: Macmillan.
17. Lyden P, Brott T, Tilley B, Welch KMA, Maacha EJ, NINDS TPA Stroke Study Group. Improved reliability of the NIH Stroke Scale using video training. *Stroke* 1994;25:2220–2226.
18. Hier D, Mondlock JJ, Caplan L. Behavioral defects after right hemisphere stroke. *Neurology* 1983;33:337–344.
19. Photographs for recognition (Benton Facial Recognition Test) can be ordered from Oxford University Press, 2001 Evans Rd., Cary, NC.
20. Caplan LR, Hedley-White T. Cuing and memory dysfunction in alexia without agraphia: A case report. *Brain* 1977;97:251–262.
21. Caplan LR. Signs and symptoms and their clinical localization. In LR Caplan (ed), *Posterior Circulation Disease: Clinical Findings, Diagnosis, and Management.* Boston: Blackwell Science, 1996;73–130.
22. The pictures of the Boston Naming Test can be ordered from either Lea & Febiger, 600 Washington Square, Philadelphia, PA 19106, or from Psychological Assessment Resources, Inc. P.O. Box 998, Odessa, FL 33556.
23. DeRenzi E, Vignolo L. The token test: A sensitive test to detect receptive disturbances in aphasics. *Brain* 1962;85:665–678. (The Token test is in the public domain. Tokens, forms, and answer sheets can be obtained for a fee from the Psychology Clinic, University of Victoria, Victoria, BC V8W 3P5.)
24. Rey A. L'examen psychologique dans les cas d'encephalopathie traumatique. *Arch de Psychologie* 1941;28:286–340.
25. Osterrieth PA. Le test de copie d'une figure complex. *Archives de Psychologie* 1944; 30:206–356.

26. The Rey figure is in the public domain. The test, manual, and forms can be obtained for a fee from Psychological Assessment Resources, Inc. P.O. Box 998, Odessa, FL 33556.
27. Koh's blocks are available as part of a large, expensive test group, such as the WAIS—R, or the Boston Diagnostic Aphasia Examination.
28. Fisher CM. Abulia minor vs. agitated behavior. *Clin Neurosurg* 1983;31:9–31.
29. Luria AR. *Higher Cortical Functions in Man*. New York: Basic Books, Consultants Bureau, 1966.
30. Damasio AR. The frontal lobes. In KM Heilman, E Valenstein (eds), *Clinical Neuropsychology*. 2nd ed. New York: Oxford University Press, 1985;340–375.
31. Mardell AM, Knoeffel JE, Albert ML. Mental state examination in the elderly. In ML Albert, JE Knoeffel (eds), *Clinical Neurology of Aging*. 2nd ed. New York: Oxford University Press, 1994;277–313.
32. Drewe EA. Go-no go learning after frontal lobe lesions in humans. *Cortex* 1975; 11:8–16.
33. University of Pennsylvania Smell Identification Test. Sensonics, Inc., P.O. Box 112, Haddon Heights, NJ 08035-0112.
34. Amsler Charts Manual. Keeler Limited, 456 Parkway, Lawrence Park Industrial Estate, Broomhall, PA 19008.
35. Haymaker W, Woodhall B. *Peripheral Nerve Injuries*. 2nd ed. Philadelphia: W.B. Saunders Co., 1953.
36. Matsumoto S, Okuda B, Imai T, Kameyama M. A sensory level on the trunk in lower lateral brainstem lesions. *Neurology* 1988;38:1515–1519.
37. Baloh RW. Charles Skinner Hallpike and the beginnings of neuro-otology. *Neurology* 2000;54:2138–2146.
38. Nelson J. The minimal ice water caloric test. *Neurology* 1969;19:577–585.
39. Detippo KL. The Burke dysphagia screening test. Validation of its use in patients with stroke. *Arch Phys Med Rehab* 1994;75:1284–1286.
40. Medical Research Council. Aids to the Investigation of Peripheral Nerve Injuries. War memorandum, no. 45. London: Her Majesty's Stationery Office, 1982.
41. Tweedy J, Reding M, Garcia C, et al. Significance of cortical disinhibition signs. *Neurology* 1982;32:169–173.
42. Foerster O. The dermatomes in man. *Brain* 1933;56:1–39.
43. Keegan JJ, Garrett FD. The segmental distribution of the cutaneous nerves in the limbs of man. *Anat Rec* 1948;102:409–438.
44. Dawson DM, Hallett M, Millender LH. *Entrapment Neuropathies*. Boston: Little, Brown, 1983.
45. Kopell HP, Thompson WAL. *Peripheral Entrapment Neuropathies*. Baltimore: Williams & Wilkins, 1963.

5

Recording the Results of the History, Examination, and Investigations

When a patient says to you, "If I go half-way up a hill I'm done for," record it in your case history in those words, do not say, "The patient complains that during ambulation up a moderate incline, he suffers a feeling of impending dissolution."[1]

—E. GOWERS

Thought must be given to the clarity and conciseness of language used. One must learn to be accurate and complete, yet sufficiently to the point so that the busy physician who next reviews the chart can do so quickly, without being misled by ambiguities, omissions, distortions or misstatements.[2]

—W.L. MORGAN AND G.L. ENGEL

We urge all house officers and physicians to try the following simple experiment. Go to any ward in a hospital in which you work and randomly choose five charts. Read the doctors' hospital notes. See if you can conjure up a glimpse of the individual patients described. What are the patients like? What is their work? Can you define clearly the patients' symptoms and the doctors' findings on examination? Then go and see the patients yourself. How well do the charts convey the patients and their problems? Unfortunately, sometimes only the notes of the social worker or the psychiatric consultant and the nurses reveal anything about the patient as a person. Much of the hospital chart is filled with medical jargon, abbreviations, and meaningless automatic phrases, such as: "Normocephalic; well-developed, well-nourished; no abdominal organomegaly masses or tenderness; PERRLA (pupils equal regular and reactive to light and accommodation)." When the chart says "expressive aphasia, confused, or delirium," without further description can you tell anything about the patient? When another physician is called to see your patient at night, can she tell if the patient is better, worse or the same? Much of the handwriting in charts is also illegible.

Table 5-1   Suggestions for Recording the History, Examination, and Results
of Investigations

- Use simple, clear, concise English
- Describe the person as well as symptoms and signs
- Make it possible for the reader to visualize the patient and the patient's problem and signs
- Quantify whenever possible
- Include positive descriptors rather than negative
- Include the patient's writings and drawings in the chart
- Separate primary observations from interpretations and conclusions
- Use stick figures to show reflexes
- Record sensory abnormalities on sensory charts
- Trace or copy important images in the chart

Another educational and usually humbling experience is to be called into court to testify as a treating or consulting physician. Given the pace of our hopelessly inefficient legal system, the incident probably took place three to five years before the summons. It is seldom possible to remember the details of the case. You are dependent on your office notes, any typed or printed reports, and the notes in the hospital record if the patient was hospitalized. You are often embarrassed in court to find that your notes are woefully inadequate to describe to the judge or jury the patient's history as related to you, what you did on examination, what your findings were, your diagnosis and other conditions that you considered, the tests you ordered, the medicines you prescribed and their doses, and your explanations and discussion with the patient. We guarantee that one such court experience will greatly improve your future record keeping.

Suggestions for recording information in the hospital or your own outpatient records are summarized in Table 5-1.

USE SIMPLE ENGLISH, NOT MEDICAL JARGON

How did Marcel Proust, John Steinbeck, John Irving or any novelist convey a vivid picture of an individual, an event, or a scene? Why is at least one course in college English required for medical students? Clear, precise writing is crucial. Record the patient's history and examination as if you want the reader of the report to be able to conjure up an image of that patient, his or her complaints, and your findings. The very same rules are applicable for recording information in hospital charts, in dictating or typing office visits and consultations, and for presenting cases at hospital rounds. Include a description of the patient as well as the medical problem. Begin the description of the examination findings with a brief sketch of the patient. This should be accurate, but not pejorative.

Miss Jones is an 86-year-old retired schoolteacher. She has always been single and lives with a younger widowed sister in a small rooming house. She has always enjoyed excellent health and makes it a practice not to visit physicians unless she must. She is active in a number of church organizations and volunteers as a librarian at the hospital. She does her own shopping and cooking, but a woman helps with the cleaning twice a week; she takes care of her sister who is hobbled by arthritis and is a bit "senile." Ms. Jones handles the finances and taxes. She came today because yesterday when she awakened and tried to get out of bed she suddenly felt as if the room was spinning and turning around. She was nauseated. She felt more dizzy and ill when she moved or turned and was better if she held very still. After five minutes or so she felt better but stayed in bed for the rest of the morning.

On examination, the patient is a tall, thin, elderly, frail-appearing person. She arrived at the office an hour early and brought with her knitting and a biography of Bach. Her hair is pinned back and covered with a black hat. She is wearing several sweaters despite the warmth of the summer day. She has brought with her typed notes of her symptoms and dates of past surgeries. She also has a list of questions that she should be sure to ask. Pulse is 84 and regular, and blood pressure is 135/70 in the left arm sitting.

Similarly, describe the examination in simple English, recording the tests and examinations performed and the results. At some point in the future, you may want to review your notes for particular findings.

Suppose a 27-year-old woman consults you because of pain and blurring of vision in the left eye. Her visual acuity is now 20/25. You had seen her a year before because of a numb left foot. Your notes of the earlier visit should tell you if you had examined her visual acuity and what it was.

Suppose an elderly woman consulted you in 1998 because of transient loss of vision in the left eye. She died a few months later. Now her daughter is contesting her will, which she changed shortly before seeing you. She claims her mother was demented. The court would like to know what tests of intellectual function you conducted and how she performed on the tests. You do not recall the patient and must rely on your 1998 office notes to use during testimony. They should be adequate.

An example of clear, accurate reporting would be as follows.

The heart was slightly enlarged, and the apex impulse was a focal left ventricular thrust. There were no murmurs. Neck pulses were normal, and I heard no carotid or vertebral bruits. Mental state: Miss Jones was very alert and presented her history in an organized and detailed fashion. She wrote at my request a long paragraph about the Brookline public schools and described changes she would suggest for improving the system. She drew a clock well, but crowded the numbers from 9 to 12, having not planned well. She accurately copied a complex drawing of mine. She read a 100-word Aesop's fable with only one trivial error and gave an excellent abstract interpretation of its meaning. She was able to analyze three scenes that I showed her briefly, select the key features, and describe their approximate location and vintage. She identified by name eight of ten well-known individuals from their pictures, missing only Winston Churchill (whom she did recognize as "a former British prime minister during World War II") and Barbra Streisand (whom she knew was a modern entertainer). After fifteen minutes, she spontaneously recalled seven of the ten individuals, all three scenes, and the content of the fable she read. With contextual cues, she could remember the other three individuals. She consistently recited six numbers backwards and seven forward. Cranial nerves: Visual acuity was 20/50 in each eye with glasses measured with a hand-held card. Confrontation testing of her visual fields with a 10-millimeter white pin showed no field defect. She did not extinguish either visual field when fingers were wiggled simultaneously in each field. Her pupils were slightly irregular, measured 4 millimeters, and reacted quickly and fully to light.

Examinations that are always performed in the same way with the same equipment need not be described in such detail. If you always use a 128-hertz tuning fork for vibration sense testing and a 256-hertz tuning fork for hearing, you need not include that detail in the report. If you have an invariable routine for muscle strength and reflex testing, you might report, "strength and reflexes were normal."

Use small clear words rather than complex multisyllabic words whenever possible; for example, small words such as hop, jump, skip, sing, bump, dip, zip, sing, and pop, but long words such as obfuscate, obliterate, invalidate, discombobulate, and decompensate. Avoid words that you would not use in ordinary conversation. For example, "The patient experienced headaches." How does one *experience* headache? Experience is an excellent noun that conveys important meaning but is a rather pedantic verb. "The patient had headaches" is much preferred. Also avoid terms such as *suffer* unless you are describing torture. The patient *had a stroke* is preferred over the *patient suffered a stroke*. Suffer can have important medicolegal implications not intended by the writer.

CLEARLY SEPARATE PRIMARY DATA FROM INTERPRETATIONS AND CONCLUSIONS

Always try to record primary data from the history and the basic abnormal examination findings. In recording the history, report patients' descriptions of their symptoms using their own words. Don't translate into medicalese. Patients' words are often helpful when you retrospectively review the case notes. "My head was swimming. I was mixed up," is quite different from faint, light-headed, spinning, dizzy, or vertigo. If you have walked through the illness with the patient (see Chapter 3), record the edited salient features of the development of symptoms.

In recording past data, note important evidence whenever possible. If a patient said that she was diabetic and hypertensive, note that, "six years ago a doctor told her after taking blood tests on a routine visit that the blood sugar was a 'little high.' She should lose weight and avoid carbohydrates, but required no insulin or pills. Subsequent blood and urine sugars have been OK. She had taken hydrochlorothiazide 25 milligrams a day for ten years for what the doctor called 'slight high blood pressure.' Recently, she recalls the nurse writing down a pressure of 140/85 or thereabouts."

In the report of the examination, record primary observations, for example, "she had a droop of the left lower face, and more teeth showed on her right when she smiled," rather than "she had a left VIIth nerve weakness." "On finger-to-nose testing, she showed minor clumsiness and slowness on the left, with slight overshooting of the target" is preferable to "she had left cerebellar signs." Include with your records the piece of paper used by the patient to write, draw, copy, and make lists. When seeing a patient in the hospital or office when time constraints require brevity and speed, considerable information can be documented quickly for later dictation. Simply recording the date and place specified by the patient, objects named, figures identified, memory test objects recalled, calculations made, and so on takes little time. For example: "3/1/88 (5/1/00), place-Wegman's supermarket; names chair, key, book; recalls: paper, rose, book; cowboy story OK; repeats OK; adds quarter, dime, nickel, penny = $.41; crisp description of workplace details." This and other information can be added below a sample of drawing and writing. A more detailed note can be typed or dictated later.

After the description of the primary observations, there should be a brief paragraph summarizing the key history and examination findings and your interpretation and conclusions. Note your diagnosis and the differential diagnosis, the investigations ordered, the medicines prescribed (with their dosage), and instructions for the future (is the patient to return and when?).

QUANTITATE WHENEVER POSSIBLE

Past medical diagnoses are useless without some quantification. For example, "the patient has hypertension" conveys little of the importance of that diagnosis. The statement includes a wide spectrum of severity from patients who may have been told several times that their pressure was a little high to patients with poorly controlled blood pressures >200 systolic during a 5-year period. The duration, severity, and treatment is helpful to know, especially in a patient whose differential diagnosis includes cerebrovascular disease. "The patient has been recognized to have hypertension for five years. Blood pressures on hydrochlorothiazide have usually ranged in the 140–160/80–90 range."

Similarly, it is not possible to weigh the import of the diagnoses of atherosclerotic vascular disease, diabetes, coronary artery disease, or breast cancer without further elaboration and quantification.

Sometime in the future, you or others may want to compare subsequent findings with the present results. This will be impossible if your findings are not quantified.[3] It is also much easier to visualize quantitated results than general statements. For example, "he could lift his left thigh and hold the leg outstretched straight to a height of six inches for only five seconds, then the limb dropped" is much more vivid than "he had severe leg weakness." "On gaze to the left, there was slow-coarse nystagmus with an amplitude of 4 millimeters and a frequency of two beats per second. The nystagmus was to the left, and rotatory in a counterclockwise direction" is preferable to "there was nystagmus to the left." "The patient felt the 128 tuning fork for ten seconds in the left ankle; when he said it stopped, I could feel it for another ten seconds on my finger" is detailed and accurate. I have already described quantification of muscle strength in Table 4-2. Deep tendon reflexes should also be graded between 0 and 4, with 2 and 3 being normally active. Table 4-3 shows a sample reflex chart; a stick figure that illustrates this quantification is shown in Figure 4-15. When you can't grade the findings by numbers, use descriptors such as minimal, slight, moderate, severe, and profound.

Scales offer useful but very vague information. One may surmise from a Folstein Mini-Mental Status score of 18, an NIH Stroke Scale of 20, or a Glasgow Coma Scale of 3, that the patient has significant problems, but one can hardly visualize that patient.

POSITIVE DESCRIPTIONS OR QUOTES ARE BETTER THAN NEGATIVE STATEMENTS

After testing the patient's orientation for time, place, and person, examiners often record in the chart, "he was oriented × 1" or "he was not oriented to place or time." What do these negative statements convey to you reading the chart? On November 27, 2000, a person who gives the date as November 26, 2000 is technically disoriented to time. However, there are many gradations of errors. Many normal individuals (especially if hospitalized more than a few days) miss the date by one to three days, nearly always erring by giving a past date. Errors of giving a future date are much less common. Few normal individuals miss by a month, and none miss by a season (3 months). Occasionally, even normal people may post-date the year to 1999 from 2000. If instead of writing "not oriented to time," the examiner recorded, "on November 27, 2000, the patient said it was November 25, 2000, or November 27, 1996, or July 4, 1931," much more information would have been provided.

Similarly, in relation to place orientation, there is an obvious difference between a hospitalized patient at the Beth Israel Deaconess Medical Center thinking that he is in the Peter Bent Brigham Hospital rather than claiming that he is shopping in Filene's Basement department store, watching a hockey game in the Boston Garden, or sunbathing on the Boston Common. Reporting what the patient said gives so much more information in the same space and time than recording a general negative statement.

When describing the verbal output of an aphasic patient, quoting the exact words used conveys much more than a general description of the patient's language. "I went soma alga nop, then kot restaurant dinnet." Who went with you? "My husbet." Or "the patient gave the following names for objects shown: spoon—spoon, comb—coma, watch—a time tella, scissors—no answer." The replies made can be analyzed later and are more informative than recording "there were naming errors" or "he failed to name three out of five objects."

USE CHARTS OR SIMPLE DIAGRAMS TO ELABORATE ON THE FINDINGS, NOT TO SUBSTITUTE FOR WRITTEN DESCRIPTIONS

Some physicians keep in their offices or at the workstations of the hospital wards charts of muscle testing, sensory charts, and other preprinted materials that can be filled in. These are often helpful in quantifying and localizing findings. We often use a very simple hand-drawn stick figure for recording reflexes (see Figure 4-15). If you use such a figure, make sure it is large enough to see clearly, and right and left should be marked. An alternative is a simple chart of the reflexes (see Table 4-3). Figure 4-16 shows a sensory chart. In general sensory charts and stick-figure reflex cartoons are easier for readers to interpret quickly than verbal descriptions.

We do not approve of using only fill-in-the-blank or checklist forms in lieu of a description of the findings. These forms are usually checked mechanically with little enthusiasm and less thought. Their informational value is quite low. There may be a situation that warrants their use. The new Medicare evaluation and treatment codes define the complexity of evaluations on the basis of numeric criteria that would allow an unsophisticated auditor to reject claims based on the note written. As of this writing an effort is being made to have a more rational way of rating the evaluation but this has not yet been accepted. The presence in the record of a brief form that shows 4 aspects of the present illness; past medical, social, family history; a 10-item system review; and 8 organ systems examined are relatively painlessly checked off for billing compliance. This can defend the level of service billed while a meaningful note can be dictated for patient care.

DO NOT INCLUDE IN YOUR NOTES OR RECORDS PEJORATIVE STATEMENTS ABOUT THE PATIENT OR OTHER CAREGIVERS

Even if you feel negatively toward the patient or critical of prior or concurrent care, do not criticize in the chart. Simply record the facts, as you understand them without comment.

The patient took the prescribed Dilantin for three days, taking one pill each night. (I had prescribed one in the morning and two each night and those are the directions on her pill bottle.) She stopped because, after talking over her symptoms with her Aunt Bessie on the phone, she decided that the medicine was not good for her and that she did not need treatment. She visited Doctor A after three blackouts. She reported that he told her that she was a very nervous and troublesome woman and should immediately get rid of her black cat, which she was probably allergic to.

TRACING IMAGES IN THE CHART

Dr. Denny-Brown taught L.R.C. a very useful technique that he had never seen described in writing. Denny-Brown (and later L.R.C.) instructed his neurology residents to trace abnormal angiograms and pneumoencephalograms in the patient's medical record. This is done by simply removing a lined progress note page in use or a plain sheet of white paper, holding the film and the page up to a lit viewbox or a bright window pane, and tracing the outline of the abnormalities onto the page, which is then labeled and returned to the chart (Figures 5-1, 5-2, and 5-3). The traced image conveys much more than the written description by the radiologist. ("A picture is worth a thousand words.") During later admissions, it is often difficult to quickly retrieve old films from storage or microfilm, and a picture in the chart is very useful for reviewing previous imaging abnormalities. Computed tomography (CT) and magnetic resonance imaging (MRI) scans, angiograms, vertebral X-rays, electroencephalogram (EEG) and electromyogram (EMG) portions, and evoked response abnormalities (if not included in the chart) can all be traced. Copying machines are commonly available and can later save much time tracking down older data. Digital transmission of radiographs is increasingly common but requires too much memory to allow this means of storage in office records. Key findings can also be included in outpatient records if the patient is seen in the office or clinic.

PHOTOGRAPHS

We have for more than a decade tried to persuade various hospital chief executive officers to include in the front portion of the patient's hospital chart a face frontal-view photograph of the patient. This can be taken during the admissions process. The photography would be quite inexpensive compared with other "routine" laboratory procedures that have relatively low yield. A photograph of the patient's face is an excellent form of identification. The availability of digital photography has led a colleague to include a patient facial photo in all his records. Typing is generally done on computer and the image can be stored with the patient data (Figure 5-4).

Facial expression and detail yield a wealth of information to the seasoned clinical neurologist. Ptosis, a Parkinsonian facies, acromegaly, a Wilsonian expression, an early hint of corrugated frontalis muscles (Hutchinson's sign of

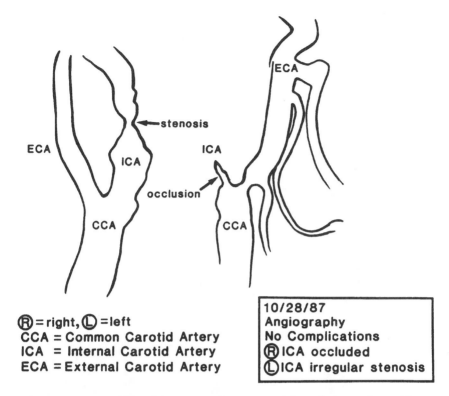

® = right, **Ⓛ** = left
CCA = Common Carotid Artery
ICA = Internal Carotid Artery
ECA = External Carotid Artery

10/28/87
Angiography
No Complications
® ICA occluded
Ⓛ ICA irregular stenosis

Figure 5-1 Tracing of films from a carotid angiogram. The right internal carotid artery was occluded. The left internal carotid artery had a moderately severe stenosis above the origin.

early ptosis), a myasthenic snarl or facial droop, Horner's syndrome, and proptosis are only a few of the myriad findings available from a picture. Review of old records could show changes and transformations in the eyes, lids, and face, differentiating congenital abnormalities from acquired disease. Neurologists often request that patients bring in old photographs for review to see if there has been a change.

Why not routinely include this valuable data in the patient's chart? Is a photograph for the patient's hospital record any more intrusive than the obligatory snapshots required for driving licenses, passports, and college and medical school applications? It is already routine in many hospitals to photograph decubitus ulcers present on admission. Hospital records are already protected as privileged private records.

SCALES

Research needs have led to the generation of large numbers of scales. An individual physician's practice may make some of these scales particularly useful.

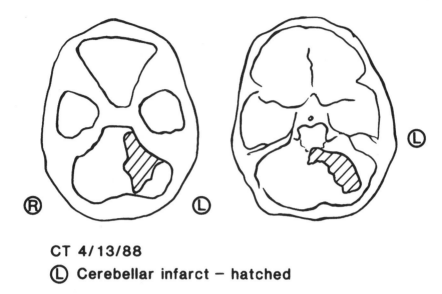

CT 4/13/88
Ⓛ **Cerebellar infarct – hatched**

Figure 5-2   Tracing from 2 views of a CT scan that showed a left cerebellar infarct.

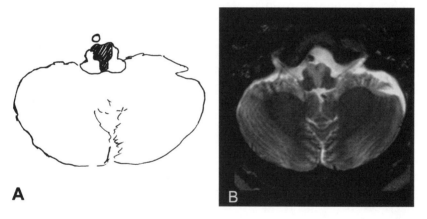

Figure 5-3   A, Tracing of the T2-weighted MRI shown in **B.** The patient had a bilateral medial medullary infarct caused by a vertebral artery occlusion. Note only the flow void of one vertebral artery is seen.

At the Rochester General Hospital, the nurses on the stroke unit utilize the NIH Stroke Scale rather than the "neuro checks" used elsewhere in the hospital, which are nothing more than the Glasgow coma scale. A physician with large numbers of multiple sclerosis patients may wish to use an MS-specific disability scale or another may use a Parkinson's disease scale or a headache scale. In all of these scales, there is a precise method of scoring and it requires a little effort to learn each scale. These scales will not be of general use in routine office practice but

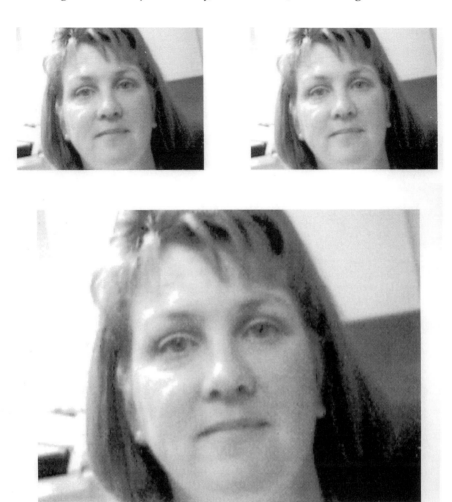

Figure 5-4 Sample photographs of a Rochester General Hospital Neurology Unit secretary taken with an inexpensive digital camera. The larger image allows assessment of pupil size and the presence of a minor asymmetry of the nasolabial folds.

may well be useful to an individual whose practice has become weighted in a particular area. Herndon[4] has not only assembled many of these scales in a book, but a diskette is included that facilitates usage. The new edition of this book should also include headache scales.

WATCH YOUR HANDWRITING

Illegible notes are useless and can lead to harm. Whenever possible, notes should be typed or dictated for transcription. We would like it to be mandated (with appropriate funding) that dictating phones and transcriptions be used routinely for hospital records as they are now used for descriptions of surgical procedures. This is increasingly available in hospitals as many hospitals gradually move to a computerized medical record system. If you must write, take special care to ensure that others will be able to read your notes. We recently had a case of an order written on a medical chart where no one was able to either decipher the order or the name of the order writer. This is not only discourteous, but it is also dangerous. Notes should always be dated, and hospital entries should carry an appropriate time of day.

REFERENCES

1. Gowers E. Medical jargon. *The Practitioner* 1958;181:338–344.
2. Morgan WL, Engel GL. *The Clinical Approach to the Patient.* Philadelphia: W.B. Saunders Co., 1969;175.
3. Fisher CM. Quantification of deficits in clinical neurology. *Trans Amer Neurol Assoc* 1969;94:263–265.
4. Herndon RM. *Handbook of Neurologic Rating Scales.* New York: Demos Vermande, 1997.

6

Ordering and Interpreting Tests

For when the cause of the complaint's unsure
Twould be a miracle to find a cure.[1]

—Cervantes

Recall that there is a great deal of difference between accumulating clinical data and acquiring definitive clinical information. Many studies will supply an abundance of the former and none of the latter. . . . Before performing a particular study, one should ask the question: "How likely is this study to give me definitive information about this patient's disorder that will not be subject to a variety of interpretations and will the result carry significant weight in allowing me to determine the probable causes of this patient's sickness?" Once I have the answer from this study, will I be appreciably nearer to understanding what is wrong with this patient, or will I simply have more nonspecific data?[2]

—P. Tumulty

History and the physical examination provide the essential basic facts for diagnosis. Facts obtained by other means may be superfluous or even misleading. When the results of tests cannot be correlated with the facts disclosed by the history and physical examination, they should be considered subsidiary to the main issue. In spite of the crucial significance of the ancillary examinations in many cases, it seems important to emphasize that skill in differential diagnosis is not determined by one's ability to assemble and correlate laboratory reports.[3]

—A.M. Harvey and J. Bordley

After the history and general and neurologic examinations, the clinician must plan laboratory investigations and further diagnostic tests. When the patient is seen as an outpatient, planning of tests must begin almost immediately; the patient expects directions as to the next step before leaving the doctor's office. As the outpatient examination proceeds, the physician weighs possible diagnostic and treatment options in order to plan what information to tell the patient. The clinician must decide if any investigations are needed and,

105

if so, what, when, and where. With hospitalized patients, the situation is quite different. Some investigations are prescheduled. There used to be more time and opportunity for discussion and planning unless the patient was acutely ill. Now most patients are admitted through the emergency department. In the hospital, decisions concern which tests, in what sequence, and how urgently they are needed. Current health care reimbursement considerations introduce goals that conflict with a sequential, reasoned evaluation. Reducing length of stay becomes a hospital fiscal imperative when hospital reimbursement is Diagnostic-Related Group (DRG) based. Managed care systems demand efficiency when hospitals are reimbursed on a per diem basis. A logical, sequential evaluation will require close monitoring of results and scheduling issues may prompt ordering multiple tests concurrently in an effort to control costs and length of stay. It may be cheaper to order a study that may prove unnecessary rather than extend the stay in the hospital. The physician must balance the conflicting demand for efficiency while trying to approach the clinical problem in a logical, sequential manner.

FACTORS TO BE CONSIDERED

Table 6-1 lists the most important questions to be asked when a physician is considering ordering a test.

How Sick Is the Patient?

In general, the more ill the patient appears to be, the more the physician feels pressed to investigate urgently and treat. Hospitalization is usually suggested for patients who are acutely ill or unable to function. Theoretically, the decision to hospitalize and the decision to investigate are separate. In practice, accurate diagnosis should precede specific therapy, and hospitalization strongly facilitates rapid and definitive investigation to fully evaluate the patient's ill-

---

Table 6-1   Questions to Be Asked When Considering Ordering a Test

- How sick is the patient?
- How certain or uncertain is the diagnosis?
- Is the condition tested-for treatable?
- Will the test provide a baseline that will be useful later?
- Are the test results likely to be worth the cost?
- Is this the best time to order the test?
- What clinical hypothesis is being tested?
- How sensitive is the test?
- How specific is the test for the disorder being considered?

---

ness. Meningitis, paraplegia, acute hemiplegia, or acute and severe paralyzing neuropathy or myopathy, are examples of acute conditions in which hospitalization and urgent testing are mandated. Less acutely ill patients with more slowly progressive myopathy, neuropathy, or mental failure can often be investigated on an outpatient basis.

Some patients, although not acutely ill or disabled, nevertheless have very serious disease with a poor long-term prognosis. A 60-year-old man who consults a physician because of slight weakness of the right thumb is found to have fasciculations of the tongue and muscles of the arms, legs, and back, and hyperreflexia. Though he has noticed few symptoms, this patient has a serious disease, and most physicians would feel compelled to confirm the diagnosis of motor neuron disease and exclude by investigations other possible diagnoses even of low probability. This type of outpatient is one of those most likely to be referred for another opinion.

Is the Disease Treatable?

Physicians fear missing the diagnosis in a patient with a treatable disease. Some of the greatest moments of physician satisfaction are derived from finding a condition that can be cured or at least greatly ameliorated by specific treatment. We recall with pride and satisfaction a patient with myxedema coma brought back to life with a small dose of thyroid, and another patient with mental changes and altered gait whose symptoms and signs were reversed by vitamin B_{12} treatment of her pernicious anemia. In these types of situations, draw the blood and treat. Although therapy in neurology has shown remarkable advances, we still have too few patients we can successfully treat. When the most likely diagnosis is not specifically treatable, we must be sure to exclude remediable conditions that could mimic the more likely diagnosis. A very small percentage of patients with acute hemiplegia have subdural hematomas, but the potential reversibility of the disorder makes its exclusion very important.

How Certain or Uncertain Is the Diagnosis?

The more uncertain and unknown the diagnosis, the more likely the doctor is to seek help from various investigations. A "shotgun" approach of ordering multiple and diverse tests may adversely affect the patient's confidence in the doctor. Patients respond well to a brief discussion of the rationale for the approach taken. The time and money spent on needless and negative tests raises the patient's anxiety level and sometimes evokes distrust and anger. Computed tomography (CT) or magnetic resonance imaging (MRI) of the lumbar spine and nerve conduction velocity measurements and electromyography will not be helpful in the evaluation of thoracic cord compression. Too often physicians are like the legendary wise men of Chelm who looked for a dropped purse where the streetlight was brighter rather than where it was dropped. The ease of ordering a test should not be its sole indication. In neurology, in which tests are often disease- or anatomically specific, diffuse investigations without well-thought-out hypotheses (a so-called fishing expedition) are seldom effective in making a diagnosis. Many neurologic disorders remain clinical diagnoses rather than absolutely definable by a single test. Often a pattern of test results may make or break the diagnosis. The neurologist should have a sense of what the test might show and what he or she expects to learn from the study before ordering it. It is often better (if the patient is not acutely or seriously ill) to wait until the differential diagnosis, or at least the anatomy and pathophysiology of the symptoms and signs, is further clarified by the later course of the illness. If the diagnosis is very uncertain and the patient is ill, consultation is important before needless tests are ordered. When the physician chooses consultants carefully and keeps patients and their families in the loop, the patients' trust in the physician's interest in their well-being is enhanced.

Is It Important to Document the Diagnosis and Stage of the Illness?

Verifying and documenting the diagnosis and severity of illness are often useful for a variety of reasons. If the disease is serious and potentially disabling or fatal, the patient and family must be given a diagnosis. That diagnosis should be as firmly established as possible. Robert F. Loeb told his third-year medical students at Columbia of an illness he had while a student at Harvard College. Jacques Loeb was notified that his son Robert was dying of leukemia. He cancelled his engagements and took the train to Boston. On arrival, he discovered that his son's leukemia was mononucleosis and he had already begun to recover. It may be necessary to transmit bad news to a patient or family, but it must be true. Specific predictions about duration of life ("he will be dead in six months") are fraught with error.

Some patients and families without severe disease need reassurance that the illness is not serious. This may be difficult if the physician has not been careful and thorough in documenting the correct diagnosis. The anxiety level of the patient and family may dictate the need for urgent tests to document or exclude diagnoses. These may be fanciful concerns or directly derive from incorrect information previously given by others. The Internet offers patients and their relatives much useful information but also much error. Even when the information presented is from an authoritative source, the layman can easily misinterpret that information. It is best to address the specific areas of concern raised by what they have found on the Internet or learned from a friend. When confronted by such patients, it is necessary to define their understanding of the situation to allow you to correct any misinformation they may have obtained.

The present medicolegal climate induces a special concern. Occasional litigious patients and some indiscriminate and greedy lawyers have clearly influenced physicians to increase the number of tests. Unfortunately, all too often, doctors will worry, "How will it look in court if I have not ordered this or that test?" For legal reasons, some physicians feel compelled to order skull and cervical spine X-rays and CT scans for patients with relatively trivial head injuries. "Defensive medicine" clearly increases the number of investigations. Occasionally, unexpected findings on these tests lead to further proliferation of tests to explain the abnormalities. A cascade of anxieties, clinically inappropriate tests, and even therapies may ensue. Patients devoid of neurologic symptoms or signs may be told that the MRI shows multiple sclerosis, multiinfarct dementia, "brain atrophy," or a brain tumor. The "multiple sclerosis" may be a few minute white matter lesions in a patient with migraine; the multiinfarct dementia may represent minimal periventricular white matter hyperintensity in a cognitively unimpaired individual; the "brain atrophy" may represent slightly more spinal fluid in cerebral sulci, the "brain tumor" might be a 1 cm convexity meningioma.

In a teaching hospital, documentation is often important for instructing students, house officers in training, and staff. We all learn by imprinting in our memory the signs, symptoms, and laboratory findings of patients with known verified diseases. Experience with five patients with well-documented syringomyelia, along with reading of the literature, familiarizes a neurologist with the usual findings in this unusual disease. This knowledge helps the clinician recognize the significance of the signs and symptoms of other patients in whom syringomyelia or other spinal cord disease is suspected. But what if several of the five patients did not have syringomyelia, but instead had another disease process? The wrong reference memory pattern would have been imprinted. We must continuously document and test our hypotheses if we are to learn, teach, and advance neurologic knowledge.

Documentation is often needed to stage a disease or for a baseline determination to judge future improvement or progression of disease. The diagnosis of brain tumor may be secure and even the histology known from biopsy, but the size and location of the tumor must be documented before treatment in order to measure the effects of the treatment and the course of the illness. In a patient with early dementia, neuropsychological tests seldom secure a specific diagnosis but provide a baseline to gauge subsequent change and may provide the family a better understanding of the patient's ability to accept responsibility for self-care.

Economic Considerations

The cost of health care in the United States has escalated so rapidly that it has become a very central consideration for all concerned with evaluating and treating patients. The pressure from all parties (patients, families, doctors, medical trainees, lawyers) to document the diagnosis and the severity of the disease has led to a proliferation of testing, some very expensive and some invasive, carrying potential for further risk to the patient.

Some doctors profit directly from tests that they order and perform or interpret in their offices. These tests include electroencephalogram (EEG), electromyogram (EMG), CT, MRI, noninvasive vascular tests, and others. The ethical physician will be concerned over self-referral and whether the decision to order a particular study was truly motivated by patient need. Doctors often rationalize ordering unnecessary tests by citing one of the factors already mentioned: medicolegal, patient reassurance, patient or family demand. Furthermore, doctors know that most patients do not pay for these tests directly out of pocket. Third-party payers (health insurance) and government agencies, in the case of Medicare and Medicaid, foot the bill. Unfortunately, there is no free lunch. Doctors and the public all pay in the end because unnecessary tests increase the total health care bill and stimulate governments, employers, and third-party payers to demand and legislate control over all aspects of medical care in order to control costs of testing. Doctors lose their autonomy. A few avaricious physicians can wreck the entire system.

How should physicians decide on the investigations to be performed? We suggest using the Golden Rule. If the tables were turned and we were the patients and we had the symptoms, signs, and background psychosocial and environmental characteristics of the patient, would we want testing to be done? Which tests, when, and where? What if the patient was your mother, father, child, spouse, or sibling? If you would not order the tests for yourself or your loved ones, they should not be ordered for the patient.

Timing of Tests

Is it important to make the diagnosis now? In a number of circumstances that we can readily visualize, the patient and family may be worse off when an early diagnosis is made and shared with the patient.

Let us illustrate this point about the importance of the timing of diagnosis with three patient examples from our own experience. A 59-year-old administrator had a series of Jacksonian seizures beginning with jerking of the right hand. Later, right facial and mouth muscles contracted rhythmically, the head turned to the right, and the patient stopped speaking. Postictally, he was aphasic for ten to fifteen minutes. Examination long after an attack was normal except for a right extensor plantar reflex and right hyperreflexia. He was able to return to work and, according to his wife and coworkers, he functioned normally. An EEG showed focal slowing in the left central suprasylvian region. A CT with and without contrast showed no mass or definite abnormality, but sulci were less prominent in the left central region. The most likely diagnosis by far was a glioma. Metastatic tumor, meningioma, or brain abscess would probably have shown on CT. Stroke seldom causes Jacksonian seizures, and he had no risk factors for stroke. Serious occlusive vascular disease can be sought by outpatient duplex ultrasound of the left carotid artery and transcranial Doppler (TCD) ultrasound testing of the intracranial carotid and middle cerebral arteries. Intensive investigation with MRI or angiography or both might allow the diagnosis of glioma but to what end? If a glioma is verified by investigations, it will be very difficult not to biopsy or operate on the lesion, and radiotherapy without a diagnosis should not be seriously considered. If surgery is performed, there is a real risk that the patient will become aphasic and unable to work or function optimally at home. With time, if the patient has a glioma, the diagnosis will become evident. Spells will become more difficult to control; motor, sensory, visual, or cognitive abnormalities will appear; and the CT will become positive. When the patient develops a disability, diagnosis and treatment can be pursued with less risk of further harm. Three to six months of relatively well-preserved function in a patient with a high-grade glioma, or years in patients with low-grade lesions, may be gained by waiting. We suggest treating the patient's seizures with anticonvulsants but no aggressive tumor workup. No patient has been cured by early treatment of a glioma. Even when gliomas are unexpectedly found in specimens of temporal lobe removed for seizure control, the outcome has not been good.[4] Results in the few long-term survivors of high-grade gliomas are discouraging and most are more or less severely incapacitated.

A 74-year-old widow consulted one of us (L.R.C.) because of weakness of her left leg and a change in her gait. She occasionally lost control of her urine. Examination showed slight weakness of the left lower extremity, a hyperactive left knee jerk, and a left extensor plantar response. Despite a limp, she was able to continue working and to lead an active social life. L.R.C. saw her in the pre-CT era and was clever enough to diagnose by angiography her right parasagittal meningioma. After successful removal by an excellent surgeon, she never quite bounced back to her former state. This fiercely independent woman had to give up work and move in with her sister. Later, she entered a nursing home and was very unhappy. Did L.R.C. do her a favor by diagnosing and suggesting treatment for her meningioma when he did?

A 34-year-old married man with three children consulted one of us (L.R.C.) because he had found out that his father, demented and "shaky" for years, had been diagnosed with Huntington's disease at autopsy. He was appropriately worried that he might be carrying the gene for Huntington's disease and that he and his children might develop the disease. He had read extensively about new tests to detect which asymptomatic patients at risk will be affected. Pharmacologic provocative exposure to L-dopa, MRI, positron emission tomography (PET) scan, and genetic analysis were all potentially available but difficult to arrange, possibly expensive, and not foolproof in their predictive abilities. Should he have these tests? If so, when and after what counseling and precautions? Suicide was a real risk if the tests predicted that he carried the gene. Caution, controversy, and debate still surround individual patient's decisions about genetic testing for Huntington's disease and other familial disorders even though now genetic testing is more reliable than at the time this patient was seen.[5,6]

One of the most common situations in neurologic practice is the early diagnosis of multiple sclerosis. This is a fluid situation in which advances in therapy have made the proper approach subject to ongoing modification. A 24-year-old young mother of one child comes to your office because of tingling of the left foot, which had gradually spread to the left thigh, trunk, and arm and to the right foot during a period of three weeks. The symptoms followed an upper respiratory infection with a cough and sore throat. She has no pain, and examination shows only an asymmetrical decrease in vibration sense, worse in the left limbs. There are no motor, reflex, sphincter, or autonomic abnormalities or spine tenderness. By far, the most likely diagnosis is a demyelinative attack. The neurologist might be able to document dissemination of lesions within the central nervous system by MRI (especially using gadolinium-DPTA enhancement, or magnetization transfer imaging[7]), high-dose contrast-enhanced CT, or testing with visual, brainstem auditory, and somatosensory-evoked responses. Lumbar puncture with analysis of immunoglobulins and a search for oligoclonal bands might document immunological findings suggestive of multiple sclerosis (MS). These tests cannot definitely establish the diagnosis of multiple sclerosis since the important criteria of dissemination of lesions over time cannot be met.[8] This patient's symptoms and signs might reflect a mild monophasic illness such as acute disseminated encephalomyelitis or a transverse myelitis. The patient who has a single relatively benign event is probably not one in whom therapy is warranted at this stage in our understanding of the disease, although this subject is debated.[9] This is a patient in whom follow-up is important.

Positive findings on MRI, evoked response testing, or oligoclonal bands might allow the physician to tell the patient that there is a high likelihood that she has or will develop multiple sclerosis. But what would be gained? The patient's symptoms and signs are trivial and ordinarily would not require treatment. We have seen several patients with scenarios similar to that described who have been told that they have a high likelihood of multiple sclerosis. They had two or three years or more of anxiety and agony waiting for the axe to fall. They understandably feared serious disability because they had read about or knew wheelchair-bound and disabled young people with multiple sclerosis. Some delay having children they otherwise want. Some postpone or cancel plans for marriage, careers, or further education or training because of the prospect of disability. In most such patients, the medical prognosis is very good. They may have some spells of numbness or parasthesiae, visual symptoms, or other attacks, but the likelihood of severe disability is relatively small. After five to ten years of relative well-being, most such patients who were given an early diagnosis of multiple sclerosis realize that all their anxiety was for nought. They could have planned and lived their lives normally if the doctor had not told them they probably had multiple sclerosis.

In the patient described, is there any real hurry in arriving at the diagnosis of demyelinating disease? Clearly not. Following the patient over time would help exclude most serious and important diseases within the differential diagnosis. Simple serological tests might exclude or confirm active viral infection with cytomegalovirus (CMV) or Epstein-Barr virus (EBV) or the presence of Lyme disease. If the patient had had paraplegia, a disabling cerebellar ataxia, or blindness in one or both eyes, the situation would be quite different and diagnosis would become very important.

The development of immunotherapy with beta-interferons and glatiramer acetate (copolymer) has made early diagnosis of and prophylactic therapy of multiple sclerosis much more important. The development of clinically definite multiple sclerosis may be delayed by prophylactic therapy.[10] One should have a valid diagnosis before embarking on what may be very expensive lifelong therapy. The patient who has a clear event such as optic neuritis or paraparesis probably warrants an MRI at our present level of understanding. It is not clear that one can definitively predict the development of multiple sclerosis from any laboratory study. The finding of an MRI showing multiple lesions in this context may still leave the diagnosis in doubt, but a case can be made for early institution of immunotherapy to reduce the likelihood that clinically significant MS will develop.

One of the major factors that will influence physicians in their ordering of tests is the ability and willingness of the patient to be closely followed. *One of the best diagnostic tests is tincture of time.* Demyelinative plaques improve, tumors worsen, and the symptoms and signs of many illnesses allow ready recognition with time. The seriousness of the symptoms and the anxiety level of the patient, his or her family, and the doctor often dictate when tests will be done.

Not all tests need to be scheduled at once. In the young mother with parasthesiae just described, if spinal cord compression is seriously considered, an MRI of the spinal cord might be performed, but cranial MRI, evoked response testing, and lumbar puncture can be deferred. In an elderly patient with slight dementia, thyroid function tests, drug screening, and B_{12} blood levels might be ordered after the first visit in order not to miss treatable conditions. CT or MRI to detect early Alzheimer's disease can certainly be delayed and may lack utility. Available therapy for the diseases concerned will influence the timing of investigations. At present, since gliomas, Alzheimer's disease, Creutzfeldt-Jakob disease, and motor neuron disease are not curable, there is little to be gained by very early diagnosis. The risk of erroneously giving one patient one of these diagnoses probably outweighs any benefit of many such correct diagnoses. When and if specific treatment is found for any of these conditions, then early diagnosis may become very worthwhile.

TYPES OF INVESTIGATIONS

Ordering diagnostic tests can become so routine that many doctors do not stop and think about the reasons for the tests, their general classification (Table 6-2), and strategies for their use.

Disease-Specific Tests

Few individual tests are disease specific. Cultures, antibody titers, and polymerase chain reaction (PCR) analysis of tissue or fluids for infectious agents can identify specific infectious etiologies. Biopsies of nervous system tissues and muscle often can identify specific disease entities. Most often, however, a battery

Table 6-2   Types of Tests

Imaging—creating a picture of an anatomical structure
   CT, MRI, CTA, MRA, B-mode ultrasound, contrast angiography, echocardiography
Physiologic—displaying or measuring a nervous system function
   EEG, EMG, nerve conduction velocities, Doppler vascular interrogation
Biochemical—quantifying chemical substances in a body fluid
   antibody titers, biochemical analysis of the blood, and cerebrospinal fluid (CSF)
Pathology—morphology of tissue
   biopsy of brain, nerve, muscle
Genetic analysis
   analysis of cells for genetic patterns
Infectious disease-related
   cultures of body tissues, blood, and CSF for viruses, bacteria, fungi;
   polymerase chain reaction (PCR) of body tissues and fluids for organisms; antibody titers

of tests is required for definitive diagnosis. Examples of disease-specific testing include:

1. *Infectious nervous system disorders.* Cultures of the cerebrospinal fluid (CSF) for pneumococci, meningococci, histoplasma capsulatum in patients with meningitis; antibodies against HIV, *Borrelia burgdorferi, Listeria monocytogenes,* and cryptococci; PCR analysis of tissue or CSF for herpes simplex and herpes zoster-varicella viruses are specific for the individual infectious agents.
2. *Multiple sclerosis.* MRI, visual, and somatosensory evoked potentials, and spinal tap with analysis of CSF proteins and search for oligoclonal bands.
3. *Myasthenia gravis.* EMG with testing for decremental response, single fiber EMG looking for jitter; tensilon test; serological testing for acetylcholine receptor antibody levels.
4. *Porphyria.* Watson-Schwartz test; urinary porphobilinogen, delta-aminolevulinic acid, and porphyrin levels.
5. *Pernicious anemia.* B_{12} analysis, methylmalonic acid and homocysteine levels, inspection of blood smear (or electronic cell counters) for macrocytosis or multisegmented polyps. Schilling test, analysis of gastric aspirate for acid, and anti-intrinsic factor antibodies may clarify etiology.
6. *Pituitary tumor.* Formal visual fields, CT or preferably MRI, prolactin and other hormone levels in blood and urine, stimulation tests with pituitary trophic hormones to test responsiveness of target glands to stimulation.

Disease Mechanism–Specific Tests

Some tests are specific for mechanism of illness but are not diagnostic of an individual disease etiology. For example, paroxysmal spike and slow wave discharges point to epilepsy but usually do not yield much information about the underlying cause of the seizures. A brain image that shows hypodensity in the distribution of a single cerebral artery in a patient with the acute onset of focal neurologic signs is diagnostic of infarction but does not identify the cause of the ischemia. CSF pleocytosis suggests inflammation or infection but does not identify a specific pathogen.

Anatomy-Specific Tests

Much testing is anatomy specific. In a patient with aphasia and right hemiparesis, investigations focus on the left cerebral hemisphere. CT, MRI, duplex ultrasound testing of the left carotid artery in the neck, TCD or noninvasive angiography by MRI or CT of the left intracranial carotid and middle cerebral arteries, selective left carotid angiography, and EEG may all be ordered to give more information about the hemispheral lesion. In a patient with paraparesis of spinal origin, these investigations would be fruitless. Plain films of the spine, CT myelography or MRI of the spine at the appropriate levels, or somatosensory evoked responses could be scheduled. In the example of spinal cord disease, the physician ordering the tests must be even more specific about the anatomy and must localize the approximate level of the lesion. Cervical CT, MRI, or plain films of the neck will not detect a lesion of the conus medullaris or cauda equina. It is all too common to see lumbosacral imaging ordered to rule out spinal cord compression because the legs are weak without concern for the sensory level or the absence of spinal cord below the L1–L2 vertebrae. In disease of the peripheral nervous system, EMG, motor and sensory nerve conduction velocities, and nerve or muscle biopsies may be performed; these investigations would shed little light if the patient had cerebral or spinal cord disease.

Some anatomical tests are likely to be *definitive*. A CT or MRI might be able to diagnose a meningioma, brain abscess, demyelinative plaque, Arnold-Chiari malformation, brain infarct, intracerebral hemorrhage, cavernous angioma, and AVM with a high degree of probability. Angiography can define and localize an arterial occlusion, plaque, dissection, aneurysm, and embolus in some patients.

Pathophysiology-Specific Tests

Some tests are *functional*; that is, they most often characterize the pathophysiology without defining a specific disease entity. Diffuse EEG slowing suggests a metabolic, inflammatory, or degenerative process but is not very specific. Similarly, focal EEG slowing points to a local process but cannot reliably distinguish between tumor, abscess, traumatic hematoma, and infarction.

Small amplitude polyphasic muscle potentials on an EMG suggest a myopathy but are not specific for any single disease of muscle. EEG, evoked potential testing, psychometrics, EMG, and nerve conduction velocities are examples of tests that give functional information. Occasionally, abnormalities on these tests can be very suggestive of a specific diagnosis, for example, the characteristic EEG appearance of periodic sharp wave complexes of subacute sclerosing panencephalitis (SSPE) and Creutzfeldt-Jakob disease or the multiple fasciculations and giant motor units seen on EMG in patients with motor neuron disease.

Some tests identify *risk factors for disease,* helping the physician to estimate the probability of a given condition, but do not make a specific diagnosis. Elevated blood cholesterol and triglyceride levels slightly increase the probability of brain infarction. A hypokinetic segment of the left cardiac ventricular wall detected by echocardiography and atrial fibrillation confirmed by an electrocardiogram (EKG) greatly increase the probability that a cerebral lesion is due to an embolus of cardiac origin. However, patients with each of these cardiac conditions often have other unrelated problems that may have caused their strokes. An elevated blood sugar determination increases the probability that a patient with clinical and electrophysiological evidence of peripheral polyneuropathy has a diabetic neuropathy but does not exclude other equally important potential causes such as toxins, drugs, cancer, or thyroid deficiency. Moderate stenosis of the internal carotid artery detected by B mode ultrasound is frequently found in normal asymptomatic adults. This finding raises the possibility of an etiological relationship, but does not prove that a patient's brain symptoms are caused by the vascular lesion.

TESTS SHOULD BE HYPOTHESIS DRIVEN AND SHOULD BE ORDERED AND PERFORMED SEQUENTIALLY

We have emphasized repeatedly in previous chapters the vital importance of making hypotheses about disease mechanism and anatomy. Investigations should be planned to test and elaborate on these hypotheses. The results of initial tests help guide the choice of further tests.

We will illustrate with several case examples. A 48-year-old man is brought to the hospital by a neighbor because the patient appeared to be ill. Examination shows severe aphasia and a moderate right hemiparesis. The patient can give no account of the development of his symptoms. In this patient, the anatomy is quite clear. The patient must have a lesion in or abutting on the left cerebral hemisphere. The disease mechanism is purely speculative without further history. The initial investigation should be a brain imaging test—CT or MRI. Subsequent testing will depend on the general category of lesion found. Infarction, hemorrhage, and neoplasm are all possible. If an infarct is found, echocardiography, 24-hour cardiac rhythm monitoring, noninvasive carotid and middle cerebral artery evaluation, and carotid angiography all should be considered. If, however, the lesion on CT is an intracerebral hemorrhage, cardiac and noninvasive testing would not be indicated. Angiographic search for an aneurysm or an arteriovenous malformation (AVM), MRI testing for an AVM or cavernous angioma, and tests for a bleeding diathesis might be pursued instead, depending on the location and shape of the hemorrhage. If CT/MRI findings suggested infection or tumor, other investigations such as a chest X-ray and/or chest CT scan would be more appropriate.

A 25-year-old woman comes to the emergency ward because of a severe headache that began abruptly that day. She is vomiting, has a slight fever, a stiff neck, and is restless and agitated. The possibility of subarachnoid or intraventricular hemorrhage and meningitis are foremost in your mind. You expeditiously perform a CT scan and lumbar puncture. If blood is found on the CT or in the CSF, angiography will likely be needed to identify a possible aneurysm or AVM. If, however, white blood cells are found in the CSF without blood, cultures and smears of the spinal fluid, blood cultures, PCR analysis, and serological tests for antibodies are important, but angiography is seldom warranted.

SENSITIVITY AND SPECIFICITY OF TESTS BEING CONSIDERED

A very important consideration in deciding on whether or not to pursue an individual investigation is how powerful the test is.[11] If the individual being tested has a given condition, how often is the test likely to be positive? The true positive rate is customarily referred to as the *sensitivity* of the test. A sensitive test is likely to detect a high proportion of individuals with the condition being tested. The false negative rate refers to the frequency of negative results in patients who have the condition. Also important is the specificity of a test. A specific test has relatively few false positive results; that is, patients who have a positive test have a very high probability of harboring the condition being tested. Cultures of the spinal fluid for the tubercle bacillus are highly specific but have low sensitivity. Antinuclear antibody testing has a high sensitivity but a low specificity. Testing of the spinal fluid for the 14-3-3 protein in patients suspected of having Creutzfeldt-Jakob disease has a high sensitivity but a relatively low specificity since other conditions can give a positive result. Clinicians should be wary of tests that have a low specificity because false positives are usually more of a problem than false negatives.

SOME RULES ABOUT INVESTIGATIONS

1. *Investigations should be chosen that test or confirm hypotheses.* Residents and young practitioners should routinely write down their hypotheses; this will ensure that some important investigations are not neglected. Even experienced clinicians, faced with a difficult diagnostic problem, can profit by putting their thoughts on paper. Studying this list of ordered probabilities of plausible anatomical and mechanism of disease diagnoses may clarify the best strategy for testing. Can some of the diagnoses be excluded or established by tests?

2. *Order tests systematically. The most important issues should be studied first.* If a given sign could be due to cervical spinal cord or a cerebral hemisphere lesion, clarify the anatomical differential first before proceeding with tests of disease mechanism. *Settle first issues first.* An example of not heeding this principle was a 45-year-old woman who developed a progressive paraparesis during the preceding week. She was unsteady on her feet and had sensory loss below the rib cage. She also reported bifrontal headaches. A low-grade fever was thought to be due to a mild urinary infection when pyuria was noted. The physician reasoned that the patient probably had multiple sclerosis but the gradual onset of headache and paraparesis might be due to a parasaggital meningioma. An MRI of the head was scheduled the next week to pursue these possible diagnoses. A small convexity meningioma was found. This woman with paraparesis and sensory level could not have had an intracranial lesion that would explain her signs. Even though multiple sclerosis could explain spinal cord dysfunction, the first priority had to be the spinal cord. Despite the irrelevance of this finding to the patient's clinical presentation, she was referred electively for neurosurgical opinion. While at home she became paraplegic with back pain and fever. Urgent intervention for her spinal epidural abscess did not prevent significant permanent impairment. Addressing her clinical problem of possible cord compression might have improved her outcome by earlier appropriate management.

3. *Seek treatable diseases even when they are not the most likely diagnosis.* Missing the diagnosis of subdural hematoma, hypothyroidism, pernicious anemia, chronic paroxysmal hemicrania, hypoglycemia, or bacterial meningitis in one case is far more serious than missing ten cases of glioblastoma, motor neuron disease, and Creutzfeldt-Jakob disease.

4. *If the anatomical and disease mechanism diagnoses are very uncertain, either wait for clarification by the evolution of clinical symptoms or signs, or obtain a consultation from one of your colleagues.* If either the anatomy or mechanism can be assigned a differential diagnosis, then proceed with the diagnostic evaluation.

5. *Do not give the patient mixed signals.* If you tell the patient the diagnosis is secure, do not order lots of tests, searching for other diagnoses. These tests make the patient worried that your opinion may be insecure or wrong. Your assurances to the patient that you are certain that she has migraine are contradicted by intensive investigation even if you tell the patient the tests are "just to be sure." *Do as you say.* If you tell the patient you are uncertain of the diagnosis and that tests will be needed to clarify the problem, then proceed with investigations. If you tell the patient the diagnosis is secure but minor features need to be tidied up and quantified by tests, then selectively order a limited number of tests that will elaborate on the diagnosis. The patient should rest assured that the doctor is certain about what to do.

6. *Explain the tests to the patient, but do not let the patient trap you into giving a list of possible diagnoses.* Laundry lists of potential diagnoses are never helpful to the patient and are very alarming and anxiety provoking. The patient

may be collecting diagnoses from well-meaning but uninformed friends or exploring the Internet to help maintain control of the medical situation. This may lead to questions about a specific disease, for example, a brain tumor. It is best to answer honestly that a tumor is a possibility if that is the case. The patient should know what a specific test will entail and what type of information it provides.

7. *Recognize the strategies of investigation you are using.* In playing the game Twenty Questions, the inquisitor can narrow down the possibilities by asking general questions, for example, if a number is sought, "Is the number between 100 and 150?" Alternatively, the questioner can "go for it" by guessing 123, but if the guess is wrong, no information about the correct diagnosis has been gleaned and a question has been wasted. Similarly, ordering B_{12} levels, acetylcholine receptor antibodies, or searching the urine for cytomegalovirus does not further the diagnosis if the tests are negative. An EEG may not make a specific diagnosis but may limit the process to the right frontal region, thus targeting further tests.

8. *Interpret the laboratory findings with respect to the findings from the history and neurologic examinations.* An elevated creatinine phosphokinase level must be interpreted quite differently in a patient with a hemiparesis and a patient with diffuse proximal muscle weakness and muscle pain. Moderate stenosis of the right internal carotid artery found by B mode ultrasound in a patient with transient spells of left hand weakness is much more significant than the same test result in a patient with a peripheral neuropathy.

INTERPRETING TESTS

Many investigations are merely extensions of the examination. These types of tests include EEG, EMG, nerve conduction velocities, evoked response testing, Doppler ultrasound of the extracranial and intracranial arteries, X-rays of the skull and spine, myelography, CT, MRI, and angiography. The electrophysiologic tests are almost always performed by a neurologist (often yourself). Depending on your own expertise in interpretation of these tests and the skill and experience of the neurologist reporting the results, you may or may not want to review the records yourself. On the other hand, the imaging tests, by custom, are most often interpreted formally by radiologists. It is essential that every neurologist have training in interpreting and reading roentgen and neuroimaging films. Nearly always, the responsible clinician should see the films in addition to reading the radiologist's interpretation. The neurologist has the advantage of knowing the clinical data in order to correlate the imaging results with the hypothesis generated from the clinical information. When there are questions or disagreements in interpretation, the films should be reviewed with the radiologist. These are neurologic tests, not simply radiological procedures. When the films are read by a general radiologist, rather than a neuroradiologist, the anatomy and pathophysiology may be much more familiar to a neurologist.

When interpreting a test, for example, CT, it is best to initially look at the films without detailed knowledge of the case. This will ensure that you see what is on the film and not what you hope to see. The films should be reviewed systematically; in reading a skull X-ray, follow the convexity, look at the base, the orbits, the sella, the craniocervical junction, and so on. Your eyes automatically go to the most obvious lesion. Discipline is required to examine all areas and remember to look at all the films. After the initial review, learn the details of the case, and then reexamine the films, examining more closely the areas of most interest. Prematurely focusing in on one area can cause the physician to miss unexpected abnormalities elsewhere. On the other hand, failing to analyze the regions of maximum clinical interest closely would be equally wrong. In many patients, you will already be aware of the clinical findings before you see the films.

COMMUNICATING WITH AND SUPERVISING OTHER PHYSICIANS WHO PERFORM TESTS

All too often, the test results are inadequate to make clinical decisions. Sometimes the wrong tests are done. More often, the correct test was done, but it did not include important regions of interest. Examples include a lumbosacral MRI that may well have been too low to visualize the conus medullaris region in the low thoracic region in a patient with abnormal sphincter functions; a carotid angiogram in a patient whose deficit consists of only a homonymous hemianopsia may not visualize the posterior cerebral artery, most often a branch of the basilar artery. Inadequate tests are a large problem. They can lead to legal suits. Moreover, it is an embarrassment for the neurologist to tell the patient that the test will have to be repeated or was inadequate to guide therapy. Who is responsible for these goofs? Usually not just the radiologist. It is the obligation of the responsible neurologist to communicate clearly the area of interest and the clinical problem with the radiologist or other specialist who will perform a procedure and supervise or interpret films.

Neuroradiologists are well-trained individuals who should be treated as consultants. Contact them directly about the test, the chief areas of interest, and your working diagnosis. Also discuss with them the next step after the initial investigation, for example, "I think this patient has a tumor; if the plain CT or MRI is normal, use contrast enhancement." The neuroradiologist may offer suggestions on choice of imaging techniques. The same courtesy is important for electrophysiological tests to be performed by other neurologists or physicians. What are you looking for? What is bothering you? Are there issues or inconsistencies that are nagging you? Are there any special tests you want to include, any routine procedures you want to omit?

NEUROLOGIC TESTS

Electroencephalogram

Undoubtedly, EEG has become less important since the advent of modern neuroimaging technology. Its major function now is in the diagnosis of seizure disorders. In patients with altered consciousness, it may be the only way to recognize nonconvulsive status epilepticus. It is a functional test, giving information about how the brain works, not what it looks like. EEG can also be helpful in following patients with metabolic encephalopathy, coma, organ failure, and toxic disorders. EEG is useful in making the diagnosis of brain death. EEG during sleep can also identify abnormalities of sleep, though unfortunately, to date, we have too little information about the boundaries of "normal" sleep. The proper assessment of sleep disturbances requires utilization of the polysomnography laboratory to quantitate such disturbances as obstructive sleep apnea and its response to a CPAP mask. Does the patient really have narcolepsy or merely want easy access to certain medications?

Electromyogram and Nerve Conduction Velocities

These electrophysiological tests are an extension of the neurologic examination. They are useful in elaborating and quantifying clinical impressions. They are not a substitute for a careful examination. It has been said that the true neurologist is one who can make a diagnosis during a power failure. Few neuromuscular diagnoses are made solely on EMG findings, and had we no EMG machines, relatively few important diagnoses would be missed by careful, experienced clinicians. Most often, the electrophysiological results serve to document the diagnosis. Care must be taken not to overinterpret EMG results. The test is very sensitive and some abnormalities are common in older patients who do not have active neurologic disease or neurologic symptoms. Denervation in paraspinal or leg muscles could be old and is not necessarily due to acute lumbar disc disease. Too many EMGs are performed for remunerative reasons. Also, too many physicians are performing EMGs. To be done expertly, electrophysiologists should have fellowships of at least six to twelve months. EEG and EMG laboratories should be run by trained, experienced electrophysiologists.

Evoked Response Testing

This technology has grown dramatically during the last decade. Results are beginning to tell us a great deal about the function of the nervous system, but clinical indications are very limited.[12] Abnormalities in evoked response testing in clinically uninvolved regions in patients suspected of having multiple sclerosis can help establish the diagnosis. Remember that slowed responses are not specific for any one disease. Many of the indications that were quite important a few years ago have receded because of the dramatic advances in neuroimaging. The frequency of usage has generally declined except in some sites where remunerative considerations lead to too many tests done for inadequate indications. Because these studies are physiologic in nature they have a role in intraoperative monitoring during various neurosurgical procedures. These studies sometimes provide support for the suggestion that a patient may have psychogenic blindness or deafness.

Noninvasive Vascular Studies

Duplex ultrasound studies of the neck arteries have a mature technology that combines a B mode image with a Doppler frequency analysis. This testing is highly operator dependent but in good hands is accurate in the 90+ percent range. The neurologist not performing these studies should be aware that the reports give ranges. If the velocity indicates a 60–79 percent stenosis, it may really be 55–65 percent if the velocity is at the laboratory lower limit for that degree of stenosis. The use of power Doppler and color-flow Doppler imaging enhance the analysis of flow in the carotid and vertebral arteries in the neck. The study should be tailored to the clinically relevant question. Routinely, technicians analyze in detail only the carotid artery bifurcations—the most common site of atherosclerotic disease. But in patients suspected of having carotid dissections, the pathology may be well above the carotid bifurcation. In other patients the proximal vertebral arteries should be the focus of the ultrasound examination.[13-15] Accreditation by the Intersocietal Commission on Accreditation of Vascular Laboratories offers the referring physician some security that the results are meaningful. *Know your laboratory!* How many patients are studied each week? Have the studies been correlated with pathology found at surgery or with standard angiography? Have the results been calibrated against other established reference laboratories?

Transcranial Doppler study of the intracranial arteries is even more operator dependent than ultrasound of the neck arteries.[13] Intracranial arteries are insonated using a small probe placed at positions on the skull where there are foramina or natural soft spots. The usual windows are the orbit, foramen magnum, and temporal bone. TCD probes are placed parallel to arteries, for example, the middle cerebral arteries, while the technician or physician performing the test listens for a characteristic pulsatile swooshing sound indicating that the probe is correctly placed. The computer allows the person performing the TCD examination to view Doppler spectra at successsive 5mm depths along an insonated artery.

A commonplace analogy helps individuals understand the meaning of Doppler spectra.[16] Most people have had the experience of trying to wash a pavement or patio with a garden hose. Figure 6-1A shows the water flowing from the hose when the spigot is turned fully on and the nozzle is not turned. When the nozzle of the hose is turned, a stronger, more targeted water spray is generated (Figure 6-1B). Turning the nozzle reduces the size of the lumen at the end of the hose. The velocity of flow in the water jet is inversely proportional to the luminal size until a critical luminal size is reached, at which time flow is reduced. If the nozzle is turned fully, then water stops flowing or dribbles out the end of the hose (Figure 6-1C). Similarly, if an insonated neck or intracranial artery is stenotic, then blood flow velocities are increased at the site of narrowing. If an artery is occluded by an embolus or in-situ thrombus, then no or very low signals are obtained.

The use of a probe to create a B mode image of intracranial blood vessels is possible but proves unsatisfactory in many patients. TCD has revolutionized

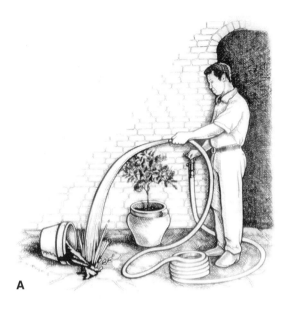

A

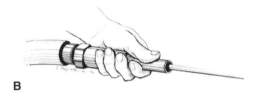

B

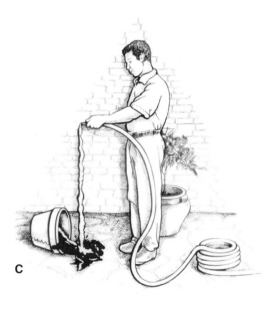

C

Figure 6-1 **A,** Drawing of a man cleaning a patio with a hose. The water spigot is opened fully and the nozzle is wide open. **B,** The nozzle is turned, making the lumen of the hose smaller and narrowing the jet of water. **C,** The nozzle has been turned nearly fully, obliterating the lumen of the hose. Only a dribble of water escapes from the hose. (Drawn by Dari Paquette. Reprinted with permission from Caplan LR. Brain embolism. In LR Caplan, JW Hurst, MI Chimowitz (eds), *Clinical Neurocardiology.* New York: Marcel Dekker, 1999.)

the study of stroke patients at the bedside. TCD can accurately detect important atherostenotic lesions within the major basal cerebral arteries—the intracranial internal carotid arteries, middle cerebral arteries, intracranial vertebral arteries, and the proximal and middle portions of the basilar artery. TCD is also helpful in showing the hemodynamic effects of extracranial occlusive lesions of the carotid and vertebral arteries in the neck on velocities in the intracranial arterial branches of these arteries. Duplex scanning of the neck arteries and TCD effectively screen for severe occlusive lesions within the anterior circulation. The combination of continuous-wave Doppler, color-flow Doppler, and TCD is very effective in screening for major occlusive lesions of extracranial and intracranial arteries within the posterior circulation. Vascular narrowing due to vasoconstriction, and augmented flow through collateral channels and through AVMs all increase blood flow velocity. TCD can be used to monitor vasoconstriction in patients with subarachnoid hemorrhage. Most radiologists are uncomfortable with a technique that gives physiologic information without a picture and so this technique is mostly performed by neurologists and some neurosurgeons. Monitoring of intracranial arteries using TCD can detect microembolic signals, and their distribution may suggest a carotid or more proximal (cardiac or aortic) embolic source.[14,16]

Computed Topography

More than any other single advance, the advent of CT in the early 1970s revolutionized neurologic diagnosis and care. The introduction of MRI and advances in both CT and MRI methodologies require continued reevaluation of their relative utility. Until the development of gradient echo-planar MRI, CT was unparalleled in its ability to differentiate recent hemorrhages from other lesions. CT allows excellent delineation of the location, size, and shape of intracerebral hemorrhages and whether the hemorrhages have drained into the ventricles or produced pressure shifts in brain contents.[17] CT is superior to conventional MRI in imaging subarachnoid blood. CT is also an excellent modality for studying bone. When proper films are ordered, skull fractures, bone erosion, size of the sella turcica, paranasal sinus disease, and diseases of the skull and vertebral column are well shown. Axial tomography of the lumbar spine is an excellent means of studying lumbar disc disease and spinal stenosis, especially when the level of root involvement is known. CT is more readily available in many sites and may be the only test available for patients with pacemakers.

A few general rules concerning CT:

1. Whenever possible, order a plain CT before one that is contrast enhanced. Contrast enhancement can render some hypodense lesions such as infarcts isodense and no longer easily visible. The presence and degree of contrast enhancement are helpful diagnostically. Without a precontrast film, the degree of enhancement of a lesion cannot be determined.

2. Be sure to make it crystal clear to the radiologist what you are looking for and if you want any special views or contrast. Lesions at the cranio-cervical junction, within the posterior fossa, involving the sella turcica, the skull base, orbits, cavernous sinus, and other regions can often be shown by CT when the proper films are taken but will easily be missed without special views. Helical technology and multi-slice imaging has allowed high-quality CT angiography. These angio-grams with volume rendering three-dimensional processing allow for high-quality images that can be rotated and clarify subtle vascular anatomy such as aneurysm necks and venous sinuses. A significant contrast bolus must be administered. These matters must be planned. The neuroradiologist cannot read the physician's mind. The responsible clinicians must either write clearly on the requisition what is wanted or directly contact the radiologist. In hospitalized patients, sometimes the requisitions are filled out by the most junior caregivers, and as a result studies are suboptimal.

3. Too many CTs are performed on an emergency basis when patients arrive in the emergency ward or hospital. Many emergency department CTs are performed for marginal reasons to protect the ordering physician from malpractice risk. This swamps the imaging unit and impairs the radiology staff's ability to perform needed studies in a timely manner. Many of these emergency CTs are ordered by junior house staff. In general, emergency studies are less carefully performed and less complete. Special views are not easily obtained. Moreover, early ischemic lesions are seldom evident, and contrast infusion is often not feasible in emergency situations. Technicians as well as nurses are in short supply, and calling in technicians during the night often heavily taxes staff resources. Many patients who have emergency CTs require subsequent imaging later during their hospital course. The stated reason for many emergency CTs is to exclude hemorrhage, especially if anticoagulant therapy is to be given. In our experience, when these cases are reviewed, anticoagulants have usually not been prescribed even when the scan showed no hemorrhagic lesion, and in fact, a more senior neurologist would probably not have seriously considered acute heparinization. Many of these so-called emergency scans could have waited for the next regular work day, and discussion of the case with more senior clinicians often obviates the need for the emergency study. Some patients will require urgent CT to rule out hemorrhage when the use of thrombolytic agents (intravenous or intraarterial) is being considered. If the patient is ill enough to require urgent investigations, then the gravity of the problem is such that a more senior physician should be told about the case and decide with the house staff what should be done. Frequently, this will require the senior neurologist to come to the hospital and examine the patient. A CT scan is not a substitute for a history and physical examination.

Magnetic Resonance Imaging

Unquestionably, MRI is superior to CT for imaging many central nervous system lesions. There is, however, more technical complexity involved in obtaining and interpreting the films. The myriad sequences of the scans and the relative T_1 and T_2 components can make the difference between detecting or missing pathology. It is said that the right combination of TE and TR can make most tumors disappear. Water content greatly influences magnetic resonance of tissues. Edema and Wallerian degeneration may be very difficult to differentiate from the primary disease process, for example, hematoma, tumor, or infarction. Fluid attenuated inversion recovery (FLAIR) allows much better visualization of T_2 abnormalities near the cortical or ventricular surfaces by turning CSF black.

The advent of echo-planar imaging has greatly advanced the capability of magnetic resonance imaging.[18] Susceptibility imaging using echo-planar MRI allows for even early detection of brain hemorrhage.[19] Diffusion-weighted imaging (DWI) shows areas of altered water diffusion and allows visualization of an infarct less than an hour after the ictus. Combining this with perfusion-weighted imaging and magnetic resonance angiography greatly enhances understanding of the clinical situation in stroke patients in relatively few minutes. The discrepancy between the areas of diffusion and perfusion abnormality may define the ischemic penumbra and the area of brain at risk early in a stroke.

The ability to image the central nervous system in multiple planes simultaneously—coronal, horizontal, sagittal—is a great advantage. Bone density and calcifications produce less magnetic resonance and so the skull does not interfere with brain images as much as in CT. This allows much better definition of lesions along the base of the brain near the skull base, diseases affecting the posterior fossa, and processes involving the cranio-cervical junction and the spinal cord. White matter disease such as demyelinating plaques, leukodystrophies and myelinolysis are exquisitely seen. Contusions and vascular malformations such as cavernous angiomas are seen better with MRI than with CT. MRI is also clearly superior in delineating brainstem lesions.

A moving column of blood also affects magnetic resonance so that vascular lesions can be imaged by MRI. Magnetic resonance angiography (MRA) is an evolving group of techniques (saturative, subtractive, and luminal opacification) with many techniques to be refined. One can see large intracranial vessels and large aneurysms. The sensitivity of this technique for intracranial stenoses relative to TCD and invasive angiography has not been established but adding this to an MRI only adds a small amount of time. This technique generates maximum intensity projections (MIPS), which look like vessels but are highly sensitive to turbulence and lead to overestimation of stenoses. The source images are harder to deal with but are more reliable. Venous MRA is excellent for venous sinus thrombosis. Cervical MRA is most useful combined with axial cross-section MRI in evaluating arterial dissections of neck arteries.

We emphasize that MRI, like CT, is a neurologic procedure. Knowledge of neuroanatomy and neuropathology and understanding of the clinical context are needed for optimal interpretation. The neurologist must either personally perform or interpret the procedures or communicate before the scheduled examination with the individual who will perform and interpret the MRI scans. In many centers, because of the technical complexity of magnetic resonance and because of its wide and increasing use in scanning most other body organs, the individuals who supervise the lab are radiology specialists who may not be fully trained neuroradiologists. They need guidance to plan the scans and interpret them. Contact with the radiologist before or during the scan may avoid disappointment, embarrassment, and even anger when the scans do not contain the desired information.

Catheter, Dye Contrast Angiography

Some time will be spent discussing cerebral angiography because, in our experience, inadequate studies are the rule and not the exception. Often, unnecessary films are taken, and, frequently, key arteries are not opacified. The fault is not with the radiologist, but with the clinician who has not worked directly enough with the radiologist. Since other technologies now show the brain well, the major indication for angiography is cerebrovascular disease. Some general rules and principles govern the performance of angiography, irrespective of the location of the lesion and the clinical setting.[20]

1. *Angiographic results will only be useful if they answer a clinically relevant question.* That question will be derived from the clinical symptoms and signs, the background and past history of the patient, and the results of other tests. Faris and Poser analyzed angiographic results from supposedly neurologically intact prisoners with no neurologic symptoms.[21] A large percentage had significant occlusive vascular disease. The mere presence of an occlusive lesion does not mean that this lesion is the cause of clinical symptoms. The main purpose of angiography is to determine the vascular cause of symptoms or, in the case of asymptomatic patients, to clarify and quantitate findings suggested by other, usually noninvasive tests such as duplex ultrasound, TCD, computed tomography angiography (CTA), or MRA.

2. *Complexity of angiography dictates that the procedure should be performed by a specialist with training and experience in cerebral angiography.* Most often that specialist will be a neuroradiologist. Angiography should be considered as a consultation. As in any other consultation, it is imperative that the consultant know what questions the clinicians are asking. The angiographer also must know all data relevant to the procedure, for example, the presence of prior contrast allergy, renal disease, or claudication caused by occlusive disease of the lower extremity arteries. The neuroradiologist cannot read the minds of the clinicians, and frequently the case notes in the hospital chart are not clear or detailed enough to capture the thought processes of the clinician responsible for the patient's care. *Nearly always, the responsible clinician and the angiographer should talk to each other before the procedure;*

they should discuss the major questions and the information needed from the angiography. They should also agree on the first step.

3. *In deciding on the first step, follow Sutton's law.* Willie Sutton was a notorious bank robber. When Sutton was asked why he kept robbing banks, he replied: "That is where the money is." The first procedure should be the one most likely to answer the key question. In medicine we must "go where the money is." For example, a 56-year-old white man with a history of coronary artery disease has an attack of weakness of the left face and arm. His background (age, sex, past vascular disease) makes him a likely candidate for occlusive disease of the large arteries, and the clinical localization is most probably the right cerebral hemisphere, making atherosclerotic stenosis originating in the right internal carotid artery by far the most likely diagnosis. This lesion would also have the most impact on treatment. The first questions should logically be: Is there disease of the right internal carotid artery origin and, if so, what kind and how severe?

The radiologist might find when trying to catheterize the arteries from the arch (in this hypothetical case) that the catheter has slipped into the left common carotid artery. The angiographer recognizes that if the right internal carotid artery is stenosed, the clinicians will want to know the status of the contralateral internal carotid artery. Some angiographers might reason, "Well, we are already there. Let's film the left internal carotid artery while the catheter is in place." Unfortunately, all too often and unpredictably and for a variety of reasons, the angiographic procedure must be terminated prematurely. In that case, the data derived might be very tangential to the main question. The temptation to get ancillary data before the primary goal has been attained must be resisted.

4. *The clinician cannot always predict what will be found at angiography.* Sometimes, the first results are unexpected. The initial results will, to a large degree, determine what should logically be the next step. In the absence of subarachnoid hemorrhage so-called four-vessel studies are not necessary in most patients. The complication rate increases with the complexity and duration of the procedure and the amount of contrast used. Decisions on what to study should be sequential; *the second step depends on the results of the first step.* The neurologist should always be available to discuss the second step during the procedure, unexpected findings or complications. Let us return to the example of the patient with the left face and arm weakness. If the right internal carotid artery bifurcation and the intracranial internal carotid artery and its middle cerebral, anterior choroidal, and anterior cerebral artery branches are normal, intrinsic nonembolic occlusive disease of the large vessels in the anterior circulation can be excluded. The normal condition of large arteries would not, of course, exclude penetrating small artery disease in the anterior circulation, because these penetrating arteries are too small to image reliably. Left hemiparesis could have been caused by a right vertebral artery lesion. The next step should be right vertebral artery injection.

If the right internal carotid artery injection revealed a tight stenosis of the right internal carotid artery, this might warrant surgery. If there was no important right intracranial occlusive disease, the surgeon would want to know about the left internal carotid artery and the extent of its contribution to the supply of the right cerebral hemisphere.

If, instead, the lesion were a right internal carotid artery siphon occlusion and a superficial temporal artery-to-middle cerebral artery shunt was being considered by the neurosurgeon, he would need to know if there was significant external carotid artery disease, the size and status of the superficial temporal artery, and whether patent middle cerebral artery branches could be seen either from ipsilateral leptomeningeal collaterals or from collaterals from the left cerebral hemisphere. External carotid arterial opacification using a common carotid injection would, in that case, be the next step.

Optimally, the angiographer and the clinician should talk after the initial results, especially if they are unexpected, to plan the next steps. If this is not possible, the various likely possibilities should be discussed beforehand so that a "game plan" for the study can be generated. If surgery is contemplated, the surgeon who will operate should be consulted before or during the angiographic procedure to ensure that all necessary data have been acquired.

When close communication lines during the procedure between the angiographer and the clinicians are not maintained, the angiograms, though technically satisfactory, sometimes do not produce the information desired by the clinicians who care for the patient.

5. *"Arch" studies should not be routine, and in our opinion are seldom warranted.* Arch injections require a side hole catheter and a large bolus of contrast and have an accompanying increase in complications. Opacification of individual extracranial arteries is often suboptimal, and arteries are frequently superimposed. The films are rarely sufficiently precise to allow definitive treatment decisions. The intracranial arteries are not opacified well on arch injections. Information about the origin of vessels found in the arch can usually be obtained fluoroscopically when the arteries are being catheterized. If a significant lesion is found, selective films can be taken. If the aorta is dilated and tortuous or the vessel cannot be found, then an arch injection is reasonable. Also, if the more common lesions are not found, the origin of the artery from the arch can and should be studied at the end of the study. For example, if a patient with left hemiparesis and sensory loss has a lesion demonstrated by CT in the paracentral right cerebral hemisphere and the internal carotid artery and its branches are normal, then the common carotid artery should be studied and filmed at the end of the procedure. Some vascular radiologists (not neuroradiologists) pride themselves on how quickly they can do an arch injection and be finished. Arch studies often do not address the clinical questions and do not allow sufficient opacification of intracranial arteries. Intracranial views are usually not obtained or are inadequte. When the neurologist becomes involved, the patient may be resistant if a second angiogram is suggested.

6. *The angiographer should talk to and examine the patient after each bolus of contrast.* If the posterior circulation was injected, the ability of the patient to see and form new memories should be determined. If the injection

was into the left internal carotid artery, the patient's ability to speak and understand speech and use the right arm and leg in the same way as before the procedure must be checked. *Complications will not be found unless looked for.* An adverse effect should trigger consultation with the clinician, and a joint decision should be made as to whether the procedure should be terminated.

7. *A high-quality brain image should precede angiography.* Even though the clinical history and findings seem to indicate occlusive cerebrovascular disease, occasionally patients with brain tumor, subdural hematoma, AVMs, intracerebral hemorrhages, and aneurysms may have findings indistinguishable from occlusive disease on purely clinical grounds. Even in a patient with transient ischemic attacks (TIAs) and a carotid bruit on the appropriate side to explain the symptoms, a CT scan may reveal unexpected findings such as multiple lacunae, subcortical lucencies, or cortical infarcts. CT or MRI is also performed in the patient with an established stroke to define the location and extent of infarction and to exclude intracerebral hemorrhage. Knowing the location of infarction helps in planning the arteriographic strategy. Ordinarily, noninvasive vascular studies (MRA, CTA, or ultrasound) should precede catheter angiography. These tests will suggest regions of abnormality and, by showing normal vessels, can limit the angiographic study to the arteries most likely to harbor pathology.

In patients with massive infarction or hemorrhage, CT or MRI scans are important. Angiography will have risk and not alter treatment plans. It should be deferred and the patient treated on the basis of the clinical findings and brain imaging.

8. *In any stroke patient, the shorter the time interval between stroke onset and angiography, the more likely the angiogram is to explain the clinical syndrome.* Emboli will tend to break up and the pathogenesis of the ischemia may be missed.

9. Selective arterial digital subtraction angiography has achieved high quality and has become commonplace. It is less expensive than cut film angiography and safety is enhanced because it requires half the volume of contrast agent used in conventional angiography. Rotational angiography is allowed in some digital subtraction units and can enhance the information gathered. If biplane digital subtraction angiography is available, it can be used in place of conventional biplane angiography.

TEST ORDERING

Those paying for medical care (federal and state governments that administer Medicare and Medicaid, third-party payers, HMOs, etc.) are focusing on doctors' test-ordering behavior. Tests, especially those that use high technology, are perceived as expensive. Tests are not done unless physicians order them. Payers are exerting pressure on physicians to reduce expensive testing as a way to control the rapidly escalating costs of medical care. *He who pays the piper calls the tune.* Yet physicians know that technology clearly can lead to vastly improved diagnoses and more effective and rational treatment. Patients often link tests with quality, and will sometimes demand the application of modern technology to their cases. Managed care organizations may require precertification or, more perniciously, they may retroactively deny payment to the test provider and penalize the ordering physician.

Physicians should become more self-conscious and more aware of their test-ordering behavior. Laboratory, imaging, and physiological evaluations should be *planned to test hypotheses* derived from the history and examination. Tests should be *sequential.* The results of early tests will impact on selection of subsequent tests. Some routine testing may not be very effective and probably could be eliminated. Another consideration in hospitalized patients is the pressure to discharge patients quickly. This may compromise the ability to be completely sequential in testing, but does not free the physician from planning and the need for ongoing evaluation of the data as it becomes available. Before ordering tests, physicians should ask themselves, "What am I looking for? What is the most effective way of deciding between the diagnostic possibilities and avoid missing treatable causes of the symptoms?" Physicians must expeditiously review the tests and the results in order to interpret them within the context of the patient's problems.

REFERENCES

1. Miguel de Cervantes Saavedra. *The Adventures of Don Quixote.* London: Penguin Books, 1950, part l, Chapter XXIII.
2. Tumulty P. *The Effective Clinician.* Philadelphia: W.B. Saunders Co., 1973;105.
3. Harvey AM, Bordley J. *Differential Diagnosis: The Interpretation of Clinical Evidence.* Philadelphia: W.B. Saunders Co., 1955;8–9.
4. Rasmussen T. Surgery of epilepsy associated with brain tumors. In D Purpura, JK Penny, and RD Walter (eds), *Advances in Neurology,* Vol. 8. New York: Raven Press, 1975;227–238.
5. Wexler NS. Disease gene identification: Ethical considerations. *Hospital Practice* 1991;26:145–152.
6. Hersch S, Jones R, Koroshetz W, Quaid K. The neurogenetics genie: testing for the Huntington disease mutation. *Neurology* 1994;44:1369–1373.
7. Filippi M, Grossman RI, Comi G. Magnetization transfer imaging in multiple sclerosis. *Neurology* 1999;53 (Suppl 3):S1–S53.
8. Poser CM, Paty DW, Scheinberg L, McDonald WI, Davis FA, Ebers CC, Johnson KP, Sibley WA, Silberberg DH, Tourtellotte WW. New diagnostic criteria for multiple sclerosis: Guidelines for research protocols. *Ann Neurol* 1983;13:227–231.
9. Caplan LR, Hauser SL, Achiron A. What to tell patients with their first attack of multiple sclerosis. *Eur Neurol* 1996;36:183–190.
10. Jacobs LD, Beck RW, Simon JH, Kinkel P, Brownscheidle CM, Murray TJ, Simonian NA, Slasor PJ, Sandrock AW, CHAMPS Study Group. Intramuscular Interferon Beta-1a therapy initiated during a first demyelinating event in multiple sclerosis. *N Engl J Med* 2000;343:898–904.
11. Cox, K. *Doctor and Patient. Exploring Clinical Thinking.* Sydney: University of New South Wales Press, 1999;113–116.
12. Kimura J. Abuse and misuse of evoked potentials as a diagnostic test. *Arch Neurol* 1985;41:78–79.

13. Caplan LR. Laboratory diagnosis. In LR Caplan (ed), *Caplan's Stroke: A Clinical Approach*. 3rd ed. Boston: Butterworth–Heinemann, 2000;73–113.
14. Tegeler CH, Babikian VL, Gomez CR. *Neurosonology*. St Louis: Mosby, 1996.
15. Caplan LR. Diagnosis: Clinical, imaging, and laboratory. In LR Caplan (ed), *Posterior Circulation Disease, Clinical Findings, Diagnosis, and Management*. Boston: Blackwell Science, 1996:131–161.
16. Caplan LR. Brain embolism. In LR Caplan, JW Hurst, MI Chimowitz (eds), *Clinical Neurocardiology*. New York: Marcel Dekker, 1999;35–185.
17. Tanenbaum, LN (guest ed). CT in neuroimaging revisited. In BP Drayer (consulting ed), *Neuroimaging Clinics of North America*. Philadelphia: W.B. Saunders Co., 1998;497–708.
18. Heiserman, JE (guest ed). Fast scan and echo planar MR imaging. In BP Drayer, (consulting ed), *Neuroimaging Clinics of North America*. Philadelphia: W.B. Saunders Co., 1999;227–396.
19. Linfante I, Llinas RH, Caplan LR, Warach S. MRI features of intracerebral hemorrhage within two hours from symptom onset. *Stroke* 1999;30:2263–2267.
20. Caplan LR, Wolpert SM. Angiography in patients with occlusive cerebrovascular disease: A stroke neurologist and neuroradiologist's views. *AJNR* 1991;12:593–601.
21. Faris AA, Poser CM, Wilmore DW, Agnew CH. Radiologic visualization of neck vessels in healthy men. *Neurology* 1963;13:386–396.

7

Physician Information Giving and the "Dismissal Interview"

The interview, in my view, is the most powerful, sensitive and versatile instrument available to the physician. The interview serves many functions. Through it a relationship is initiated, the conditions and requirements for communication are established, roles and obligations are defined, the information necessary to delineate disease and to characterize the patient and his life circumstances are collected, data are processed, the patient and his family are prepared for decisions and judgments, are instructed in care and a human contract between patient and physician is achieved.[1]   —GEORGE ENGEL

The patient shouldn't be given too much advice at once for he is easily confused and will forget much of what he is told. At the first conference the general features of the program should be outlined and the most important items stressed in detail. At subsequent conferences the basic features should again be reviewed and more details stressed. In other words, the patient is indoctrinated regarding the program in a stepwise fashion, adequate opportunities for reinforcement of its details being afforded.[2]   —PHILLIP TUMULTY

The truth can be exaggerated when the doctor talks to a hopeless patient. There are no two cases alike. Judgment, tact, and compassion can be the only guides; and external circumstances must be taken into account. In some cases, the cold truth may bring panic and serve no useful end whatever.[3]   —HANS ZINSER

Courts of law divide doctors into experts without direct interaction with the patient and "treating physicians." The common goal, the raison d'être of medical care, is treatment of the patient. In our medical system, except in very unusual circumstances, patients have the right to choose whether they will or will not accept suggestions and medical advice, whether they will agree to medical procedures and interventions, and whether they will comply with suggested and prescribed treatment. Physicians must obtain the respect and cooperation of patients if they are to influence them to follow their best advice. This can only be accomplished by effective doctor-patient communication. Transmission of information and patient education are important functions of the effective clinician. Physician-patient communication is especially important in neurology because of the seriousness of many neurologic illnesses; effective communication is particularly challenging in neurology because patients often have some perceptual or cognitive impairment. Gone are the days of paternalism (or maternalism) when the doctor could simply tell the patient "do as I tell you" or defend suggestions by answering "because I think it's best for you." Patients have a need and a right to know about their illnesses. Clinicians have an obligation to tell patients in simple terms what's wrong with them, what they advise them to do about it, and what alternatives are available.

HOW WELL DO DOCTORS TRANSMIT INFORMATION TO PATIENTS AND HOW IMPORTANT IS THIS FUNCTION?

The evidence is clear: Doctors in general transmit information poorly. In one study, the comments of 450 patients discharged from one hospital during an eight-month period were analyzed (every fifth discharge was interviewed).[4] Sixty-three percent said that they were not given specific instructions about their care and sixty-four percent were given no time for instructions. On average, primary care internists spent about 1.3 minutes of a 20-minute encounter on information giving; furthermore, they usually overestimated the time spent by a factor of nine.[5] Patients are dissatisfied especially when neither their expectations nor their main worry are given attention. As a fourth-year student on rotation to a tuberculosis facility, one of us (J.H.) met a man who spoke only Lithuanian but was very cooperative with all treatments only to become very agitated and hostile at discharge. After review of the problem with an adequate interpreter, the reason for his anger became clear. He had presented himself for medical care because of concern about a large shoulder lipoma. A history of bright red blood per rectum prompted a barium enema for which a chest radiograph was inadvertently substituted. Cavitary tuberculosis was noted and he was admitted for further evaluation and treatment. He remained compliant in the misguided notion that we were addressing his complaint but could not understand discharge when nothing had been done about his lipoma. Keep the patient's complaint in mind, even if other medical issues are of greater concern to physicians.

One of the most important reasons for poor communication is failure to explain concepts in terms that the patient can understand. Patients have much less knowledge of medical terminology than most doctors think. Even a college education is not sufficient for understanding most medical terms.[6] Doctors assume that most patients understand very elementary anatomy and physiology, but they don't. Surveys have repeatedly shown large percentages of people still think stroke a problem of the heart and not the brain. Many family members ask repeated questions about whether a stroke had caused brain damage. They thought of "brain damage" as dementia as opposed to a large area of dead brain. Most stroke patients with hemiparesis do not understand that the problem is in their head, not in the weak limbs. They do not know that the contralateral hemisphere controls voluntary movements of the arm and leg. Patients certainly do not know that pain, tingling, or prickling in a limb or other body part can be due to disease of the nervous system outside the affected part. Introductory college biology classes are frequently crowded with driven premedical students and are avoided by others. Colleges that provide "physics for dummies" often do not provide equivalent courses in biology. Our premedical and medical curricula emphasize biomedical sciences. Most college and medical school tests are multiple choice or short answer responses. Some medical school graduates are very poor at verbal and written communication. English, history, economics, and social sciences have traditionally been seriously underemphasized in the training of physicians. Moreover, few young physicians have had any instructions about how to communicate with patients. Few have been present during a dismissal interview given by a concerned and experienced clinician. When residents are given intensive training in interviewing and communication techniques, their skills and patient satisfaction improve measurably.[7]

The fault, however, does not rest completely with doctors. Patients are often ill, tired, anxious, unaccustomed and inexperienced in the role of a sick person, or cognitively impaired. Patients, like other normal folks, hear what they want to hear and ignore what is unacceptable or unwanted. Patients forget about one-third of what doctors say to them, and their recall of instructions or advice is less than 50 percent.[8] In a study of information recall by sixty-four consecutive outpatients, 74 percent recalled some information about further tests, but only 45 percent recalled instructions, and only 31 percent remembered the explanations given about the disease or its treatment.[9] There was about 50 percent loss of information even when the patient was interviewed immediately after seeing the doctor, whether or not the patient was articulate. A friend, an educator, called in great distress because his wife had just had a breast biopsy positive for adenocarcinoma. The friend asked very basic questions that should have been covered by the surgeon, a compassionate man who spent considerable time with patients. J.H. asked the friend what the surgeon had told him. He explained that the surgeon spoke to him at great length but he had been unable to comprehend anything after the word cancer had been mentioned.

Even using optimal techniques, patients and families often do not get the thrust of the information transmittal the first time. Doctors tend to assume that "message sent" is "message received" but all too often the patient is just not ready or able to take in the import and details of what is said.[10] Information giving is a long-term, recurrent task. Repeat and reinforce information, and give the patient the opportunity during subsequent visits to ask more questions. Cox commented, "I don't know what I've said until I hear the response to it."[10] Butt introduced a novel and probably effective way to reinforce information given in the dismissal interview.[8] He taped his own dismissal interviews, including the discussion and his directions, and gave patients the cassettes to review at home. Most patients had ready access to a cassette player. On a questionnaire given to his patients during a three-month follow-up, the great majority (91 percent) said they thought the method helped them to understand the physician's instructions and discussion, 75 percent found it helpful to have their spouses or relatives listen to the tape, and most preferred the tape to a formal letter.[8] We write instructions on a prescription and find that it significantly reduces (but not eliminates) errors in medication or diagnostic plan. We also write out the diagnosis, so patients can talk to family or friends not present with them. We also find it useful to have the family present during the dismissal interview so that all are told the same information together. If there is something private we want to say just to the patient, this can be done outside of the family interview.

The cardinal rule is to be honest.

Most patients want more and better communication from their doctors. Patients seek a larger role in decision making and more involvement in their care. In one study, 210 hypertensive patients were questioned about their care.[11] Forty-one percent wanted more information about hypertension. Clinicians underestimated patients' wishes to be involved in decisions about therapy: 53 percent of these hypertensive patients wanted to participate actively in treatment decisions. Studies show that doctors, in general, spend more time giving information to women and older persons. They also spend more time and effort communicating with patients with whom they've had a longer relationship and those in higher socioeconomic classes who have more educational background.[12] But expectations and needs are just as high in men, younger patients, and those who have different cultural and educational backgrounds.

Failure of communication has serious consequences. If the doctor cannot influence the patient to follow suggestions and advice, the doctor's time and effort have been wasted. The most elegant diagnosis and the most advanced and elaborate medical knowledge are for naught when they are not effectively transmitted to the patient. Noncompliance is also a common outcome of failure to communicate. Failure to comply with treatment is very common and can often be traced to poor instructions or understanding.[13] Clearly, doctors' prescriptions do little good if they're unfilled or lie unused on bathroom shelves. Another increasingly frequent result of poor communication is litigation. Patients sue when they have not understood the nature and natural course of their illness and have false expectations of what their doctors will be able to accomplish. Lack of detailed communication, not medical-related injury, is the primary reason for medical malpractice suits in the United States.[14]

WHEN IS THE BEST TIME FOR INFORMATION GIVING?

Teaching and transmission of information are integral parts of the doctor's job and occur to some degree throughout the patient relationship. Be wary of giving impressions and opinions too soon. L.R.C. vividly recalls going to a consultant periodontist whom he told that he had a recurrent infection in his left lower molar tooth. Before any further questioning or examination, the dentist told L.R.C. that he must be biting and grinding his teeth at night. He proceeded to lecture L.R.C. on the subject of night teeth clenching. L.R.C. immediately "turned off" and distrusted everything the dentist later said because of the clear perception that he had come to a firm premature conclusion with inadequate data. A premature guess or impression relayed to the patient can do immeasurable harm later if the initial hunch proves erroneous. The traditional time for the most concentrated and intense information giving is during the so-called "dismissal interview." We often refer to this session as the denouement because it is the culmination of the doctor's initial diagnostic activities and it is so critical for further doctor-patient interaction and treatment.

The dismissal interview should occur when the diagnostic data is fairly complete. When the patient is hospitalized, the responsible physician should sit down with the patient and the family after the initial investigation results are available and a preliminary diagnosis and plan of treatment have been chosen. If further treatment or tests will be performed while the patient is still hospitalized, then another information session should coincide with discharge from the hospital. When the patient is seen as an outpatient, the physician should sit down with the patient after the results of investigations are known. Most often, this will be at the end of the second visit. At the end of the first visit, the doctor should discuss at least briefly the proposed tests and the initial impression and plan. Sometimes the diagnosis is evident at the first visit and no important investigations are needed or planned; the "dismissal" session might then occur at the end of that visit. When the physician visit is a consultation, the physician should exercise more caution in deciding what to tell the patient. Too many cooks spoil the broth, and too many doctors telling the patient different things only cause confusion. Yet, you owe the patient some explanation. What the consultant tells the patient will vary with the wishes of the referring physician, the patient, the nature of the problem, and the consultant's style and findings. The topic of consultations will be discussed in Chapter 12.

We have already remarked on the fact that the patient is often, for a variety of reasons, a suboptimal learner. Whenever the formal dismissal interview occurs, the information must later be repeated and reinforced. Time must be spent repeatedly answering questions and determining if the patient has understood what you have said. Repetition and reiteration are integral parts of any teaching and learning experience.

THE DOCTOR'S "STYLE" DURING THE DISMISSAL INTERVIEW AND OTHER INFORMATION SESSIONS

The method of transmission of information is almost as important in gaining the respect and cooperation of the patient as the content. How is as critical as what. We have already used the phrase "sit down with the patient." We mean this literally. It is important that all parties in the session have a chair or bed to sit on and that they are positioned near each other. In the hospital, the patient's bed is his world. It may be necessary to sit on the bed to have this conversation but the patient's consent for this should be sought. By standing, the doctor transmits two unspoken messages—that he or she is superior and is in a dominant position above the patient and that there is some time pressure so that the physician needs to be in a position to exit quickly at any time.

At all times, the doctor should appear calm and concerned. The atmosphere of the interview should appear unhurried. These are very important matters for the patient, sometimes involving life and death; they cannot be handled precipitously. The session should be a dialogue, not a monologue or a lecture. There must be ample time for questions, discussion, and interaction. After the information has been delivered by the doctor, the patient should be given time to react.

Most important, the doctor must always be honest. This does not mean precipitously or cruelly confronting patients with stark realities that they are unprepared for. Truths can be delivered gradually and sensitively. Honesty does mean that you should not tell the patient anything that you know is false. Families and friends will sometimes pressure the physician to conceal an unfavorable diagnosis or finding and substitute a more favorable impression or prognosis. Resist this pressure. The foundation of the doctor-patient relationship is respect and mutual trust. One lie can undermine the patient's respect and trust in you as a physician and confidante. Patients somehow sense when a doctor has been less than honest with them. They will distrust anything that doctor later tells them.

Lawsuits are instituted because patients and their families do not realize the seriousness of the prognosis and the expected course of the illness. False expectations also surround procedures and treatments. We urge physicians to emulate the tactic of the wise football coach who traditionally "hangs crepe." "Our team doesn't belong on the same field as our opponents. We will be lucky to get out of the game without serious injuries, much less score a touchdown." If the team does even passably well, potential critics will be silenced. Similarly, we believe that, when the patient's illness or condition is serious, the gravity of the situation must be impressed on the patient and family. They must be told the limitations of your ability to treat the disorder successfully. They must also be told about potential complications of the disorder and the treatment. Be honest, but at the same time be kind and sensitive. Patients are legitimately concerned about complications of tests and the side effects of medications. Handing a patient the list of potential side effects from the package insert may answer the question, but a frank discussion of the more common serious side effects is more helpful.

Understanding the components of doctor-patient dialogues, and the factors that affect them, lays important groundwork for improving patients' (and doctors') satisfaction and for improving patient outcomes.[15] Studies show that

(1) patients recall best the first subject covered in the session, (2) recall decreases according to the length of the interview; the longer the session, the lower the percentage of material remembered later, and (3) patient understanding and compliance also decrease with increasing complexity of discussion and amount of medical terminology. It follows logically that clinicians should keep the data-giving aspects brief, use very simple, commonly understood words and examples, and begin the session with the most important information. The material will need to be repeated, elaborated on, and reinforced later in order for effective transmission.

WHAT TOPICS SHOULD BE DISCUSSED DURING THE DISMISSAL INTERVIEW OR LATER?

Diagnosis

Patients have a need and right to know their diagnoses. The diagnosis should be told to the patient gently and in a sensitive manner when a serious illness is present. Clinicians vary in their style of transmitting the diagnosis. We usually relate the information in steps, letting the patient digest and adjust to the information gradually. Though we usually do not volunteer feared terms such as cancer, Lou Gehrig's disease, or multiple sclerosis (MS) during the initial interview, we are very careful to be certain that what we do say is true and honest, if not the full grim story.

We illustrate the method with several examples. A 23-year-old woman consulted L.R.C. because of tingling in the legs that had developed during the past three weeks. She described a peculiar shocklike electrical feeling in her arms and back when she gradually flexed her neck. Four years ago, she had an attack of decreased vision in the right eye diagnosed as "optic neuritis" from which she recovered completely after two months; and two years ago she had tingling in her right arm, leg, and trunk similar to her present paresthesiae. These cleared during one month. Her examination showed only a slight afferent pupillary reflex abnormality in the right eye and slightly decreased vibration sense in the feet. This patient has MS. The neurologist may or may not choose to confirm the diagnosis by magnetic resonance imaging (MRI), lumbar puncture, or evoked response testing; this issue was discussed in the preceding chapter on tests. Now we are concerned with what to tell the patient about her diagnosis. We would tell her that she is having a "reaction" in her nervous system, probably in her spinal cord in the neck. We draw her a picture showing a nerve cell, an axon, and the surrounding myelin sheath. We use an easily understood analogy comparing the structures drawn to an electrical cord that is made up of a wire and insulation. We explain to her that the insulation around her nerves in the local affected region, which is called myelin and is analogous to insulation around the electrical wire, has undergone a reaction. We tell her that we do not know the cause of these "demyelinating reactions" but do know that they usually occur in young people and more often in young women than men. They often follow infections, injections, or injuries but can occur without obvious precipitants. Individuals that have had one reaction often have recurrences, and the fact that she has had three attacks makes it likely that at some time she will have a fourth one and possibly a fifth attack or more. Subsequent attacks usually follow the pattern of the initial reaction: if the early attacks are mild, the later attacks are usually not severe. We would reassure her that, in her case, the previous two episodes resolved completely, and her present examination is almost entirely normal. The findings that are present are slight and should cause her no handicap and have a high likelihood of resolving or at least improving. L.R.C. would tell her that he was confident that she would do well in the future. J.H. worked in an MS clinic seeing about 75 patients with established MS with significant deficits. Most resented physicians who had not been frank with them about the diagnosis earlier in their disease. J.H. would explain that some controversy about the management of these disease processes exists at the present time. J.H. explains to the patient that she may have a benign form that will not need therapy but prefers to perform some studies to confirm the diagnosis and consider therapy. He will usually order an MRI to assess the body burden of demyelination and consider prophylactic treatment.

Most patients, after questioning, will assimilate the information. On subsequent visits, they will ask new questions and ask the clinician to repeat and elaborate on some features already discussed. Almost inevitably, bright patients will read and inquire about "demyelination" and will bring up the term "multiple sclerosis." Many referring physicians have already broached the possibility of MS. Many patients think that multiple sclerosis and muscular dystrophy are the same, while others may have seen the fund-raising literature for MS showing wheelchairs. By that time, the patient's symptoms have usually improved. We can then discuss multiple sclerosis in a calm and dispassionate way, explaining the wide range and spectrum of the illness. We emphasize that the description we have given them is accurate. If the patient had brought up the term "MS" in the initial session, we would not deny the diagnosis but would strongly emphasize the spectrum of severity of the attacks, the variable prognosis, and the benignity of the course in her case. We would also stress that studies show that patients who do well and have no disability after two years, and especially after five years, seldom develop serious handicaps. If, instead of paresthesiae, she had a paraplegia and could not walk, we would have handled her case quite differently. In that circumstance, we would have hospitalized her, pursued a definitive diagnosis, given her treatment, explained her condition as multiple sclerosis, and discussed prophylactic therapy with her. Even then, we would prepare the patient gradually, initially telling her of worry about her condition because of the severity of her present symptoms. We would emphasize that multiple sclerosis, though not a benign condition, may still be preferred to other potentially more grave conditions within the differential diagnosis.

A 17-year-old boy was seen because of an episode witnessed by his father. His dad came with him to the appointment and described the spell. A conversation about baseball was suddenly interrupted when his son looked blank, fumbled with buttons on his shirt, and did not respond to questions or to gentle shaking. This spell lasted two minutes. Afterward, he seemed groggy and could not recall the topic of conversation. The boy said that he had had several similar brief "blackouts" during the past year. Upon questioning, he recalled that three years ago he was surprised upon awakening in the morning to find that he had wet his bed during the night and his mouth and limbs felt unusually sore as if he had been exercising vigorously. Neurologic examination was normal. An electroencephalogram (EEG) showed spikes and intermittent theta slowing in the right anterior temporal leads. MRI showed that the right temporal horn was significantly larger than the left.

The diagnosis in this case is epilepsy, more specifically, partial complex seizures most likely secondary to sclerosis of the right Ammon's horn. What should the patient and his family be told? We usually tell the patient that he has seizures. We proceed to tell him and the family that the nervous system is composed of millions of electrical connections and circuits. Everyone has the capacity to have a short circuit called a seizure if given a sufficient stimulus such as a blow to the head, an electric shock, too much of certain medicines or drugs, withdrawal from alcohol or addictive drugs, very high fever, or very low blood sugar. All people have the potential to have a seizure if provoked by exposure to sufficient provocation. Some people are a bit more susceptible and others a bit more resistant to seizures than the average person. If the boy or his parents are sophisticated about science or math, we mention the concept of a bell-shaped curve distribution of susceptibility, explaining that he is a bit more vulnerable than the average person but is much less susceptible than others farther to the periphery of the bell-shaped curve. We indicate his relative position on the curve. Put differently, his seizure threshold is slightly reduced and medications should be able to raise the threshold so that the seizures can most likely be well controlled. The concept that seizures are not a binary, that is, black and white phenomenon, that there is a continuum ranging from normal to abnormal is helpful to patients. It is not as if they have a dread disease that distinctly separates them from average folks. They merely are slightly different in their tendency to have something happen that any "normal" person might experience under certain circumstances.

At a later visit we may introduce the analogy of a seizure to ignition of a fire.[16] Spontaneous combustion occurs if the firewood is dry enough and the environment conducive (analogous to a generalized seizure due to metabolic, hereditary, or toxic disorders); alternatively, the fire can be started by a local match (analogous to a focal lesion). His case is like the match. A local area in the brain, too small to cause any abnormal function or handicap, and possibly so small that it can only be seen with a microscope, is the site of short circuits that spread to the rest of the brain. We do not volunteer the word "epilepsy" on the initial visit. Invariably, some time later he will hear the word epilepsy in relation to his attacks. Sometimes a careless pharmacist filling his anticonvulsant prescription will ask if he is epileptic. He might hear the word from another doctor, on TV, or from friends. At that time the term can be discussed in light of the previous information that we have given him. We might also explain that epilepsy is an old term often used by laymen, and neurologists usually use more specific descriptions such as partial complex seizures. Epilepsy is a lay term while physicians tend to refer to the epilepsies as a large group of disparate disorders sharing only a recurrent seizure as a feature of the illness. Some patients will later want to discuss genetic aspects. We often mention that there are now new medications that have a lower frequency of behavioral side effects. Precipitous use of the term "epileptic" can be very difficult for some patients and their families to handle. With time, experience, control of the spells, and your information, the illness, no matter what you call it, becomes more palatable. Straightforward discussion of issues such as compliance with medication regimen, driving, and other potentially hazardous activities, are usually presented in terms of the seizure itself not being something terrible but the potential for injury if control is lost. Driving is a major limitation for patients in communities with limited public transportation. When presenting this, it is important to stress that the restriction is probably temporary and seizure control will allow resumption of driving.

A 55-year-old man had a focal seizure beginning in his left hand and spreading to his left arm and leg. He had been having headaches for several weeks and his wife had been concerned because he simply "has not seemed himself recently," uncharacteristically impulsive and careless. Examination showed a slight left hemiparesis and motor impersistence.[17,18] Computed tomography (CT) showed a moderate-sized, poorly delineated area of mixed low and slightly high density in the right paracentral lobule. After contrast, there was patchy enhancement of the lesion but not in a gyral pattern. A low-density region of edema surrounded the lesion and there was early compression of the right lateral ventricle.

This patient most likely has a high-grade glioma. What should we tell him? We convey to him and his family that we are very worried about him. The test (CT) indicated something very definitely wrong in an area consistent with his symptoms and with the abnormalities found in his examination. The CT cannot establish a definitive diagnosis, but the abnormality does not look typical for a stroke. He needs further tests and treatment. If he or his family press for a more specific diagnosis and use the words "tumor" or "cancer," we admit that some kind of a tumor is possible. In fact, the lesion looks more like a tumor than anything else. When we discuss performing further procedures such as angiography, MRI, or biopsy, we tell him that there is a small chance that the lesion might be an unusual local infection, inflammatory reaction, unusual vascular malformation, or stroke. We recommend the procedure to make a definitive diagnosis so that we can be sure he is given all indicated treatment and is not given treatment that he does not need. If the biopsy confirms the initial diagnostic impression, then he should be told that he has a glioma. We have slowly prepared him for the diagnosis.

In each of these examples, we have gradually informed and educated the patients about their problems. What we have told them at each step is true, but we have shielded them from a hasty confrontation with stark reality. The technique is rather like gradually explaining sex to young children.

Certainty of the Diagnosis

Don't be afraid to admit when you do not know exactly what is the matter with the patient. Doctors are human and you are not infallible. If the symptoms are worrisome, you will need more tests before you can say much about the diagnosis. An alternative to extensive testing is a consultation with, or referral to, another specialist. Cox notes that doctors tend to use four main management strategies: treatment, reassurance, wait and see, and referral to another doctor.[10] Don't let the patient or family pressure you at this point for a laundry list of differential diagnoses. You should, however, ask if the patient is concerned about one or more specific diseases. Sometimes the patient identifies an illness not even worth considering in the differential diagnosis, for example, muscular dystrophy or myasthenia in a patient with central nervous system symptoms or signs. You will then be able to reassure the patient that he or she does not have these conditions, but that further testing will be needed to make a diagnosis. If the patient's symptoms are minor or trivial, a reasonable alternative to extensive testing is to wait and watch for further developments. The future course of the illness may clarify the problem and reduce the number of tests needed to make the diagnosis. Patients usually have no problem with this approach if they are assured of a revisit at some future time.

When you are secure in your diagnosis, be sure to convey this to the patient. Sometimes you are reasonably sure but need some tests to be absolutely certain and document the diagnosis. We recommend telling the patient how confident you are of the diagnosis.

Explanations of the Mechanism of the Symptoms or the Illness

Explaining the mechanism of their illnesses and their symptoms to patients in terms they can grasp has a number of important salutary effects:

1. Patients recognize that the doctor has pinpointed what is wrong with them. This greatly increases patient confidence in the physician.
2. Understanding the mechanism improves compliance with treatment, especially if patients understand why the doctor has prescribed certain treatments and given other advice.
3. Understanding the nature of their symptoms brings patients out of the state of limbo and into reality. The patient learns what the enemy (the disease) is and what it isn't. Unrealistic medical fears are a great problem and are often not relieved by a physician simply naming an illness or phenomenon that the patient does not understand. Explanation may help the patient understand why you have ordered certain tests.

Using analogies and diagrams helps in explanations of disease. We illustrate with some explanations that we often use for three common neurologic problems. Vertigo and dizziness are extremely common symptoms. Vertigo is a very uncomfortable symptom and alarms many patients. People depend on having their feet firmly planted on terra firma and a precise awareness of where their head and body are in space. False sensations that the environment or they are moving are very disconcerting. If the vertigo is due to peripheral vestibular disease, by far the most common localization of disease in patients with unaccompanied vertigo, we use the following explanation and diagram (Figure 7-1):

In each inner ear, sheltered by bone, there are canals that look something like tires. These canals contain a fluid that moves when the head turns. When you move to the right, the fluid in the right ear canal moves quickly in a counterclockwise direction, while at the same time, the left ear fluid moves in the opposite direction, as diagrammed. When the fluid moves, it pushes on hairs and other sensors or receptors that protrude into the canals from the walls of the "tires." The hairs and other receptors are connected to nerves that send messages immediately to your brain telling you where your head and body are in space. Each ear sends different information that is coordinated in your brain. Normal function depends on the two canals working in a coordinated fashion. When one or both canals give imprecise information, you feel as if you are moving or rotating when you are not. The message sent to the brain is normally very precise, like a Swiss watch, even when your motion has just lasted a few fractions of a second. The message tells you exactly when you start to turn, in what direction, how fast, and when you have stopped moving. When there is a problem with the system, false information is transmitted. The abnormality is sometimes caused by trauma, a virus, inflammation, allergy, and numerous other, usually self-limited, problems. False information coming from the problem in your ears is the cause of your vertigo. We emphasize that this is an ear problem, not a brain problem. Thank

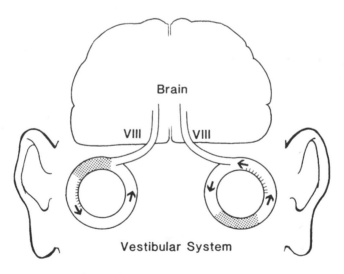

Figure 7-1 Diagram used to explain vertigo to patients. (Drawn by Harriet Greenfield.)

goodness this is not a serious problem like a stroke. Although it may cause you to have unpleasant feelings, it is not risky or dangerous to your health. The symptom, vertigo, is a bad nuisance. Normal people have similar feelings when they are seasick, or temporarily when they emerge from a rapidly moving merry-go-round or revolving chair or door.

J.H. explains the presence of two balance systems in the inner ear. One has three perpendicular tubes sensitive to motion in different directions (like yaw, pitch, and roll for sailors) responsive to fluid motion bending hair cells, the other with little stones glued to hairs that bend in response to gravity. Dizziness occurs when an abnormal ear gives an inappropriate signal of motion to the brain. Since the ears are paired and only one is abnormal, the brain gets two conflicting signals. Since both ears are fixed in the head and one cannot be still while the other is spinning, the brain understands that the message is spurious and is ignored and dizziness subsides. When patients understand that the dizziness is self-limited and they can make it go away faster, they are less terrified and can bear with the symptoms. This also allows an explanation of the very common benign paroxysmal positioning vertigo, in terms of a loose stone from the gravity system getting trapped against the motion hair cells. This makes the motion system inappropriately responsive to gravity, producing a burst of dizziness when the head is put in certain positions. This can lead to an explanation of how the Epley maneuver[19,20] might help them by shaking the stone loose.

Syncope is another very common and very alarming symptom. Patients who have temporarily lost consciousness are often frightened that it will happen again, perhaps in embarrassing or dangerous circumstances. Explanations help the patient understand the mechanism, the need for tests when indicated, and ways of preventing recurrence. We explain to patients that, when they begin to faint, there is not enough blood going to the brain. Supplying the brain with blood can be likened to an easily understood plumbing situation in a home or dormitory. If there was a shower on the third floor, an effective plumbing system would require that water be delivered under high enough pressure to operate the shower (Figure 7-2). To work effectively, the system needs (1) a full tank of water (if the tank is too low, there is insufficient fluid in the system to maintain pressure), (2) a normally functioning water pump to pump the fluid under pressure, (3) open pipes between the pump and the shower, and (4) adequate water pressure in the system. We explain that the head is comparable to the third-floor shower and is located above the pump (heart); the pipes are analogous to the blood vessels leading to the head, and water pressure, of course, is similar to blood pressure. If the tank is too low (hypovolemia, bleeding, dehydration), or if the pump works irregularly or with inadequate force (heart failure, arrhythmia), or if the blood pressure is too low (hypotension, especially postural), or the pipes are badly blocked (severe extracranial occlusive disease), then blood can't get up to the "third floor." We also try to explain the effects of quickly standing on blood pressure and blood flow. Were the shower on the same level or below the pump, flow would be a lot easier. This explanation helps patients understand the

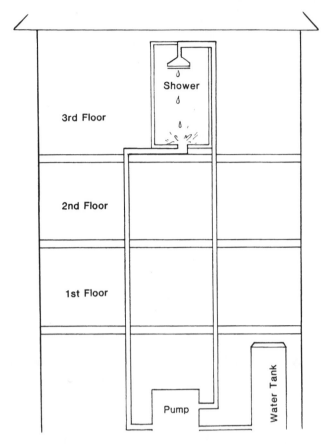

Figure 7-2 Diagram used to explain syncope and ischemic stroke to patients. (Drawn by Harriet Greenfield.)

need for some tests. It also helps them understand the reason for your advice to put their head down or level to avoid syncope.

The same diagram (see Figure 7-2) is also often useful in patients with focal transient ischemic attacks. In that circumstance, water pressure in one of the third-floor bathrooms was temporarily diminished. Study of the pipes that lead to the bathroom might show partial blockage. Alternatively, a small particle could have broken loose from the tank or main pipe in the basement. This diagram and explanation helps the patient understand the need for tests that study the heart, aorta, and major arteries that supply the area of the nervous system that temporarily did not function normally.

Headache, especially of the vascular type, affects at some time nearly 20 percent of the population. Most neurologists see many headache patients. In patients with migraine, L.R.C. uses the analogy that blood vessels are like very elastic rubber hoses. They can constrict or dilate, depending on many factors, including the volume of water going through them. When vessels constrict, less blood goes through them, and visual, tactile, or other neurologic symptoms can develop. When dilated, the expanded vessel stimulates nerve endings on the surface, causing pain. J.H. usually tells the patients that there is evidence for a hereditary component to migraine with a less stable nervous system. In response to a variety of factors, such as stress or menses, patients may have an attack that causes nerve irritation and headache or transient shutdown of some brain circuits giving them the aura. These explanations help patients better grasp the use of prophylactic agents and triptans.

We know that the analogies described are grossly oversimplified. In some ways, they are inaccurate. Remember, you are not giving a science lecture. You are merely giving patients some insight into very complex subjects. If you have helped them understand their symptoms, you have taken a large step toward cementing a doctor-patient relationship and facilitating compliance with medical advice.

Prognosis

If allowed just one question, most practical patients would probably ask the doctor, "What will happen? What will be the outcome of my illness?" They are asking the doctor to tell them their medical prognosis. We have two general rules for discussing prognosis with patients at the time of their initial visit or dismissal interview. First, in most circumstances, do not give extensive information about prognosis at this time, especially if the outlook is poor. There will be ample time for elaboration later. Second, what you do say should be guided by the mood you want to set. If the patient's disorder is trivial, mild, or is likely to be self-limited or easily treatable, be upbeat. Emphasize the benignity and optimistic outlook of the problem. On the other hand, if the prognosis is very poor, set a serious tone but avoid giving specifics during the early interview. Statements such as "I am worried" or "I am concerned and disappointed about how things seem to be going" transmit an appropriately serious tone and demonstrate your own involvement and concern. We find it counterproductive and unnecessary to transmit the fact that the disorder will be fatal or that there is limited time left, or to share grim statistical probabilities with the patient during this initial session. We consider it virtually never wise, except perhaps when the patient is obviously in extremis, to share predictions on how much time is left. These guesses are almost always wrong and can undermine the confidence of the patient and family in your medical wisdom and judgment.

There are several exceptions to the rule of not discussing the details of a bad prognosis at the time of the initial or dismissal interview. Some patients seek your advice as a second opinion, and others are sent by their doctors for consultation, desiring your opinion about a treatment, investigation, or course of action. In order to discuss a procedure or treatment, it is often necessary and important to discuss with a patient the naturally expected prognosis if the procedure is not done and the probable outlook if the procedure is done or a specific treatment plan is followed. Another exception is when you, as the principal physician for the patient, are suggesting a specific plan of action and must describe the prognosis in order to help the patient decide on consent. J.H. was caring for a patient with motor neuron disease who was a successful politician up for reelection. He was deteriorating rapidly and asked if he could finish his term. J.H. had to frankly share grave doubts that he would survive his term of office if elected. A patient may need to have enough information to allow intelligent future business or financial planning. The family may need to be told more specifically than the patient about the poor prognosis.

One of the most difficult situations that physicians, patients, and families face is the discussion of "do not resuscitate" (DNR) orders for patients with very serious or disabling medical and neurologic diseases and terminal illnesses. Physicians should prepare families for these issues as early as possible. Ask patients about their desires if they are capable of participating in this type of discussion. If the patient cannot contribute, ask the family if the patient has discussed medical treatment previously. Has the patient made his or her philosophy about these matters known? To help prepare for the DNR decision, the patient or the family must be given some indication of the prognosis and the likelihood of discomfort and suffering from the illness and its treatment.

Time teaches patients more than physicians' words. If your statement of the expected prognosis differs from what the patient wants to hear, your opinion will usually be ignored or denied or received with great anxiety. When patients begin to perceive and realize that they are failing or improving, then discussions of prognosis are more appropriate. Wait until the patient introduces the subject. Even then, answer first by asking patients what their perceptions are. Be honest but sensitive and kind.

Description of Tests to Be Ordered

If tests are planned, it is wise to discuss the nature of the tests, why you suggest ordering them, and the risks and complications if any. Some investigations such as EEG, evoked response testing, noninvasive vascular tests, and psychometrics are harmless. Regardless, to allay anxiety you should describe briefly what the patient should expect. Anything that you relate about the tests will be appreciated, even things that may seem trivial to you, for example, that the patient may have to wash his or her hair after an EEG because of the paste used on the electrodes. Some tests are innocuous but are unpleasant or involve minor discomfort, such as blood drawing, electromyography (EMG), electronystagmography (ENG), and MRI. If these tests are unfamiliar to patients, you should warn them of the discomfort so that they know what to expect. Some patients feel very enclosed or claustrophobic inside CT or MRI scanners. In regard to potentially invasive tests such as CT with contrast, angiography, and myelography, you must tell patients about the risks and complications of each procedure. If they are reluctant to consent to the tests, you must tell them about alternative procedures or means of evaluation or treatment. Various organizations have literature describing investigations. You may prefer to give this literature to patients rather than taking the time to explain the tests yourself. In that case, be sure to tell patients that you will be glad to answer any questions after they have read the materials.

Let us illustrate with a discussion that we might have with a patient who has had a transient ischemic attack (TIA) or minor stroke for whom we have suggested catheter angiography.

DOCTOR: "I want you to have an angiogram so that I will know exactly where the problem is in your blood vessels. This test will also tell me how bad the problem is and what is the best treatment."

PATIENT: "Who will perform the test and what will they do?"

DOCTOR: "Specialists in neuroradiology do the test. They put a little injection of novocaine or a similar local anesthetic in your groin to numb the area. Then they put a small tube called a catheter into an artery in your leg. While watching a monitor screen that looks like an ordinary TV, they thread the artery to the blood vessels in your neck. They then put dye into the blood vessels and take pictures. The dye makes the arteries look opaque on the pictures. With these films, I will be able to see how the blood travels through your arteries and whether there are any regions of blockage. You will feel warm when the dye is injected, and the picture taking sometimes makes a lot of noise."

PATIENT: "Are there any risks?"

DOCTOR: "There are some risks. In most centers like ours where specialists do the tests and the most modern equipment is available, complications of any importance occur in one or two patients in 100. The major problems are something breaking loose from inside the blood vessels and causing a stroke; when that happens, often the symptoms are just temporary. You can have an allergic reaction to the dye, and rarely the artery in the leg where the catheter is inserted can be injured and the leg can be deprived of blood. I have not seen that happen in my experience with over 2,000 patients who have had arteriograms."

PATIENT: "What if I don't want the test to be done, how would you treat me?"

DOCTOR: "We have done all of the other tests we can. You recall the ultrasound tests on your neck and the Doppler tests listening through your eyes and the side of your head to determine where and how bad the blockage is. We have also done an MRI with an MR angiogram. Unfortunately, these tests haven't given us enough information to know exactly what is wrong with the arteries to your brain. If we didn't do the arteriogram, I could guess on the best treatment—aspirin, blood thinners, or surgery. I could guess right or I could guess wrong. If I were wrong, that would mean that you would be given treatment you didn't need or I didn't give you a therapy that was indicated. Of course, the surgeon might not operate without being more sure of what was wrong."

PATIENT: "What would you do, doc, if it were you?"

DOCTOR: "I would have the test. Your chances of having a stroke are pretty high if you had no treatment—maybe around 10 to 20 percent within the next few years, depending on which study you read. I'm not confident that I can choose the best treatment for you unless I have more information about your arteries that supply the region of the stroke. The small risk factor, 1 to 2 percent for angiography (and by the way, in my own experience there has been a lower risk of important complications—less than 1 percent), to me is well worth being sure I've given you the most logical treatment. I would have the angiogram."

This discussion has been abbreviated and might contain more detail, depending on the patient and his or her problem, background, and desire for detail. A similar type discussion would also be important before a brain biopsy or other invasive diagnostic procedure.

Treatment

We will consider the issue of selection of treatment in the next chapter. Here, we are concerned with how to tell the patient about the treatments that have been prescribed and any upcoming therapeutic procedures. Since patients often forget, it is important that the doctor write down specific instructions, that is, the name of the pills, directions for dosage, and how long the pills are to be used. This is especially important if the dose of a pill (such as Sinemet, amitriptyline, lamotrigine, or baclofen) will be gradually escalated. The doctor should also document directions somewhere in the outpatient records or the hospital chart. Some patients get very mixed up with multiple medications and as a result are noncompliant. Take time during one of the visits to help the patient, or the family, organize medicine taking with pillboxes labeled for the days of the week. Before the week starts, the patient should place the prescribed number of pills in each compartment. At dinner on Wednesday, if the patient sees there are two carbamazepine pills left instead of the scheduled one, he will know to take an extra pill. Even better are cardboard boxes with multiple compartments for each day, providing a separate space for each pill (Figure 7-3).

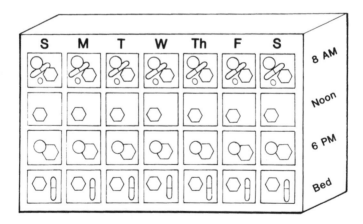

Figure 7-3 Drawing of a pillbox compartmentalized by dosage for days and times of day. (Drawn by Harriet Greenfield.)

Alternative strategies like crossing off or noting on a schedule when pills have been taken can be explored. Try to simplify the schedule as much as possible; it's easier to take pills at home on arising or retiring than carrying them along during the day. Have patients bring all their pills with them and ask them on return visits what medicines they are taking. You may have in your records a listing of what you told the patient but that may bear little relation to what is really happening.

In discussing medications or procedures with the patient, it is essential that you relate the potential serious side effects of the treatment. Try to allay anxiety by emphasizing the rarity of complications, when appropriate. We often divide problems with medicines into three groups:

1. Allergic reactions (usually a rash) that patients can develop with almost any pill and serious hypersensitivity responses, especially with certain medications.
2. Dose-related toxic side effects such as drowsiness and ataxia that occur with high blood levels of phenytoin or carbamazepine. These symptoms improve with reduction in dose. These medications and others require titration to arrive at the optimum therapeutic dose that will give the least side effects.
3. Idiosyncratic severe toxicity that will require stopping the pill. Liver necrosis with valproate and phenytoin, leukopenia with carbamazepine, and thrombocytopenia with ticlopidine are examples that are fortunately rare.

Patients should be told of the need for routine testing for drug levels and toxic side effects when this is part of your treatment plan. The American Medical Association and other organizations publish tear sheets containing important information about frequently used medications that can be given to patients in lieu of a long discussion. Do give patients a chance to ask questions after they have read the material. In my experience, the printed inserts that accompany most medicines are too complex and contain details about side effects that alarm or worry many patients. If you rely on these inserts to educate patients about the treatment, allow time to review the information with them, especially features that are worrisome to them. The same general advice applies to information obtained from the *Physician's Desk Reference* (PDR), which many patients somehow gain access to. Pharmacists may try to be helpful by giving patients long lists of side effects and by informing the patient about the indications and proper use of medications. Headache patients might find it disconcerting to be told they are taking heart medicine (propranolol) or anticonvulsant drugs (valproate). It is best to anticipate these types of problems when discussing the prescriptions given.

When the treatment advised is a surgical or invasive diagnostic procedure, the neurologist, as well as the surgeon or physician who will perform the procedure should talk to the patient. You must inform patients of the risks of the procedure and their relative likelihood of occurrence. You should document these discussions in your office notes or the hospital chart. When patients sue because of a bad outcome, they invariably sue the neurologist and other physicians as well as the surgeons. Never cajole, persuade, or push patients to have operations they don't want even when you think they are needed. Impress your firm opinion on patients and their families, but do not use any form of coercion. A prominent English surgeon said that he will not operate on a patient unless the individual virtually pleads for the surgery. Again, the tactic of hanging crepe and being conservative, if not pessimistic, about the outcome is useful. It seems that it is always the cases in which the physician or surgeon has pushed the patient to have surgery that turn out disastrously and have a high rate of litigation.

Alternatives

One of the most important roles that the physician plays is as adviser and educator. The patient should feel that you have dispassionately weighed alternative tests and therapies before coming to your decision. Especially when the disease you are treating is likely to be very serious, be certain to inform the patient and family about other types of approaches and why you have elected a different course.

A common example is brain tumor. If you have suggested a biopsy followed by radiation therapy, explain to the patient and family why you do not favor a more aggressive course, such as surgery, chemotherapy, or other, newer alternative treatments. If you have selected a consultant or a surgeon, explain to the family why you have chosen that physician. When doctors convey to the family all the viable alternatives and the reasons for selecting a particular plan, patients usually appreciate the doctors' concern and wisdom.

Some patients have an effective information network; Aunt Bess, Uncle Joe, the *New York Times*, television, the Internet, medical journals, or some other source of information always seems to offer the patient a new form of treatment or a cure. Uncle Charlie's coworker's friend was cured by chemotherapy. An acquaintance was given intracarotid treatment with carmustine (BCNU). When patients or family members bring such information to the physician, it may appear to them that the doctor has been less than thorough and is perhaps not fully informed. Anticipate requests for information, alternative suggestions, and consultations. The physician should appear to be informed and in control. If a procedure or treatment is suggested with which you are unfamiliar, say so and agree to look into it. If the patient has printed information from the Internet or clipped an article from a news report, read it and discuss it with the patient.

WHAT IS THE NEXT STEP?

Before patients leave the office, they should know what is planned and if they are supposed to take any actions. Should they make the next appointment now? Or should they call you instead to report their progress? If so, when, and what should they be looking for to report? The patient should have a list of instructions that includes the next doctor-patient contact. When patients are seen for a single visit or consultation, make it clear to them that they do not need to see you again. Under what circumstances, if any, should they call or see you again? Should they return to their primary physician?

If you have specific times or guidelines for phone contact, inform patients so that they know how best to contact you. I sometimes find it very useful at the end of visits to ask patients to repeat to me what I expect them to do, so that I am sure they have heard and understood.

ALLOW SOME TIME FOR QUESTIONS

Patients must feel they have been heard. Your discussion may not have answered some of their questions. They may be concerned about misconceptions or misinformation that you can readily correct, reassuring them that they have no reason to worry. With some patients, time simply does not permit in-depth discussion of all their questions. If the queries are not urgent or pressing, urge patients to call or visit later when you will be able to answer their questions. Some patients who talk incessantly can never be quelled. Explain to these patients, who habitually dominate your time, that today you have time only for one or two very important questions. An alternative way of dealing with these patients is to ask them to send you a letter or an e-mail listing their questions, assuring them that you will either reply by mail or answer the questions during one of the next visits.

LITERATURE AND REFERRALS TO OUTSIDE ORGANIZATIONS

Literature concerning the patient's illness can be very helpful, but you must be careful what you give the patient and when. Various organizations such as the Muscular Dystrophy Association (MDA), the Amyotrophic Lateral Sclerosis Society (ALSS), the American Heart Association (AHA), and others have booklets describing muscular dystrophy, motor neuron disease, stroke, multiple sclerosis, Parkinson's disease, and Tourette's disease. These are helpful to patients who have accepted their illnesses and to patients and families who want information. However, premature information, especially regarding a poor prognosis, can be a setback for patients. Reading in an ALSS booklet that extreme disability and death are imminent can be counterproductive in the early stage of the disease. Later, the same information may help the very same patient understand what he or she and the doctor are up against. Read a booklet first before recommending it to patients.

Sharing literature conveys to the patient the doctor's willingness to consider any steps that might be of help to the patient. We often refer patients to books written for the general public about their illness. A good example is

Episode by Eric Hodgson[21] in which the author, a well-known popular writer, shares his experiences during and after his own left hemisphere stroke. We also often refer patients with serious illnesses to general books that may help them to understand their illnesses and their reactions. *When Bad Things Happen to Good People* by Harold Kushner is an outstanding example of such a book.[22] Rabbi Kushner had a son who died in his early teens of a rare progressive disease, progeria. Like Job, Kushner asks the usual question: "Why me?" Kushner's answers to this and other questions can be very useful to some people, especially those with important religious beliefs, regardless of affiliation.

At the proper time, with the appropriate patient, a referral to an outside specific disease-oriented organization can be very helpful. Sometimes, however, a visit to such an organization can have adverse effects. Let's use local multiple sclerosis chapters as an example. In general, patients who are active in MS chapters are those with significant disabilities and handicaps, for whom the disease is an important, ever-present problem. Also, in order to raise money, these organizations tend to emphasize the seriousness of multiple sclerosis ("the crippler of young adults"). For a patient with only minor or intermittent symptoms or episodes, attendance at a meeting of the local MS society can be very depressing and may needlessly arouse anxieties that are not applicable to that individual patient. For other patients with significant disability, the society and its members might be very helpful.

Organizations can be helpful in a number of different ways:

1. They can provide more information about the disease and the nature and availability of various treatments. This information can then be discussed with the patient's neurologist. Education is most important for patients so that they can better understand and cope with the illness. Your referral to the organization signifies to patients your willingness to do all that is possible to help them and to consider the recommendations or approaches of others.
2. The members can often provide concrete practical suggestions from their own experience. Patients with motor neuron disease or other chronic neuromuscular conditions and their family members can provide advice about specific aids such as utensils, special shoes or clothing, brace makers, shower apparatus, and equipment about which most doctors know little. Stroke support groups, where members are usually stroke patients and their families, can give practical advice about recovery and can also be an important source of motivation and emotional support. Talking with patients who have "made it back" after a stroke can be inspiring to a patient and may help much more than hearing the physician's words of encouragement.
3. Organizations can provide other types of information, for example, which buildings in town have special facilities for the handicapped (toilets, ramps, etc.), how to get handicapped driver car stickers, and so on. Sometimes legal information is useful: What are the laws con-

cerning discrimination against patients because of epilepsy and other handicaps? Some organizations even provide tangible help with job selection and have contact with key employers.

4. Volunteering to work in an appropriate organization may help the patient psychologically. Doing for others with similar problems enhances feelings of self-esteem and self-worth at a time when they may be low.

The American Academy of Neurology can serve as a source of information about various organizations concerned with neurologic diseases, and the American Heart Association has information about stroke clubs and other stroke-related resources. In general, physicians tend to underutilize organizations. When patients contact such organizations, they may feel that they are doing so behind your back, that you may be unconcerned with offering this type of help, or that you may be unwilling to consider alternate approaches. It is far better to make the referral yourself.

Information exchange is probably the single most important product that the patient and family receive directly from the physician. Naturally, patients and families tend to judge the doctor by what he or she does and tells them. That is all they have to use. Like an examination in school, the teacher or grader sees only what the student has said or written. They have no other information that would help decide what the student knows or what has been done to prepare for the examination. Yet of all physician activities, information transmittal is the least well taught, and many doctors spend precious little time or effort in improving their communication skills. Premedical curricula, traditionally dominated by science courses and multiple-choice tests, do not prepare physicians well for skillful communication.

We urge physicians to become more self-conscious and aware of their own information-giving activities and skills. In a test week, keep track of the relative amount of time spent with each patient on this activity. Also analyze several patient encounters for the content of the interaction. Which of the subjects discussed in this chapter have been covered and how completely and effectively? How comfortable does the physician feel while giving information? Have the patients and families understood what was said? Better physician-patient communication will lead to more satisfied patients, better compliance with advice and prescriptions, and fewer lawsuits generated by unhappy families and patients.

REFERENCES

1. Engel CL. The best and the brightest—the missing dimension in medical education. *The Pharos* 1973;36:127–133.
2. Tumulty P. *The Effective Clinician.* Philadelphia: W.B. Saunders Co., 1973.
3. Zinser H. *As I Remember Him: The Biography of R.S.* Boston: Little Brown and Co., 1940;141.
4. Nickerson H. Patient education. *Health Eth Man* 1972:95–97.

5. Waitzkin H. Information giving in medical care. *J Health Soc Behav* 1985;26: 81–101.
6. Tring EC, Hayes-Allen MC. Understanding and misunderstanding of some medical terms. *Br J Med Educ* 1973;7:53–59.
7. Smith RC, Lyles JS, Mettler J, et al. The effectiveness of intensive training for residents in interviewing. A randomized controlled trial. *Ann Int Med* 1998;128: 118–126.
8. Butt HR. A method for better physician-patient communication. *Ann Int Med* 1977;86:478–480.
9. Ley P, Spelman MS. Communication in an out-patient setting. *Br J Soc Clin Psych* 1965;4:114–116.
10. Cox K. *Doctor and Patient: Exploring Clinical Thinking.* Sydney: University of New South Wales Press, 1999.
11. Strull WM, Lo B, Charles G. Do patients want to participate in medical decision making. *JAMA* 1984;252:2990–2994.
12. Waitzkin H. Doctor-patient communication. *JAMA* 1984;252:2441–2446.
13. Davis MS. Variations in patients' compliance with doctors' orders: Analysis of congruence between survey responses and results of empirical investigations. *J Med Educ* 1966;41:1037–1048.
14. Levinson W. Physician-patient communication: A key to malpractice prevention. *JAMA* 1994;272:1619–1620.
15. Roter D, Hall JA. *Doctors Talking with Patients/Patients Talking with Doctors: Improving Communications in Medical Visits.* Westport, CT: Asuburn House, 1992.
16. Caplan LR, Kelly JJ. *Consultations in Neurology.* Toronto: B.C.: Decker Inc., 1988;46–48.
17. Fisher CM. Left hemiplegia and motor impersistence. *J Nerv Ment Dis* 1956;123: 201–218.
18. Hier DB, Mondlock J, Caplan LR. Behavioral defects after right hemisphere stroke. *Neurol* 1983;33:337–344.
19. Epley JM. The canalith repositioning procedure for treatment of benign paroxysmal positional vertigo. *Otolaryngol Head Neck Surg* 1992;107:399–404.
20. Caplan LR, Brandt T, Troost BT, Baloh RW. Management of acute peripheral vestibular disorders. *Eur Neurol* 1993;33:337–344.
21. Hodgson E. *Episode: Report on the Accident inside My Skull.* New York: Athenaeum, 1964.
22. Kushner H. *When Bad Things Happen to Good People.* New York: Schocken Books, 1981.

8

Treatment: What Neurologists Can Offer Patients

This big stout fellow had simply melted away. He had cares and worries, a great many. He came up from the country moribund. Doses of optimism lavishly administered by a house physician cured him.[1]

—WILLIAM OSLER

What must it be like to meet strangers who immediately confess to you their bodies' most brutal secrets, who come to you openly acknowledging their need for help? What must it feel like to be able to help, to cure them on occasion, to touch them reassuringly on the shoulder, to put their minds at ease? How would it feel to fail?[2]

—R. MARTIN

Ordinarily, people think of physicians as diagnosticians who tailor the treatment to the patient's condition. By this definition, treatment is usually conceptualized as medication or surgery. But the treating physician is or should be much more than a person who selects the correct drug or procedural intervention. In truth, most illnesses that patients bring to neurologists are curable neither with drugs nor surgery. The clinician neurologist has many roles to play in order to treat the patient optimally.

CLINICIAN ROLES

Confidante and Listener

Illness and its attendant woes exact heavy tolls on individuals and compromise their performance as parents, spouses, and workers. Many sick and discouraged people have no ready place to turn for support. Strangers aren't interested in the details of their problems; they have enough of their own. The old adage "don't ask him how he feels, he may tell you" is all too true. Many are reticent about burdening their friends or families with their concerns for

157

fear of upsetting or altering their present relationship with them. They consult their doctor, hoping for an attentive ear and objective analysis and advice. Sometimes just listening to what patients have to say somehow lightens their load. Thinking about their problems and organizing the details for presentation to the doctor sometimes give patients insights that prove helpful.

Teacher

One of the most important functions of any doctor is to teach patients about their illness and its treatment. The word doctor originates from the Latin verb *docere*, "to teach." Most patients come to the doctor naive about their health and often not very knowledgeable about the workings of their bodies. The neurologist can educate epileptics to recognize the warning signs before their seizures, to avoid circumstances that precipitate seizures, and about what to do should a seizure occur. Instruction on the use and side effects of the anti-convulsant medications prescribed for them can also be very helpful. For patients with muscular dystrophy and their families, fostering understanding of the limitations created by the disease and helping them to adapt to their handicaps is very valuable. We used to spend considerable time teaching myasthenics about the manifestations of their disease and side effects of anticholinesterase drugs. Often, patients would become so proficient in recognizing the signs that indicate the need for more medicine, and those indicative of cholinergic excess, that they could titrate their own dose of prostigmine or pyridostigmine. Just like insulin-dependent diabetics, the myasthenics could adjust their medicines, depending on the timing and severity of weakness. Now thymectomy, steroids, and plasma exchange have greatly diminished the importance of anticholinesterase drugs. Parkinsonian patients should be taught to recognize the side effects of L-dopa–containing compounds and to recognize when they need more or less medicine.

In some of these conditions, patients can be taught to construct charts documenting the timing and severity of their symptoms. These charts help doctors regulate the dosage and periodicity of the medicines prescribed and improve assessment of the patient's response to therapy. Seizures, headache, myasthenia, and spells of any type lend themselves well to patient-maintained records and calendars.

Teaching is not necessarily limited to the disease for which the patient has consulted you. Physicians can help patients understand why some of their activities and habits are good or bad health practices. Preventive medicine is an obligation for all physicians. Advice about smoking, exercise, losing weight, and relaxing more may be as important as specific treatment for illness. Some patients who neurologists take care of have little close personal contact with other educated persons and may benefit from their advice on other nonmedical matters that have an impact on their health and well being.

Source of Information and Interpretation

We live in an era dominated by the media. Television, radio, magazines, and newspapers are ubiquitous; advances in medicine are big news. Many of the stories that reach the press contain misinformation. Some results are released prematurely. Patients look to their doctors for interpretation of what they have heard and read. They also expect you to watch carefully for any advances that could improve their condition. This is especially true if they have a disease for which there is no or inadequate treatment.

Some patients have seen more than one doctor about their problem. Invariably, there are some differences of opinion about their diagnoses or treatment. The patient may ask you as a consultant to explain the reasons for the different opinions. What are the facts that are known? What is unknown and simply represents differences of interpretation and style?

Ombudsman

You are the patient's advocate. You are on his or her side. This is especially important in treating patients with diseases for which there is no known cure. Physicians often sit behind a desk or stand above the patient at the bedside. The physician occupies a superior position, both practically and figuratively. The patient looks *up* to the doctor. Just as citizens envision their rulers to be larger than life, patients sometimes invest their doctors with superhuman attributes and capabilities. Patients depend on the wisdom of doctors to cure them. This traditional reverence for the physician undoubtedly has a therapeutic effect. A good part of the placebo effect relates to the belief that their doctor will make them better.

But what if you can't make them better? Their continued expectation of a cure or at least some progress is in stark contrast to what is actually happening; they are getting worse, and your therapeutic endeavors have been impotent. Faced with this situation, patients become frustrated and impatient and begin to doubt their doctor. The physician, in turn, becomes frustrated. Some doctors handle this situation by discharging the patient from their care, informing them that there is nothing they can do. Other physicians suggest that the patient seek medical care elsewhere.

In this situation, when you as a physician know that there is little effective treatment and your ministrations are very unlikely to work, we find it useful to "turn the tables." Come out from behind the desk and sit alongside patients. Tell patients honestly that together you are fighting against the odds. You do not have anything in your bag of tricks that you know will have a major salutary impact on their disease. But you are willing to fight with them. The enemy is the disease. This tactic changes the terms of the struggle in the patient's mind. The patient is no longer questioning the doctor because of disease progression. Instead, the patient is working with the doctor as a team against the illness. You are willing to listen to and interpret any information the patient gleans. You will do your utmost to seek out possible advances in research and treatment. You are willing to try remedies that have even a slight rationale as long as they are not likely to harm the patient. You are willing to persevere despite your own frustrations at not being able to offer a cure.

Healer

Physicians, including neurologists, are sometimes able to heal. They may cure the disease or alleviate the impact the disease has on the patient or both. Of course, responses to treatment are not always binary—black and white, cure or failure. Some treatments help the symptoms and the disease. Patients may achieve only slightly improved feelings of well-being, but they can be advised on how to best adapt to their problem and not let it conquer them.

Some patients become distraught and decompensate over relatively minor problems. Tingling, minor pain, leg discomfort after walking six blocks, tinnitus, and benign positional vertigo that occurs only on retiring and arising are examples. Perhaps patients view these symptoms as a sign of ill health or loss of capability or aging. Explore with these patients ways of avoiding or improving the symptoms; for example, exercises that induce vertigo often allow resetting of the brain's response to vestibular stimulation and enhance recovery. Suggest ways of masking the symptoms, for example, having patients with tinnitus sleep with a radio on. The doctor can also allay patients' misconceptions about their body images. Help patients manage the symptoms; then the irrational overresponse to the discomfiture can be quelled.

Friend

No one ever has too many friends. Let patients know you like them and care about them. An impersonal, cold, and detached demeanor is countertherapeutic. Take a few minutes during each visit to shoot the breeze. Make patients feel that you care about them as people, that they are not just specimens or examples of a disease. Learn about their families, hobbies, work, and concerns. They are not just clients or consumers (to use the language of health economists).

Referee and Arbiter

Differences of opinion among physicians are extremely common and create confusion for the patient. It often falls to the primary caregiver to sort these differences out for the patient. We will have more to say about this problem in the discussion in Part III, Chapter 12 on consultations.

Also, disputes between patients and their spouses, children, and parents are often brought to the doctor. Everyone in the family seems to know exactly what the patient should and should not do. In the circumstances of an ill young person especially, some parents believe it is in the child's best interest to restrict and control activities. Children with seizures are not allowed to participate in sports, or go out alone or with their friends. We have seen similar limitations placed by well-intentioned children on their aging parents. Life is to be lived. The caretakers of the sick person often need help in allaying their own fears and guilt feelings. Physicians often find themselves in the center of these discussions and disagreements, serving as referees or judges who must rule with the best interest of the patient as the major criterion.

Source of Referral

Neurologic and medical care is growing even more complex, and subspecialization even more pronounced. Intercurrent medical and surgical problems often develop in patients with nervous system disease, especially in the older age groups. Diseases of the central and peripheral nervous system are extremely common among the geriatric population. Few patients over eighty have no neurologic symptoms, signs, or findings when examined by a careful neurologist. Patients have respect for various specialists, and, in my experience, they often place neurologists a peg above other consultants. They often come to neurologists as a source of referral for other problems unrelated to the neurologic disease. Their neurologic problems often necessitate referral to other neurologists, neurosurgeons, cardiologists, and psychiatrists or nonphysician health workers such as social workers, speech and occupational therapists, nutritionists, and even fitness counselors.

Do not be parochial in your referral. Send patients to professionals that you know are competent and have a caring style. There is a passage in the book *Heart Sounds*, by Lear, that is very humorous but at the same time quite pathetic.[3] The patient, a physician, has been having serious psychological problems and asks his cardiologist if he can suggest a psychiatrist for "one of his friends." The patient consults the psychiatrist and finds him wanting. He tells his cardiologist who replies, "Oh my goodness. I didn't realize you were asking for yourself. He was looking for referrals and I wanted to help him out. He's my wife's cousin." Refer the patient to the best and most humane caregiver. It should not matter if the physician or other health professional is affiliated with your own institution or is a friend or an acquaintance of yours. If you yourself had the same problem, whom would you consult?

The same considerations apply to patients under your own care. If patients have a problem outside your usual areas of expertise, and better care could be administered conveniently and economically nearby, then you have an obligation to patients to refer them. Never keep control of patients because they are interesting or might be a case report for a journal or for economic reasons. Care for the patient only when you are well qualified to do so.

Psychologist

The practice of medicine and neurology is more than 50 percent psychology or psychiatry. Hysteria, malingering, and exaggeration or feigning of symptoms and signs often mimic organic neurologic disease. The more senior and professorial a neurologist becomes, the more likely referred patients are to be either very ill or to have no organic disease at all. Psychoneuroses are very common in the general population and invariably some of these neurotics develop neurologic disease and consult a neurologist. Nervous system disease and sickness are profound psychological stresses on most patients' and families' adaptive capabilities. Most patients need some psychological help from their physicians, especially their neurologists.

In most circumstances, we have not had success in referring patients with organic neurologic disease or hysteria with conversion signs to psychiatrists.[4] Because psychiatrists seldom, if ever, examine patients and usually do not inquire into the details of their pain, weakness, and so on, many patients have been unwilling to accept their assurances that the symptoms are psychological or functional. After all, psychologically ill individuals also get physical illnesses just like everyone else. To be effective, physicians must care for mind and body; they must analyze symptoms, examine the symptomatic region, and pay a great deal of attention to the patient's problems, stresses, and maladaptive behavior.

Team Leader

Patients with neurologic disease, especially the elderly, often have multiple medical problems and require a team of physicians. During the acute neurologic illness and when the major chronic problem is neurologic, the neurologist may have to coordinate the various physicians and caregivers to assure maximum cooperation and effectiveness. The role of coordinator should usually rest with the patient's family physician or internist in most other circumstances.

CATEGORIES OF TREATMENT

The details of and indications for specific neurologic therapies are clearly beyond the scope of this chapter. We can, however, organize treatments into various categories. We find it useful to ask ourselves what is the purpose and intent of the treatment or procedure. Surgical procedures may be (1) diagnostic, for example, various biopsies; (2) curative, such as tumor removal, clipping of an aneurysm, insertion of a shunt for hydrocephalus; (3) palliative, such as tumor debulking, rhizotomies and tractotomies to control pain; or (4) preventative, such as a carotid endarterectomy in a patient with an asymptomatic stenosis, or aneurysm repair for an asymptomatic unruptured aneurysm. Similarly, most medical therapies can also be thought of in the same categories. Some medicines, such as pyridostigmine for myasthenia gravis, phenytoin for seizures, and triptans for migraine, are rather specific for certain indications. Therapeutic trials of these agents can be helpful diagnostically. Most drugs are palliative, but a few such as B_{12}, penicillin and other antibiotics, and hormone replacement therapy can be curative. Immunizations and penicillin prophylaxis of endocarditis in a patient with valvular heart disease are examples of preventive medicine.

Medical and surgical treatments may be aimed at treating the symptoms, others at controlling or remedying the disease. In the case of myasthenia gravis, anticholinesterases merely improve the symptoms, while thymectomy, plasma exchange, and immunosuppressants are used to battle the production of antibodies against the acetylcholine receptor. In Parkinsonian patients, dopaminergics replace deficient production of dopamine in the nigrostriatal pathway. The use of L-dopa does not cure the pathogenesis, and, when the drug is stopped, patients return to their former state. Carbamazepine for pain and baclofen or tizanidine for spasticity are used to treat some patients with multiple sclerosis, but they do nothing to retard the disease process.

Physicians should also categorize treatments by their general acceptability. Is a medical or surgical procedure established, widely used, and considered effective? Or is the therapy in common use, but its effectiveness as yet unproven and uncertain? Or is the treatment still experimental? Questionnaires from drug companies often inquire of physicians whether they use a drug as soon as it is marketed, after encouraging reports and some experience, or only after years of experience and results.

Treatments should also be categorized as to their degree of risk. Is a medicine or procedure very safe, with only extremely rare serious side effects? Is there some but relatively minor risk, or is a drug or procedure very risky? Are the risks of the drug related to dosage or length of use? Are most of the important idiosyncratic side effects likely to occur soon after starting the drug or is close surveillance necessary for the entire time it is used? Is the drug a newly released agent like felbamate or tolcapone, or has it been around long enough so that its spectrum of side effects is well known?

In treating any prolonged or severe illness, the clinician should try to make the patient aware of the category of treatment (affects symptoms or course of disease, risk, acceptability) used and realistic chances of success. Misconceptions and false hopes breed mistrust, resentment, and lawsuits. In most minor, self-limited, and functional neurologic disorders, there is also a definite placebo effect with any treatment prescribed. In that circumstance, lengthy discussions about the limitations of the treatment defeat the placebo effect and are unnecessary. Doses of optimism and confidence given liberally with prescriptions do wonders.

SELECTING TREATMENT

We firmly believe in the autonomy of the individual patient. It is hoped that physicians are educated, experienced individuals who select what they feel will be the best treatment and so advise the patient. However, the final decisions should and must rest with patients, their families, and caregivers. When the patient is incapable of making decisions and no responsible family is available, the physician will have to decide for the patient, taking into consideration the patient's prior wishes if known. Courts are not good places to make therapeutic decisions.

The clinician, in analyzing any treatment, should keep in mind four major factors or concerns: decision to treat, risk/benefit ratio, expense, and discomfort

Table 8-1 Spectrum of Considerations on Whether or Not to Treat

Try something	⟵⟶	*Primum non nocere*
Benefit of treatment	⟵⟶	Risk of treatment
short-term benefit	⟵⟶	short-term risk
long-term benefit	⟵⟶	long-term risk
Inexpensive treatment	⟵⟶	Expensive treatment
Discomfort of illness	⟵⟶	Discomfort of treatment

and disability. Analysis of these concerns is not simply a yes/no, true/false matter; there are gradations. We're often asked on evaluation questionnaires to rate something on a scale from one to ten. Similarly, one can construct a scale for each of the factors, representing a spectrum of choices (Table 8-1).

Decision to Treat

"Try something" is a temptation and instinct common to patients and physicians alike. No one likes to sit idly by while a patient suffers and deteriorates. Treatment is often equated in the patient's mind with hope. But physicians have always been told *primum non nocere* (first do no harm). No one wants to make the patient worse. It would be sad indeed if treatment with little or no chance of helping the patient had sufficient toxicity to make the patient even more miserable. The physician must weigh these two dicta in reference to each treatment contemplated.

Risk/Benefit Ratio

Risk/benefit ratio should be a familiar concept to all physicians. Is the probability of success high enough to outweigh the risk? For powerful, potentially curative drugs, a real but small risk of toxicity or reaction is well worth the effect of the treatment. Penicillin can cure some examples of Lyme disease, endocarditis, and meningitis. The use of this drug in these conditions is well worth the risk of an allergic reaction. The decision to use penicillin is easy, but what if the disease is an inoperable tumor that is relatively radioresistant, such as metastatic melanoma? The benefit of treatment is dubious, and radiotherapy has important side effects at the dosage considered.

Expense of Treatment

Expense of the treatment is an important consideration for the patient. By expense, I mean dollars and time. If the proposed treatment is curative, then expense should be very unimportant. But what if the treatment will have doubtful effects? If you had a malignant glioma and your predicted lifespan was short, and at present you were functioning well, would you like to spend the greater part of six weeks traveling back and forth to the hospital for radiation treatment with uncertain prospects of benefit? Would you spend $10,000 for an implantable infusion device without proven effect on your disease if your economic resources were severely limited?

Discomfort and Disability

Discomfort and disability are "softer" phenomena, harder to quantitate and weigh than life and death. So-called "quality of life" is very important. Some patients believe that the physician's main task is to allay pain and suffering, to cure occasionally, but to comfort always. Illnesses have their own titer of discomfort and disruption of life. Treatments can also take their toll in toxicity and side effects. Patients also vary greatly in their tolerance of symptoms and their ability to carry on despite problems. Cancer undoubtedly causes suffering in many ways. So can chemotherapy. Chemotherapeutic agents are cell poisons that are intended to kill or injure rapidly growing tumor cells more than they do normal cells. Some agents may have marginally greater efficacy with major increase in toxicity. Gastrointestinal, systemic, and hematopoietic toxicities are common, especially with prolonged chemotherapy. The physician must weigh the relative effects of the disease versus the treatment on quality of life.

Decision Analysis

Decision analysis[5,6] is a field geared to assist physicians in making important diagnostic and therapeutic decisions. The analysis involves assigning numerical weights to various factors involved in the decision-making process. While we are not certain that quantification is realistic and that calculating the sum of the weights leads to a better decision, we are convinced that physicians should become familiar with the types of data used in decision analysis. Knowledge of the factors involved helps in the selection of treatment and communication with the patient about the treatment.

Decision analysis distinguishes between immediate risk and long-term risk. Would you choose a treatment that had a relatively high immediate risk, but a potential cure? What is the long-range risk of the illness? A surgical procedure, for example, carotid endarterectomy, can be used to illustrate this concept. You as the patient have an extremely severe narrowing of the left internal carotid artery in the neck. The risk of stroke is high enough to cause concern (perhaps 10 percent or more). The operation, carotid endarterectomy, has a chance of removing the lesion, thus greatly reducing the risk of stroke during the next ten years in the territory of that artery. But there is a real chance of the procedure itself resulting in stroke, heart attack, or death (a risk varying between 1 and 10 percent or so, depending on the surgeon, the institution, and details of the lesion). The risk of the procedure is short-term and immediate. If the surgery causes a stroke, it will be recognized just after awakening or in the immediate postoperative period (days). Of course, the surgery does not protect other arteries that also might have or develop serious disease. The alternative to surgery would be medicines: long-term use of aspirin, warfarin, and/or statins. The results of the Asymptomatic Carotid Atherosclerosis Study (ACAS) were not as convincing as to demand surgery for every patient with >60% stenosis. If medicines were used instead of surgery the risks of stroke and of serious side effects of the medicine are spread over a longer period of time. Do you put all your eggs in one basket and choose surgery, or do you choose medicine with less acute risk but also possibly a longer period of disease and treatment risk? There is no easy answer to this dilemma. Quantitated risks and benefit probabilities may help with a rational decision, but people are all different. Some of us are gamblers and risk takers; as Kipling notes in the poem, "If," "If you can risk all your belongings in one game of pitch and chance, and lose and start again at the beginning and never breathe a word about your loss." Some draw to an inside straight in poker, while others play the odds. Some drive sports cars at high speeds, parachute from planes or climb dangerous mountains for sport, while others are conservative and guard carefully against any unnecessary risks.

The quality and length of time spent free of disease is also important in decision analysis. Suppose a disease is likely to produce severe disability after five years. A treatment might prevent that disability but have a risk of causing another important immediate and persistent disability. How important is that five-year, disease-free interval? Referring back to an example already used, a 55-year-old administrator with a family had a disabling stroke in the immediate postoperative period after carotid endarterectomy. Another comparable patient had no surgery, chose medical treatment, and had a bad stroke five years later. The patient choosing medical therapy had five more useful functional years than the patient having the postoperative stroke. Jonas called this stroke-free interval "intact months of patient survival" (IMPS).[7] The utility of that time depends heavily on the patient's age and degree of function, the relative degree of freedom from symptoms, and the severity of the disability at either time, immediate or delayed. A similar type of consideration sometimes confronts patients with cancer: If they have cancer but feel relatively well and function normally, should they undergo chemotherapy that is palliative and has no precedent for a cure? The chemotherapy could possibly delay morbidity from the disease but would carry its own price in the form of discomfort and side effects. Should they choose chemotherapy and unpleasant side effects during the next year and perhaps lengthen their lifespan, or should they opt for getting the most out of the good time left and postpone treatment until that time when their well-being and function were compromised? Would the decision be the same if they knew that the longer they waited, the potentially less effective would be the chemotherapy? Would they choose disability and discomfort over a period of years, over preserved health for one year, followed by death? These are difficult decisions, most often without a definite right or wrong answer. These are also very personal decisions.

Physicians who are familiar with decision analysis are beginning to ask patients these knotty questions, asking for a quantitative judgment.

Role of the Physician in Decisions on Treatment

If these treatment decisions are so difficult and so personal for the patient, what then is the role of the clinician? We submit that it is not to make the decision for the patient. We must not as physicians and individuals thrust our values, morals, and ideas on our patients. We should be caring, knowledgeable advisers. The neurologist should transmit enough information to patients and their families to allow them to make a decision. In most instances, this information should include numbers and approximate percentage probabilities, if available. The factors outlined in this chapter—costs, risks (both immediate and long term) of the disease and the proposed treatment, alternative therapies—should all be discussed. A useful, simply understood way of handling the discussion is to use "what if?" exigencies. ("What if you choose not to have the treatment (for instance, surgery), what can be reasonably expected to happen? What if you do choose treatment, what are the risks and benefits?") If there are multiple possibilities, outline the relative probabilities of each, if you can. ("What if you do choose therapy? What if instead, I prescribe treatment X?") Information about discomfort and morbidity should be included.

Given the full complement of data, still only a small minority of patients will be able to make a rational decision unaided. Most will need help and advice. They will often ask what you would do if you were in their shoes. When you as the treating clinician feel that the decision is rather clear-cut, you should be definite about your advice. When the choice is a toss-up, you should avoid heavily influencing the patient one way or the other; impress upon the patient that there is no known clear advantage to either or any of the alternative treatments available. Some patients have difficulty analyzing data and do not want to know the details. They seek a strong, authoritarian declaration from the physician, such as "you need the surgery" or "surgery would be bad, you should instead take aspirin and lose weight." Even when a very directive mode is used, you still must tell the patient the risks of the treatment you have endorsed and obtain informed consent.

Give advice, but do not judge the patient. Doctors often admonish and cajole patients to lose weight, moderate their alcohol consumption, reduce the amount of cholesterol and animal fats in their diet, exercise, stop taking birth control pills, stop smoking, avoid addictive drugs, and so on. This advice is sound and natural for physicians who have the patients' well-being in mind. Some patients follow this good advice. Others politely listen and go about their daily activities and habits as they did before. For those patients who ignore your advice, it is very reasonable to repeat your admonishments and marshall strong arguments to support your position. It is unreasonable and wrong to strongly control the patient or judge them if they do not listen. Their bodies are their own. Some people make unwise, even very stupid, decisions at various times in their lives. All parents have agonized over irrational, ill-considered decisions that their children made, but, once parents have given their advice, they cannot accept all the blame for their childrens' foibles. Similarly, physicians should not blame themselves for what they feel are wrong decisions on the part of patients. The physician cannot consider an unwise patient decision as a personal failure or an affront. Equanimity and dispassionate calm are important attributes of the effective clinician.[8]

Neurologists usually have been considered therapeutic nihilists. Their surgical and medical colleagues might say that they are bright, cognitive, scholarly folks who think a lot but do nothing. Young physicians considering entering the field of neurology are often discouraged from doing so by other physicians who argue, "so what if you make an exotic neurologic diagnosis, you can't do anything for it." Fortunately, now there are neurologic diseases that can be effectively and specifically treated and the future bodes bright for further therapeutic advances. But we believe that the concept of treatment is usually considered too narrowly to refer only to curative remediation. If treatment was considered in the larger context of activity helpful to patients, there are countless ways that doctors can help and do help. In fact, there are very few patients with neurologic disease in whom the neurologist cannot make a contribution. Neurologists can and should play many different therapeutic roles as discussed in detail in this chapter. No other health providers have the neurologist's knowledge of the disease and the patient. As with diagnosis and testing, the physician should try to analyze systematically the management of each case. What are the goals of treatment? Can some symptoms be relieved? If the physician cannot help the patient get well, can he or she help the patient and family understand the illness and adapt and adjust to the problems?

REFERENCES

1. Bean WB. *Sir William Osler's Aphorisms*. Springfield, IL: Charles C Thomas, 1951.
2. Martin RM. *Grey and White*. New York: Henry Holt and Co., 1986;5.
3. Lear MW. *Heart Sounds*. New York: Simon and Schuster, 1980;88.
4. Caplan LR, Nadelson T. The Oklahoma complex: A common form of conversion hysteria. *Arch Int Med* 1980;140:185–186.
5. Pauker SC, Kassirer JP. Decision analysis. *N Engl J Med* 1987;316:250–258.
6. Kassirer JP, Moskowitz AJ, Lau J, Pauker SC. Decision analysis: A progress report. *Ann Int Med* 1987;106:275–291.
7. Jonas S. IMPS (intact months of patient survival): An analysis of the results of carotid endarterectomy. *Stroke* 1986;17:1329–1334.
8. Osler W. *Aequanimitas: Valedictory remarks to the graduates in Medicine of the University of Pennsylvania, May 1, 1889*. Philadelphia: W.E. Fell and Co., 1889.

9

Case Examples Illustrating the Method

We've got to learn to surrender to them—to our patients. They have stories to tell too—lives of poetry in them; bad dreams and good ones; pictures to give us—of their wounds, and their smiles, and the deep worry-lines on their faces.[1]

—W. Carlos Williams

The case histories that follow are each taken directly from my files. I offer them in all humility with the desire that the reader may derive some happiness, comfort, amusement, or hope from what is in them and that he, or she, may perhaps be aided a little further in the understanding of his fellow men.[2]

—J. Rodney

To restore the human subject at the center—the suffering, afflicted, fighting, human subject—we must deepen a case history to a narrative or tale; only then do we have a "who" as well as a "what," a real person, a patient, in relation to disease—in relation to the physical.[3]

—O. Sacks

We have sprinkled excerpts from individual patients throughout the first two parts of the book. Some patients were cited in the chapter on history taking and some in the chapter on the general and neurologic examination, but none of the patients has been described in depth. Trainees and experienced physicians alike learn neurology case by case and stroke by stroke. General rules and guidelines are best grasped with reference to the care of individual patients. For this reason, we conclude the second part of this book on the doctor-patient interface with more detailed examples from five individual patients seen during the last three decades by us. They are presented in the first person as each of us experienced the interactions as we now recall the events and our thoughts.

PATIENT 1 (L.R.C.)

M.G. was 30 years old when he first consulted me. He was referred by a Vermont physician for inpatient evaluation at the New England Medical Center in 1983 because of the development of aphasia and tingling of his right face and hand.

He was a high school graduate who worked as a welder for a large company. His wife also worked to help ends meet. They had two small children. M.G. had had no important neonatal, early life, or adolescent health problems except for "infectious mono" at age 16. He was always strongly right-handed. He considered his health to be good until 18 months before this hospitalization when he noted one day that his left face and hand were weak and tingled. He reported no headache or other symptoms. After an evaluation in a Vermont hospital, which he said included computed tomography (CT) and angiography, he was treated with warfarin during the next year. Anticoagulants were stopped about 6 months ago. He thought his left limbs had returned nearly to normal.

On the day before admission to the hospital, he suddenly noticed at work that his right hand and face felt odd. When he told his foreman about the feeling, he was surprised to find that he had some difficulty saying what he intended and a few "wrong words" came out. Today, he felt no better, but the tingling in the face had diminished. He had no headache.

The patient was sitting by the bedside as I took the history. M.G. was alert and gestured naturally with his right hand. His speech output was effortless, but he said "crumb" for "thumb" and made other word and grammatical errors. He paused on several occasions, trying to think of the name of a tool at work and the name of his company. As I elicited the history, I began to think of possible anatomy and disease mechanism diagnoses.

This young man described two separate episodes of central nervous system dysfunction separated by one and a half years. I first considered the anatomical differential diagnosis. The first episode, by his description, involved sensory and perhaps some motor symptoms involving the left face and hand. The lesion would have to be somewhere above the lower brainstem (where cranial nerve VII lies). The motor and sensory symptoms paralleled each other in the same body parts suggesting a right hemisphere lesion. Leg sparing favored a more cortical or subcortical process, and, since sensory symptoms predominated, the lesion was probably parietal rather than frontal. Since some patients with interruption of sensory fibers at the level of the thalamus or thalamoparietal tracts do report clumsiness, I wondered whether the lesion was deep in the brain in or adjacent to the thalamus or in parietal white matter. I made a mental note to (1) check with the patient's physician about any other findings at the time of the first admission, such as a hemianopia, visual neglect, or drawing and copying difficulty, that would help with localization; (2) carefully examine him for right hemispheral cognitive and behavioral signs and look hard for a visual field defect; and (3) be sure to review the old CT, and a new CT that he would surely need, for any residual right thalamic or cerebral lesions.

The more recent process had to involve the left cerebral hemisphere, most likely in the parasylvian region. The presence of sensory symptoms, absence of weakness, and fluency of his speech placed the lesion posteriorly, either in the temporal lobe or, more likely, the inferior parietal lobule. I made a mental note to examine his speech, reading, and writing thoroughly and to look for signs of Gerstmann's syndrome.

Diagnosis of stroke mechanism was more difficult. Because of his youth and the separation of the lesions in time and place, multiple sclerosis (MS) came to mind first. However, both deficits seemed to begin abruptly, and aphasia is an unusual symptom in MS. His prior physician's choice of warfarin treatment meant that the findings during the initial examination did not suggest demyelinating disease. Tumor seemed unlikely because of the separation of the lesions, improvement in the initial findings, and lack of progression during the 18 months between events. The seemingly abrupt onset, prior use of warfarin, and cortical or subcortical hemisphere localization suggested strokes. But multiple strokes would be unusual in such a young person. What types of strokes could he have? Might these be small hemorrhages due to a bleeding tendency or drug use? This seemed very remote because he said he had had a CT during his first hospitalization and his doctor would certainly not have given him warfarin if a hemorrhage had been found. Multiple infarcts? The most likely causes would be cardiogenic emboli or a coagulopathy. Could this be a paradoxical embolus through an intra-atrial septal defect or widely patent foramen ovale? Could he have premature atherosclerosis due to familial hypercholesterolemia? Some uncommon diseases, some genetically determined, can be associated with premature occlusive disease of multiple intracranial and extracranial arteries. I thought of Fabry's disease, homocystinuria, and disorders of connective tissue such as Ehlers-Danlos syndrome and pseudoxanthoma elasticum. Could he have fibromuscular dysplasia or Moya-Moya disease? I began to criticize myself for thinking so early of rare and exotic diseases, but my other self objected "but this sounds unusual, and if you don't think of those conditions you will never diagnose them." I made more mental notes to listen over the neck and orbits for bruits, look extra carefully at the retina for angioid streaks and cytoid bodies, and examine the fundic blood vessels thoroughly. I would also examine the neck for unusual skin and subcutaneous abnormalities.

I returned to the history. M.G. denied chest discomfort, shortness of breath, past rheumatic fever, and palpitations or irregular heart beating. He had no history of calf or leg pain or swelling that might be compatible with leg vein thrombosis. He had no skin rashes, chest pain, fever, or other symptoms that might suggest systemic lupus erythematosus, sarcoidosis, or endocarditis (all "young people" diseases). He denied drug use of any kind and drank only an occasional beer. His father had hypertension. Two siblings were well. As far as he knew, no member of his family had any other important medical diseases, and he specifically denied hearing about strokes, heart disease, high cholesterol, or premature death in his mother's or father's families. He had never had visual symptoms suggestive of optic neuritis, or migraine.

As I prepared to examine him, I planned to look for evidence of any of the disorders I had considered and to be especially thorough in performing cardiac examination. I also planned the neurologic examination to clarify the anatomy of the two lesions. Later, I would need to speak to M.G.'s wife and physician to get more historical details and to review the clinical findings and lab results from the first hospitalization.

On examination, M.G. was thin but muscular. His skin and mucous membrane color was good, and there were no skin lesions or unusual skin elasticity or folding. His pulse was 110, blood pressure 120/75. His heart size was probably normal, but I wondered if the systolic and diastolic intervals were more nearly equal than usual, giving a tick tock like sound. There were no gallops or murmurs. The spleen was not palpable. The retina looked completely normal. There were no neck or orbital bruits.

M.G. was very alert but was quite nervous and constantly fidgeted. He was very easily distracted. Spontaneous speech was pronounced normally but contained some paraphasic errors—"tencil" for "pencil," "week" for "day." He had difficulty repeating phrases, especially "he or she are here" and "no ifs, ands, or buts" but repeated single words fairly well. His comprehension of spoken language was quite good for yes-or-no queries. He did very well on the token test of DeRenzi[4] and performed the Pierre-Marie paper test ("Here is a piece of paper; tear it in four parts and place one on the table, give one to me, and keep two for yourself.")[5] perfectly. His naming was poor. For a watch, he said you tell time with it and wear it on your . . . (pointed to his left wrist). He could not think of the names tie, button, or belt but correctly named pencil ("tencil"), key, comb, and spoon. His reading was very poor; he had difficulty understanding very simple phrases and questions when they were written but understood the same material when it was spoken. His writing was terrible. He could scarcely write an intelligible sentence and made many spelling and grammatical errors. He spelled words poorly aloud and had difficulty naming when words were spelled aloud to him. He had a very severe apraxia. He could not, with either hand, show how to salute, wave good-bye, or hitchhike. He had difficulty showing with a spoon how he would eat soup. He also had difficulty mimicking hand and arm postures. He spontaneously used utensils and writing implements correctly. Arithmetic functions were poor. He could not compute 8 + 11 mentally and did poorly with written addition and subtraction. He confused left and right most of the time on my body and limbs and got them correct only about 50 percent of the time on his own body. He identified the thumb and pinkie but not the index, ring, or middle fingers. His clock drawing was very asymmetric, with poor organization on the left, and he copied drawings very poorly. Memory was good for three objects and a ten-part story.

The only abnormalities on cranial nerve testing were a definite left hemiachromatopsia. Though he could identify a pin and finger in each visual field all the way to the periphery, he could not tell the red color when the pin was moved from the left until it reached the midline. He had slight flattening of the right lower face, and fewer teeth showed on the right when he smiled or grimaced.

Strength was normal throughout. Deep tendon reflexes were slightly exaggerated on the left, especially at the biceps and knee, and the left plantar response was extensor. On sensory examination, he could not identify objects in either hand. Point localization was also poor in both hands, but pin and touch sensation was normal. Position sense was impaired in the left hand. Vibration sense was normal. He walked quite naturally, except for slightly less arm swing on the left.

The examination helped clarify the anatomical diagnosis but gave no new clues as to mechanism. There was undoubtedly a new left cerebral lesion. The mixture of conduction-type aphasia, alexia with agraphia, and finger agnosia, dyscalculia, and left-right confusion pointed to a left angular gyrus lesion. The abnormal sensory findings meant that the lesion likely extended deeply or anteriorly toward the postcentral gyrus. The constructional dyspraxia, poor point localization, and astereognosis in the left hand and increased left deep tendon reflexes and extensor plantar reflex helped localize the right hemisphere lesion to the superior parietal lobule, with perhaps some spread into the inferior parietal lobule and very posterior frontal lobe. I was puzzled by the left visual field defect because I always had considered achromatopsia to be a feature of occipital lobe lesions. I wondered if the visual radiations could have been affected by the parietal lesion, or, alternatively there might be a third lesion in the right occipital lobe. I made a mental note to look up the localizing value of hemiachromatopsia.

The general and neurologic examinations gave no hint of mechanisms. There were no signs of systemic illness and no abnormalities of the vasculature. The only findings were a slight tachycardia and a change in heart sounds of questionable significance.

I called the physician in Vermont who said that the onset of the left limb symptoms had been abrupt. CT had shown a hypodense lesion in the right parietal lobe, and cerebral catheter angiography on day three had been normal. Cardiac and hematological evaluation had been normal. The lesion looked like an infarct, and so he had used warfarin. I asked him to please send the CT and angiography, using the patient's wife as a carrier. I promised to call the physician after the evaluation and would of course send a summary.

With the residents and the stroke fellow, I began to plan the evaluation. The CT scan needed to be repeated, with and without contrast. If the process was an embolism, angiography had a much better chance of showing an embolus if it was performed within 48 hours of onset. Since M.G. had waited a day to come to the hospital, a plain CT was planned for the next morning, followed by angiography, and then followed by a repeat of the CT scan after the contrast angiography. (Magnetic resonance imaging [MRI], magnetic resonance angiogram [MRA], computed tomographic angiography [CTA], and transcranial Doppler [TCD] were not available at the time this patient was seen. The evaluation plan would be quite different today. Noninvasive vascular screening tests of the extracranial and intracranial arteries would be scheduled before considering catheter angiography.) I spoke to the neuroradiologist, Dr. W., to plan the angiogram. He and I agreed that it would be best to opacify the left anterior circulation first, followed by a right carotid artery injection. Posterior circulation opacification would depend on the results of CT and the findings on anterior circulation angiograms. I told Dr. W. that I would stop by during the angiography to review the initial films and we would then plan subsequent studies together. I asked Dr. W. to call me when he was starting angiography. Coagulation studies, lumbar puncture, and cardiac evaluation would also be necessary. I asked for a cardiac consultation and called to explain to the consultant that I was looking for a cardiac source of embolism. I also asked the resident to schedule an echocardiogram and Holter monitoring of cardiac rhythm.

I asked the staff to be sure to tell the patient's wife to visit early that evening and to remind her to call the Vermont physician to pick up the radiographs first. I would meet the patient and his wife and talk to them together. M.G.'s wife did bring the films. A CT 8 months ago had shown a small infarct in the right parietal area that extended deeply. The lesion went out to the periphery, was very well delineated and hypodense, and there was gyral enhancement nearby after contrast. The rest of the CT was normal, and there were no abnormalities on an arch angiogram that included good opacification of the intracranial right carotid and middle and anterior cerebral arteries.

Mrs. G. corroborated that M.G.'s neurologic symptoms started abruptly. She had eaten breakfast with him on the day he developed his recent symptoms, and he had seemed normal. When she came to his work site after being called by the foreman, his speech was very abnormal. Today, she said it had improved but was not nearly back to normal. During the interim between the two events, she had recognized no new attacks or symptoms. He had recovered well from the first event but had been slightly different in his personality since then—a bit more impulsive and talkative.

I explained to Mr. and Mrs. G. that I was worried about M.G. He was very young and had already had two potentially serious episodes of brain dysfunction. At present, I did not know for certain the cause of the problem. I would need tests and wanted to proceed quickly to try to make a diagnosis and begin treatment if any was available. M.G. seemed calm and remained quiet. Most of the questions came from his wife. I explained to them the indications and risks of the angiograms planned for the next day and they consented to them.

The next day, M.G.'s examination showed no appreciable change. He made a few more errors in spontaneous speech, but was jittery about the upcoming angiogram. Later that morning, Dr. W. called to say that he had the films from angiography of the left internal carotid artery. We looked at the CT together. There was a hypodense right parietal lesion identical to that seen 18 months ago. A new left posterior parietal lobe hypodensity involved the angular gyrus and far posterior temporal lobe just below the Sylvian fissure. There was also a small but definite hypodensity in the right occipital lobe in the distribution of the calcarine artery branch of the right posterior cerebral artery. The lesions were clearly infarcts. I asked Dr. W. if he thought they could be anything else, and he said no. Angiography showed an abrupt cutoff of the angular artery branch of the left middle cerebral artery. There was delayed filling in a retrograde fashion of the territory supplied by the angular artery. The left internal carotid artery was normal in the neck and intracranially. The intracranial anteroposterior views were adequate technically and no abnormality could be seen in the mainstem middle cerebral artery or in its superior or inferior division trunks. I and Dr. W. decided that a right internal carotid artery injection was an appropriate next step. I spoke briefly to M.G. and did a cursory motor and speech examination, which showed no change. After seeing other patients, I returned to the radiology department. The right internal carotid artery run had been normal, and the right posterior cerebral artery filled from the carotid artery. Dr. W. and I agreed that enough information had been obtained and the study could be stopped. M.G. was unchanged and had no new deficits.

Hematological and coagulation studies were normal. Prothrombin time and partial thromboplastin time were normal, and he had no lupus anticoagulant or anticardiolipin antibodies. Levels of complement, protein C, protein S, and antithrombin III were normal. Platelet function studies were normal. Serum protein and immunoelectrophoresis were normal, and the erythrocyte sedimentation rate was also normal. An echocardiogram was within normal limits, but the ventricular wall thickness was at the upper limits of normal and the ejection fraction was borderline. The cardiac consultant, Dr. R., said that the heart was normal and there was no cardiac disease. I asked about a Doppler study after an injection of air bubbles to look for an intra-atrial septal defect, but Dr. R. said it had not been done and was not indicated. I asked Dr. R. to do it anyway and that the alternative was a cardiac catheterization. Dr. R. resisted, but I insisted, saying that I would go to Dr. L., the chief of the cardiology department, if it weren't done soon.

I met with Mr. and Mrs. G. the next afternoon. I had decided to put M.G. on a continuous drip of heparin 24 hours after the angiography and after the coagulation battery had been drawn. The bubble Doppler was performed and was normal. The results had been called in to me that morning by a gloating cardiologist. I told the couple that there was still no definitive diagnosis. M.G. had definitely had three separate strokes. His blood and blood vessels tested normally. I was concerned that a "particle" could have come from the heart, but so far the results of the heart tests were normal. The cardiologist had found no abnormalities and the cardiac tests so far were equivocal. I told them that M.G. might need more heart tests. I also told them that I would order physical and speech therapy and explained to them the difference between aphasia and loss of intellect.

Mrs. G. said she was worried about her husband's work. Would he be able to return to work; if so, when? I asked for more description of his tasks at work. Did his work involve much reading and writing? Was there much complex verbal communication? There were very few written directions for him to follow, but he had to give oral and written reports to his supervisors each day. I said I did not know if M.G. would be able to return to the same job that he had before. It was much too early to tell if his speech and writing would improve enough to return to the same position. I was also concerned about whether his apraxia would prevent him from returning to his old job. I was cautiously optimistic. M.G.'s wife began to cry, and asked if she could talk with me alone. Outside the room, she broke down and said that M.G. had been very difficult to get along with since his first stroke. He was impulsive and had a short fuse, often yelling at her and the children. If he couldn't work, she didn't know what she would do. I tried to console her and explain to her that most stroke patients did improve but it might take time. I was especially optimistic because of his youth and obvious drive to get better. I discussed how she might be able to help her husband.

After going back into the room, I discussed the rest of the results of the investigations and possible treatment. No definitive cause for the strokes had been found. I told the couple that I was still suspicious of a minor heart problem, but, so far, the tests had not shown any definite heart abnormality. Because of my conviction that M.G. most likely had cardiac origin emboli, I prescribed Coumadin and explained to them the risks and the need for frequent blood drawing and monitoring. I talked about the alternatives. Cardiac catheterization could be used to look further for an unusual heart defect or disease; this test had a low yield in the cardiologist's opinion and had minor risks. I could prescribe no treatment, aspirin, or Coumadin. I told them that I felt uncomfortable with no treatment, and aspirin had not been well tested for patients with cardiac origin embolization, which was my working diagnostic impression. They said they would go along with Coumadin. When M.G. left the hospital, he was given a list of medicines to avoid while on the anticoagulant. I called his doctor and told him of the results. He agreed to the Coumadin and asked if I could see M.G. again in 3 months. I agreed and said that I would be available sooner if new problems or questions surfaced. M.G. preferred to get therapy near his home and so I asked his physician to arrange for speech and occupational therapy.

When I next saw M.G., his speech was improved. He could now repeat much better and made fewer naming errors. Reading was slightly better, but he still wrote very poorly. He seemed discouraged. He admitted to being "down" because of his inability to get back to work. His wife did not come with him; M.G. said she had to take the kids "someplace." I prescribed amitriptyline at bedtime, gave him a pep talk, and told him how pleased I was with his improvement.

Mrs. G. called about 5 weeks later to say that M.G. had had an episode that frightened her. His right hand and arm began to shake, his head turned to the right, and he had a convulsion. He had gone to the local emergency ward and had been seen by his local physician who had prescribed Dilantin. He had warned them that this could interfere with the Coumadin treatment, more frequent blood tests would be needed, and the Coumadin dose would need careful supervision for a few months after Dilantin was begun. She made an appointment for M.G. to see me.

During their next appointment, M.G. looked less depressed, and his language and writing were slightly but gradually improving. Mrs. G. held back tears. She asked if she could talk to me alone after the visit. She said that she was at the end of her rope. M.G. was not working, was at home all day, and seldom went out except for therapy. He was not interested in the kids or her and was now more like one of the children than her husband and partner. The seizure had "scared the hell" out of her. She talked for some time, and I remarked that she had been very strong so far and must remain strong for M.G. and the family to return to normal. She thanked me and I asked her to call in 1 week.

Nine months after his last stroke, M.G. returned to work with his company, but was given another job to perform. He liked his new work. He had had no new seizures. A year after his stroke, M.G. told me that his wife had left him. I was not surprised, as I had had prior experience with spouses abandoning patients who seemed to them like sinking ships.[6] M.G. said he was "not too upset." He would get along.

I asked him if he would mind my repeating his echocardiogram. I had read a journal report on atrial septal aneurysms as a relatively hidden source of emboli and had asked the echocardiographer to repeat this study and review the old films to make sure that an atrial aneurysm had not been missed. The echocardiogram was again repeated and no atrial septal aneurysm, cardiac septal defects, or valvular abnormalities were detected.

As of the summer of 1992, M.G. had not changed. He is still alone at home, sees his children occasionally, and continues to work. I see him about every 4 months. He has developed no new neurologic symptoms, but he has developed effort dyspnea and further cardiac studies showed that the ventricular myocardium was thickened, indicating myocarditis or a cardiomyopathy. He remains on Coumadin treatment.

PATIENT 2 (L.R.C.)

G.A. was a 44-year-old man. He came with his wife to see me in 1982 at my outpatient office at Michael Reese Hospital in Chicago. G.A. was a Russian immigrant who spoke only broken English. His wife spoke better English, but there was an interpreter present for the first visit to be certain that the history was accurate. Mr. and Mrs. A. had emigrated from Russia under some duress 5 years before. He was a professor of archaeology. They wanted to emigrate because they had been unable to practice their Jewish religion in Russia. G.A. was incarcerated after he put in his request to emigrate and spent 4 years in a camp somewhere in Siberia. Finally, nearly 8 years after his emigration request, he and his family got their papers. They first went to Italy and then came to Chicago 18 months ago. While in Milan, Mrs. A. had noticed a change in her husband's gait. His balance was poor, and he occasionally wobbled and fell. Since then, she thought his walking had become gradually worse. More recently, his speech had become slurred. A doctor in Italy had prescribed vitamins. She felt that G.A. had not been able to find work because of this problem and his lack of English proficiency. Through the interpreter, I asked G.A. about his symptoms. He said he did not feel "dizzy in his head," but his feet and legs were unreliable. He lurched to the sides, and he had particular difficulty on turns and walking downstairs. He had not noticed any change in his speech and denied all other symptoms, including headache. I noted some dysarthria as he spoke to the interpreter. There had been no prior important illnesses, but he had had typhus fever as an adolescent in Russia. He used no medications, over-the-counter preparations, drugs, tobacco, or alcohol.

There were two major symptoms: abnormal gait and dysarthria. I began to think of an anatomical diagnosis. Cerebellar lesions are notorious for causing ataxia and dysarthria, and I thought of cerebellar tumors, malformations, and even an Arnold-Chiari malformation. I then reminded myself that abnormalities of other systems could also affect walking: posterior column lesions, spasticity due to corticospinal tract dysfunction, even Parkinsonism and other basal ganglia diseases. I should ask again about sensory symptoms, sphincter abnormalities, and difficulty swallowing. Accurate anatomical localization would have to wait for the neurologic examination; I made a mental note to look especially for pyramidal and cerebellar signs.

I turned my thoughts to disease mechanisms. Gradual worsening during 18 months sounded most like degenerative disease or brain tumor. I would have to review with the couple the course of illness. Was he really worsening, or was their situation in Milan just difficult? Were there any periods of temporary improvement during this downhill course? Multiple sclerosis can affect individuals in their forties. Men often have a gradually progressive course and can have cerebellar and pyramidal tract demyelination. Many of the degenerative diseases are genetically determined and familial so that a thorough family history would be very important. Cancer is common in the forties and can be associated with central nervous system inflammation, degeneration, and metastases. In this case, unlike the first, there were too many uncertainties in the history to form any firm diagnostic impression at that time.

G.A. denied paresthesiae in his limbs or trunk. His general health had been good. He was not aware of anyone in his family who had any walking trouble or other neurologic disease. Most of his relatives were in "the old country." I asked if he would write to his brother in Russia to find out more recent details of the family history. I explored with the couple their criteria for judging his downward course. She described worsening in some frequent activities, for example, walking up the two-stair flight to their apartment and going three blocks to the store. There had been no improvement, even temporary, in his symptoms. She had noticed no intellectual or behavioral change.

On examination, G.A. was a tall, slightly overweight, black-haired man. His vital signs and general examination were completely normal. I looked very hard for possible signs of cancer—enlarged lymph nodes, hepatomegaly, clubbed fingers—but found none. Cognitive functions were tested with the help of the interpreter and were normal. His speech was definitely abnormal. Occasional letters were elided and slurred together. The rhythm was abnormal, with poor modulation of loudness and pitch. Occasional words were almost ejaculated quickly and explosively. Other cranial nerve functions were normal. His jaw jerk was not exaggerated, and he swallowed a cup of water normally. His strength was normal, but deep tendon reflexes were exaggerated symmetrically. Plantar responses were extensor. Finger-to-nose and heel-to-shin movements were performed very clumsily but without tremor. Alternating movements, such as patting alternately with the palm and back of the hand, were done very poorly. Sensory examination was normal. He walked with a wide base and veered and lurched to either side as he walked down the hall outside the office. Tandem walking was impossible. When he stood comfortably with legs apart, closing his eyes did not cause unsteadiness. After we returned to the examining room, he pointed to his genitalia and said "nyet." We called in the interpreter who translated to me that "he could not function like a man with his wife in bed." He had been impotent for 6 months and no longer had morning erections.

After the examination, the anatomy was more clear. The speech and gait disturbances and limb incoordination were clearly cerebellar. But there were also pyramidal signs and impotence, features compatible with a bilateral corticospinal tract problem in the brainstem or spinal cord. I tried to think of a single lesion in one place that could cause these signs. An unusual posterior fossa tumor or cyst? Arnold-Chiari malformation with pressure on the spinal cord at the cervico-medullary junction? The absence of sensory signs or nystagmus made this diagnosis less likely but not impossible. I had found no signs suggesting multiple sclerosis, but the history and examination were compatible with multiple demyelinating plaques. Cancer metastatic to the posterior fossa was possible. Spino-cerebellar or olivopontocerebellar degeneration came to mind, but the findings were atypical, as was the absence of any family history. Perhaps he had a spino-cerebellar degeneration secondary to cancer.

I told the A.s that I could not give them a diagnosis at present. I was concerned. More tests would be required. I gave them the option of admission to the hospital or outpatient evaluation, explaining the positive and negative aspects of both alternatives. They opted for hospitalization. I said I would like to order a CT scan before arranging the admission, and they agreed.

Routine blood studies, including B_{12} level, were normal. CT showed no definite abnormalities, except for possible slight prominence of the sulci between the cerebellar folia. He entered the hospital a week after the office visit. A lumbar puncture was normal. There were no cells, and the cerebrospinal fluid protein was 40. No oligoclonal bands were seen, and electrophoresis of the fluid revealed no abnormalities. After consulting with the neuroradiologist, Dr. P., G.A. had an amipaque myelogram with dye taken above the foramen magnum. CT of the upper neck and posterior fossa were performed after the myelographic films were taken. No lesion was found in the spinal cord or cervico-medullary junction. We performed a thorough search for a tumor. Upper gastrointestinal series, proctoscopy, chest CT, and intravenous pyelogram were all normal. Endocrine studies, including testosterone levels, were also normal. I sent blood to New York for antibodies to Purkinje cells and also sent blood and skin to another laboratory in New York to test for glutamic acid dehydrogenase deficiency (found in some cases of olivopontocerebellar atrophy).

During the dismissal interview, we discussed G.A.'s impotence, a great source of distress to them both. I told them that the impotence was most likely a part of his neurologic disease and was not psychological. I told them that I was not sure what was wrong with G.A. We had excluded most of the usual causes for his symptoms and all the causes that were readily treatable. I gave him baclofen in gradually increasing doses to see if it would improve his potentia and gait.

The baclofen did not help. Neither Purkinje cell antibodies or glutamate dehydrogenase deficiency was found in the specimens sent to New York. During the next year, his walking got gradually worse so that he needed help or a cane to navigate at all. No new findings or symptoms developed. I tried sequentially mysoline (it had been helpful in some patients with tremor), physostigmine, and isonicotonic acid hydrazide (INH) (reportedly helpful in some patients with cerebellar signs due to multiple sclerosis) with no success. The wife worked, but G.A. stayed at home, helping care for their two children. Both G.A. and his wife independently expressed to me their frustration at this "scourge" and how much they loved and admired each other despite the illness. Did I know of any other tests or doctors who could help?

I referred him to another neurologist at a different hospital in Chicago. His impressions and reasoning were no different than mine. He suggested trying Dantrium, which I did with no success.

In mid-1983, MRI became available privately in Chicago, but G.A. had no funds to pay. With a great deal of cajoling and pressure, I persuaded the Skokie Valley Hospital near G.A.'s home in Skokie to perform cranial and spinal MRIs. This study showed atrophy of the cerebellum, a normal brain stem and cervico-medullary junction, no demyelinative plaques, and a small spinal cord. Although we had no definitive diagnosis, I told G.A. and his wife that almost surely his problem was a type of degeneration of the cerebellum and spinal cord. Although the present symptoms might continue to worsen, it was unlikely that he would develop any trouble with his thinking, senses, or feeling. Although I knew of no medicine or other treatment that I was confident would reverse his symptoms, I was willing to keep trying if a promising treatment surfaced. G.A. received testosterone injections from a doctor in Skokie at his wife's insistence. He said that these treatments made him feel better but did not improve his sexual function or his gait. When I left Chicago in 1985, the situation had not changed. Since then, I have seen two other patients with cerebellar ataxia, decreased potency, and pyramidal tract signs and could not make a definitive diagnosis in either case. They must also have G.A.'s disease.

PATIENT 3 (J.H.)

This patient (A.C.) was initially seen in 1979. At that time she was an 18-year-old student in good health, until spring when bifrontal pressure-like headaches (left worse than right) began to occur daily. They were present upon awakening but diminished and disappeared in one to two hours. In July 1979 her penmanship deteriorated and her right arm seemed somewhat weaker. She developed slurring of speech. Two episodes of loss of consciousness occurred 4 weeks apart. There was no incontinence or noticeable seizure activity. On September 26, 1979, 3 days after the second episode, she was referred to me for neurologic evaluation. At that time, she could barely use her right upper extremity for eating. In the preceding week she had noticed weakness in her right lower extremity that had caused her to stumble, and blurring of vision that she localized to her right eye. Her general physical examination was normal. She had diplopia with vertical and horizontal image separation on gaze to the right and up but I found no definite oculomotor weakness. The angle of her mouth was asymmetric. There was minimal distal extensor weakness of the right upper limb with pronator drift. A deficit in the lower limb was seen only with vigorous functional testing. Deep tendon reflexes were slightly more active on the right with a Babinski response.

I admitted her for further investigation. I considered that her problem was serious. Multiple sclerosis is common at her age and may cause slurred speech, hemiparesis, and diplopia but the course was a progressive one and headache and recurrent loss of consciousness were more suggestive of an expanding posterior fossa mass.

Complete blood count (CBC), erythrocyte sedimentation rate (ESR), electrolytes, and liver function tests, urinalysis, and stool occult blood as well as a chest X-ray were performed to screen for obvious systemic tumor or vasculitis and were normal. EEG showed only background disorganization without seizure activity. CT scans of the head, 9/26/79 and 9/28/79 showed an enhancing mass, midline near the brainstem, causing hydrocephalus. The clivus was not well defined. A cerebral angiogram on 10/1/79 showed displacement of cerebral vasculature suggesting an extra-axial mass in the anterior portion of the posterior fossa. Fine arterial sprouting supplying the mass was observed. A mass in this area might include a chordoma or meningioma arising from the region of the clivus. Lengthy discussion with the family and the patient led to referral to Dr. Charles Drake in London, Ontario, because of his considerable neurosurgical expertise.

A right temporal craniotomy, on 11/28/79 revealed a firm, highly vascular, plum-sized mass that seemed to originate from the clivus. Four clips were placed and subtotal resection was performed. The tissue was compatible with chordoma. Subsequent radiation (6,000 centigray) in 35 treatments led to an uneventful recovery. The residual neurologic signs included a slightly wide-based gait, a right lateral rectus palsy, and right ear deafness.

During the next 20 years she completed her schooling, was able to move out on her own, worked as a retail stock clerk, and developed a stable relationship with a man. Fluctuating headaches with light-headedness and anxiety were a persistent problem. Despite all of my efforts, she could not be reassured that residual tumor was not still present.

Intermittent headaches began in 11/81. The headaches were characteristically present at awakening, sometimes throbbed, and were often accompanied by light-headedness and nausea. Although aspirin did not help, ibuprofen sometimes did. The cause of the headaches was not clear. Headaches occur in some patients after skull base surgery but not usually after headache-free years. The headaches were too protracted to be chronic paroxysmal hemicrania. She would also have times when the longer duration headaches were not present but she also described brief jabs like a red hot poker that went through her right eye to the occiput. These lasted only seconds. Her ophthalmologist never found any evidence of glaucoma. There was no associated conjunctival injection or tearing suggesting Short Unilateral Neuralgiform headaches with Conjunctival injection and Tearing (SUNCT).[7] The description was more suggestive of idiopathic stabbing headache (jabs and jolts, ice pick pains). I prescribed a variety of analgesics and migraine prophylactic agents without success. Headaches were sufficiently severe in 11/84 to keep her in bed until late afternoon. Headache frequency escalated so that by 6/87 they were a daily occurrence. She missed 2 to 3 days per month of work in 6/88. I considered whether she had developed chronic daily headaches with analgesic overuse (analgesic rebound headache). Headaches disappeared in the spring of 1991, but returned in November and were continuous, changing only in severity. I first noted a dilated right pupil in March of 1991. Review of office notes from 1988 and 1990 (both mine and an ophthalmologist's) specifically denied the presence of pupillary abnormalities.

Hypothalamic-pituitary dysfunction became evident. Abnormal menses culminated in complete cessation of menses in April of 1981. Premarin and Provera therapy was instituted after endocrine evaluation. She was only intermittently compliant because of side effects. Thyroid function was normal initially, but mild hypothyroidism and adrenal insufficiency were documented in June 1993 and treated with Synthroid and dexamethasone. Headache frequency and intensity seemed to increase with job stress and with periods when she was noncompliant with hormone therapy.

Naproxen seemed to offer some relief in the winter of 1992 but headaches recurred in the summer of 1992 following an episode of syncope—"falling into the hands of a clerk at a store" after feeling light-headed. Naproxen had been discontinued because of cost. During one dizzy spell in 1990, she slipped and fell descending the stairs and was hospitalized for a week with a fractured thoracic vertebra.

A.C. came to the emergency room on 6/28/94 for uncontrollable 5 to 10 minute episodes of crying, trembling, and slurred speech. These were unaccompanied by new neurologic findings and were thought to be anxiety attacks. Similar episodes continued intermittently.

In late 1997, A.C. began having episodes of right temporal-occipital pain of different character from her previous headaches. Episodes typically began with a funny feeling and then a patch of numbness over the temple, lasting 5 minutes, culminating in 10 to 20 seconds of severe temporal-occipital pain. Pain then subsided, but a remnant sometimes persisted for up to 10 days. Dizziness was an associated symptom. Episodes were sometimes precipitated by yawning or by repeated turning of her head. On 5/11/98 her neurologic examination was unchanged. At first, episodes were bimonthly, but increased to one attack every 1 to 2 weeks over the ensuing year.

On June 22, 1998, A.C. developed left-sided hearing loss, tinnitus, and vertigo. An otolaryngologist offered no specific diagnosis but recommended a trial of corticosteroids, which was unsuccessful and subsequent hearing recovery was minimal. In July of 1999 her neurologic exam was unchanged except for the now bilateral hearing loss. Was the hearing loss related to radiation-induced vascular damage? Was it caused by an independent process?

Throughout this period, the patient was not the only one concerned about tumor recurrence. She understood that this was a possibility from the outset and periodic imaging procedures were performed. These were initially CT examinations. Despite some potential risk because of the intracranial clips, at least two MRI examinations were done with low field strength magnets. This was probably unwise. These various studies (1984–1999) showed only postoperative changes with right temporal lobe loss and right cerebellar atrophy.

At age 38 (Spring 2000), A.C. developed recurrent headaches and dizziness. Medications included Prozac for depression, Rhinocort for chronic nasal drainage, Synthroid for thyroid replacement, and Fioricet and Tylenol No. 3 with codeine for her headaches. Symptoms continued intermittently for three months until she awoke at 3 A.M. (7/15/00) agitated and screaming with a severe headache. She was brought to the emergency room where her headache and agitation resolved with analgesics. She reported no alcohol or drug use. Toxicology screen was sent. Complete blood count (CBC), blood urea nitrogen (BUN), creatinine, glucose, electrolytes, and liver function tests were normal. Head CT scan showed no change. She was said to be lethargic and not oriented to place and time. Her heart, lungs, and abdomen were normal. However, at 9 A.M., she had vomited coffee-ground material and became lethargic. A short time later she vomited several more times and became unresponsive. After some delay for an abdominal X-ray ordered to look for free air under the diaphragm, I was able to see her. She was thrashing about with all four limbs. She did not respond to voice (deaf) or gesture and called out in an unintelligible manner. In addition to bilateral blurred optic disc margins, she had marked nuchal rigidity, Kernig's, and neck and leg Brudzinski signs. Much of her medical evaluation seemed inappropriately timed and not directed at her primary problem.

Lumbar puncture was obviously in order and findings included an opening pressure of 290 mm H$_2$O, 4653 nucleated cells (95% polys), protein 613, and glucose 44. Cryptococcal antigen was negative. Gram stain showed infrequent intracellular and rare extracellular gram positive cocci. Culture grew group B betahemolytic streptococci. Antibiotic therapy was instituted and the patient recovered. She had no findings that suggested an immunocompromised state.

A significant number of problems remained: Why should she develop meningitis with an unusual organism? What, if anything did this have to do with her tumor or radiotherapy? Why was she deaf? Why did she have headaches?

Initial attention was directed at the bowel as a site of potential infection and she underwent negative endoscopy. Echocardiography failed to show vegetations or other abnormalities. After a few days she had returned to her baseline mental status and she was able to respond accurately to written questions (while her lip reading was good, we could not be sure she grasped the subtleties in questions). At first she had positionally related headache that cleared on assuming a supine position. This was dismissed as a low cerebrospinal fluid (CSF) pressure headache due to the lumbar puncture. After several days the headache was a constant ache accompanied by nausea and brief stabbing pains as she had noted previously. A repeat lumbar puncture at this time showed a pressure of 230 mm, eliminating low CSF pressure as the culprit. A review of her history indicated that she had been having intermittent watery drainage from her nose. This was a cupful at a time of clear colorless fluid, which would gush from her nose. This had occurred most recently shortly before her recent illness. At the time there was no drainage. We thought that she might well have a CSF leak as the source of her unusual organism. While there was an air/fluid level in the sphenoid sinus, there were no areas of potential leakage of CSF detected on a thin cut CT. I thought that an isotope or contrast cisternogram might clarify the source of the leak, but decided to delay this study until she had resumed leaking. We knew that she was reporting nasal drainage but could not be sure it did not originate in the ear and pass through the eustachian tube to the nose. Review of the recent CT scan showed no fluid in the mastoid air cells.

The cause of her headaches remained obscure. I thought it necessary to rule out venous sinus thrombosis due to either the radiation or the more recent meningitis. A cranial CT venogram showed no venous thrombosis and no change in right posterior fossa abnormalities. During this admission she reported a bilateral continuous headache of moderate intensity and different from past headaches. The continuous headache, the stabbing pains, and the unexplained pupillary abnormality led to a trial of indomethacin therapy.[8] She responded dramatically to 25 mg indomethacin tid. She was discharged after a 4-week hospital stay (8/14/00).

There are many unanswered questions. I do not know if she will again have copious fluid flow from her nose, but will follow its occurrence with cisternography to define a possible CSF leak. Her headache remission may only be temporary and I will have to pursue the further historical aspects of her headache for therapeutic clues. There has been no evidence of tumor recurrence. Her radiation therapy is now somewhat remote and is unlikely to be a source of further neurologic deterioration.

PATIENT 4 (L.R.C.)

N.T. was a 28-year-old teacher who lived in Brookline, Massachusetts. She consulted me in 1971 at my office at the Beth Israel Hospital because of very bad headaches. Her headaches began when she was a freshman student at Harvard. At first, they were intermittent, one or two a week, but more recently, they were nearly constant. She described them as severe and threatening to become disabling. She was very worried that the headaches would interfere with her new job. She could not give me many details of the headaches or their character. Sometimes they throbbed and pulsed. She knew of no foods or activities that precipitated her headaches and never had preceding or accompanying visual, tactile, or vestibular symptoms. She knew of no family members with headaches. She had otherwise always been well. She took no medicines except birth control pills that she used because she and her husband had decided to "never have children."

Headaches are probably the most common problem brought to neurologists. The first step is to separate headaches secondary to serious systemic or intracranial disease from so-called recurrent problem headaches (migraine, muscle contraction, cluster, etc.). The latter group is much more common. In this patient, the very long duration, 10 years, and the complete absence of any mention of systemic or neurologic symptoms strongly favored one of the common headache disorders. I, however, needed to pursue this impression by pressing her further about systemic and neurologic symptoms and making certain on thorough examination that there were no important signs. The nature of the common headache problem was not clear from her account. These were not cluster. Moreover, the headaches had some features of migraine (pulsatility, age of onset, and initial intermittency) but other features of her headaches are found more often in patients with muscle contraction-tension headaches (constancy and lack of ability to describe the character of the headache).

She denied fever, joint pain, tick bite, weight loss, cough, or any other systemic symptoms. There had been absolutely no alterations in her concentration, thinking, recall, vision, hearing, strength, agility, feeling, or gait. She just could not describe the headache any better than she already had.

On examination, N.T. was a thin, boyish, outgoing, friendly person. Vital signs and general examination were completely normal. Her neck was supple, and there were no meningeal signs. She was alert and quick, and cortical function tests were performed normally. Cranial nerve functions were also normal. Careful attention to eye signs revealed no papilledema, and visual acuity, visual fields, and eye movements were normal. Her motor, sensory, and reflex functions were normal, and she walked naturally. The posterior neck muscles were sore and tender to palpation.

In discussing her problem after the examination, I told N.T. that I was confident that she did not have any serious problem inside her skull that was causing the headaches. I explained that her headaches were related to the blood vessels or muscles outside the brain. We spent some time discussing migraine and muscle contraction headaches and I urged her to pay more attention to the details of her headaches: precipitants, pace of onset, site, spread, character, duration, and accompaniments. I asked her to keep track of the headaches on a calendar on which she also would enter the timing of her menstrual periods and any unusual happenings of the day. I ordered some routine hematologic, serologic, and endocrine blood tests and told her to take two, five-grain aspirins for her headaches until the next visit in 6 weeks.

During the next visit, she was able to give a more complete account of the headaches. They started gradually about midday and very slowly worsened until evening when they reached a maximum. They began on the top of the head and spread to her forehead, back of the neck, face, and jaws. There were no preceding symptoms, and she had no nausea or vomiting during or after the headaches. Activity did not worsen and sometimes decreased the headache discomfort. During the headaches she was not especially sensitive to noise or light. They occurred daily, including weekends. At their worst, she also felt lightheaded. She had, at my request, asked her parents and siblings about headache, and none had had frequent or severe headache or "migraine." Headaches were not worse before, during, or after her menses. She denied any important stresses and said her spirits were excellent. She was happy at her work, felt challenged but confident, and her home life and marriage were ideal.

She had described typical muscle contraction, tension-type headaches, and examination showed muscular tightness in her paravertebral cervical region. Her blood tests were normal. The only uncommon feature was a lack of any obvious overt stresses or depression.

We had a long talk about the posited mechanism of muscle contraction headache. When muscles are continuously contracted, they begin to give off chemicals that cause discomfort, and the muscles pull on pain sensitive bony structures. I said that, in my experience, these headaches usually were caused by holding the neck in one position, neck injury or arthritis, migraine or other types of severe pain that triggered a pain-muscle spasm-pain cycle in the muscles on and supporting the head, or stressful states with anxiety or depressive feelings. I said further that, in her case, I could not be sure of the cause and I did not know her well enough to comment intelligently on any psychological factors. I asked her if she had any insights as to what could be the cause in her case. She said that she was puzzled and none of the usual causative factors applied to her case. Moreover, her headaches were "terrible and something had to be done." I prescribed a four-point program: (1) wet heat, for example, hot showers frequently to the head and neck; (2) massage with rubbing alcohol, wintergreen, or Bengay after the wet heat; (3) exercise, especially involving the trunk and neck, such as swimming, running, bicycling; and (4) Fiorinal taken regularly, one pill four times a day. I told her that the program would not work immediately, but she would have to follow it for at least 3 weeks, and at the end of that period she should call me. She seemed optimistic that the program would work and thanked me profusely.

On the next visit, she said the Fiorinal helped a little bit by taking the edge off the pain, but the headaches were still very severe. I added a muscle relaxant to the regimen. During the next 6 months, I saw N.T. four or more times. None of the medicines, including meprobamate, diazepam, amitriptyline, and imipramine had any effect on the headaches. She required more and more Fiorinal. I tried other analgesics to no avail. She always returned to see me undaunted. She always smiled and left optimistic that the next treatment would work. We got to know each other seemingly quite well. I explored with her various aspects of her work and home life. She always assured me that there were no problems. We tried physical therapy in an outpatient ward of the hospital, exercises in a nonhospital group, and biofeedback, all to no avail. She continued the Fiorinal, but I reduced the dose to three times a day. I asked an anesthesiologist to inject the insertion areas of the neck muscles on the occiput and at other times the regions of maximal tenderness. I tried nonsteroidal antiinflammatory drugs. Nothing seemed to help. Despite our failures, she always appeared at her appointments, seemed eager to see me, and approached the next treatment suggestion positively.

I often shared with her my perplexity and frustration at not being able to pin down the cause of her headaches or to treat them successfully. During the next few years, I did order some periodic tests: electroencephalogram (EEG), later CT, and blood tests, all with normal results. I continued to explore with her any stresses in her life, but she always laughed off any hint of trouble. During the first 6 to 9 months of our doctor-patient relationship, I had tense, negative feelings on the day of her appointments, and I felt anxious and frustrated, as well as puzzled, at the lack of success of any of the treatments. Of course, I had had other headache patients whom I had treated unsuccessfully, but they usually stopped coming. After a few years, I began to relax and took N.T.'s visits as a matter of course. I had fond feelings toward her and admired her courage and tenacity. I continued her Fiorinal, continued to explore gently her feelings and psyche, and halfheartedly tried different medicines, all without success.

One summer night, while I was at home writing, I received a call from the Beth Israel Hospital operator. She had an emergency call for me from Brookline, which I should answer right away because the caller was at a phone booth. I called the number and it was N.T. She sounded upset and was obviously crying. She said that she needed to talk to me. I asked her if the next morning was soon enough and she said yes. I consoled her.

The next day, she arrived early and paced the waiting room. She looked disheveled and unstrung. As soon as she got into the office and I closed the door, she began to sob. I calmed her and asked her to tell me what had happened. She related the most bizarre story. Her husband had 3 years ago developed pain in his leg after an injury. He used her Fiorinal. He also invited a male friend from work who was down on his luck to stay with them. Her husband, to her surprise, turned out to be bisexual and there developed a bizarre ménage-à-trois. Fiorinal and barbiturates became one of the prizes for participation in episodes involving the three housemates. At first she began to work in the evenings as a researcher to get away from the home situation. She loved this work and began to despise her human interrelations in her teaching job and at home. The story came out hurriedly, as if ejaculated from within. After she finished, I sat motionless, sweating. She thanked me for listening. I suggested that she and her husband needed help. She declined but said she had wanted to see me to tell me that she had decided to take no more Fiorinal. We talked about her possibly looking for a job related to research instead of her present teaching job. I continued to see her at monthly intervals. She eventually left her husband

and found a full-time research job. Six months after her confession, she told me that she didn't need to see me anymore. I learned from N.T. the importance of time, patience, and the value of simple support—being there.

PATIENT 5 (J.H.)

L.S. was a 39-year-old right-handed woman who was in good health except for a mild depression. On the morning of April 2, 2000, while going downstairs, she felt her left leg give out and she fell. Her husband heard a loud thump and found her awake but somewhat weak on the left side. She refused to have him call 911. When her weakness increased and she became more lethargic her husband called emergency medical services and she was transported to another hospital. In the emergency room there she was lethargic and had a left hemiplegia. A noncontrast enhanced CT scan showed an arachnoid cyst at the medial tip of the left temporal lobe but nothing else. I was contacted about possible IV rt-PA but was told that she had been unconscious and wondered about a possible seizure with Todd's postictal paralysis. She was transported to our hospital. At this point the history was reviewed with the patient and her husband and it was clear that she had been light-headed but had not lost consciousness. Seizure with postictal hemiparesis seemed unlikely. Risk factors included a 25-year history of smoking and the use of birth control pills.

On physical examination vital signs were normal (BP 165/55) but she was lethargic and inattentive. She could be aroused and briefly stay alert enough to obey commands and answer questions. After one or two responses she closed her eyes and required repeated stimuli to again attend. Head and eyes were turned forcefully to the right. It was difficult to distinguish visual neglect from a left hemianopia. There was no movement of her lower face on the left and her left upper limb was flaccid without movement. The left leg could be held above the gurney but drifted down. There was mild decrease in pin sensation on the left. There was neglect of the left side. Although she recognized her left side as her own she was unaware of her deficit. Further sensory examination was not considered reliable because of her lack of sustained alertness. I saw her just within the time window suggested for intravenous rt-PA but I thought that the patient had a major right hemispheral injury. Possibilities included a spontaneous internal carotid artery dissection or a major embolic occlusion. More data was needed. The angiography suites were occupied but an MRI could be obtained quickly. A moderate area of signal was seen on FLAIR and DWI in the right putamen and opercular areas and MRA showed an occlusion of the distal right internal carotid artery (ICA) and adjacent A_1 and M_1 segments of the right anterior (ACA) and middle cerebral arteries (MCA).

I considered it unlikely that IV rt-PA would help this extensive vascular occlusion. A review of reports that involved angiographic identification of sites of arterial occlusions and angiographic arterial opacification before and after intravenous thrombolysis showed that intracranial ICA occlusions rarely recanalized after intravenous treatment but more often opened after intra-arterial delivery of thrombolytic drugs.[9] I explained to the family (the patient did not seem capable of comprehending the issue) that she had a very serious problem that I thought was likely to leave her with a severe neurologic deficit—perhaps enough to render her incapable of self-care. I explained that intra-arterial rt-PA had been shown to be effective[10] but was not approved as such. I asked their permission to have an interventional neuroradiologist attempt to put "clot busters" in the blocked artery. I explained that I was worried about the area of damage shown on the MRI. Thrombolysis could result in bleeding into the site of damage. They understood the potential benefit and risks of the treatment and agreed to proceed. The interventional neuroradiologist also reviewed the problem and the plan. At about four to five hours after the fall on the stairs, 12 mg of rt-PA was infused into the right carotid, middle cerebral, and anterior cerebral arteries. The ACA (A_2 segment) was at little risk because of collateral flow from the anterior communicating artery and the MCA cortex was getting limited collateral flow from the posterior cerebral artery branches. The carotid artery and the mainstem MCA and ACA opened with rt-PA and an angioplasty balloon. There was a posterior Sylvian branch of the MCA that could not be opened. The results were gratifying and the patient's deficits resolved rapidly. There was only a slight residual left facial asymmetry and a left foot that tended to drop when she attempted heel walking at discharge 4 days later. Repeat MRI at discharge showed a 1-cm area of hemorrhage in the right putamen as well as an area of decreased density and swelling of the right basal ganglia, insula, and right temporal lobe.

The anatomic substrate of this patient's problem was clear but the mechanism remained undefined. Why had this occurred and how could another occurrence be prevented? Routine blood tests showed only an initial WBC count of 22,000 that rapidly fell to normal. Her arteries appeared normal on angiography except for the intraluminal filling defect at the top of the carotid. Her ESR and ANA were normal, which offered some reassurance about a systemic vasculitis. With a normal blood pressure and a normal 12 lead EKG she was unlikely to have an abnormal transthoracic echocardiogram so we moved directly to a transesophageal echocardiogram. There was no interatrial right to left shunt with Doppler and bubble contrast and the atria, aorta, and septum all appeared normal, as did the ventricles. A lipid profile the morning after admission was normal. A brother had had a myocardial infarction at age 44. Smoking and birth control pills were risk factors, but her young age suggested that we push forward. The possibility of a coagulopathy was next on the list even though she did not have a suggestive history. Platelet count, lupus anticoagulant, anticardiolipin antibodies, fibrinogen, protein C, protein S, antithrombin III, PCR for hypoprothrombinemia were all normal. She had reduced resistance to activated protein C but further studies showed that she did not have Factor V Leiden.

She was given Nicoderm to assist in smoking cessation. She and her husband were to meet with her gynecologist about alternate means of birth control. She was told that she probably had a rare genetic defect in coagulation.

I suggested that her two sisters be studied as well. One of the sisters tested positive. She might have factor V Cambridge or some other uncommon cause of resistance to activated protein C.[11] She was begun on warfarin therapy with a target INR of 2.5. She has two children and was worried about them. Her coagulopathy was well beyond my understanding of coagulation and so I referred her to a hematologist interested in coagulation.

She was depressed before her stroke, but depressive symptoms were much worse after the stroke. She had difficulty sleeping, with early morning arousals, and had loss of appetite. She was urged to resume more normal activity and an exercise program. Despite this she became more depressed, but her depression responded to an SSRI. Her cognitive performance seemed to be unimpaired except for some slowing of responses relative to her premorbid state.

These five case histories have explored different aspects of care of neurologic patients: diagnostic problems and reasoning, information giving, and treatment. Each patient was unique not only in neurologic condition but in personality and reactions. Each lived in a complex world that acted as an ecological backdrop to the illness. Fortunate, indeed, is the physician who is allowed, even invited, into this fascinating world of patients with nervous system diseases.

REFERENCES

1. Williams WC. Quoted by Robert Coles in *Patients, The Experience of Illness*. Philadelphia: W.B. Saunders Co., 1980;8.
2. Rodney J. *I Heal the Sick*. London: Elek Books, 1957;13.
3. Sacks O. *The Man Who Mistook His Wife for a Hat and Other Clinical Tales*. New York: Harper & Row, 1987.
4. DeRenzi E, Vignolo L. The token test: A sensitive test to detect receptive disturbances in aphasics. *Brain* 1962;85:665–678.
5. Haerer AF. *DeJong's the Neurologic Examination*. Philadelphia: Lippincott, 1992; 656.
6. Rosenberg M. *Patients: The Experience of Illness*. Philadelphia: W.B. Saunders Co., 1980;163–197.
7. Goadsby PJ, Lipton RB. A review of paroxysmal hemicranias, SUNCT syndrome, and other short-lasting headaches with autonomic feature, including new cases. *Brain* 1997;120:193–209.
8. Newman LC, Lipton RB, Solomon S. Hemicrania continua: Ten new cases and a review of the literature. *Neurology* 1994;44:2111–2114.
9. Caplan LR. *Caplan's Stroke: A Clinical Approach*. 3rd ed. Boston: Butterworth–Heinemann, 2000;124–130.
10. Furlan AJ, Higashida RT, Wechsler L, et al. for the PROACT investigators. Intra-arterial prourokinase for acute ischemic stroke. The PROACT II study: a randomized controlled trial. *JAMA* 1999;282:20003–2011.
11. VanderBorn JG, Bots ML, Haverkate F, Slagboom PE, Meijer P, deJong PT, Hoffman A, Grobbee DE, Kluft C. Reduced response to activated protein C is associated with increased risk for cerebrovascular disease. *Ann Intern Med* 1997;1326:832–833.

PART III

Types of Encounters

In the first two parts of the book, we have commented on all phases of the neurologist-patient interaction including examination, diagnosis, rapport, communication, and treatment principles. The interaction was discussed in general terms, without relation to site or other important participants, such as other physicians and neurologists, medical students and neurologic trainees, and nurses and other nonphysician personnel. In this section, we will elaborate on the site of care, consultations, and academic and educational aspects and interactions. Finally, we will touch on the growing neurologist-lawyer and courtroom interface.

10

Inpatient Care

The general wards where John Hunter received most of his tutelage in post-operative methods, hold about fifteen beds each. They were four-posters, their canopies reaching the ceiling, with heavy curtains hanging down to shut out draughts. As a further precaution against draughts, the patients wore nightcaps. One sack of coal a day was allowed to each ward in winter, half a sack in summer. By way of disinfection the floors and walls were washed down with vinegar. Twice a year a bug catcher assisted by the nurses and able-bodied patients tried to get rid of roaches.[1]

—J. KOBLER

Sights, sounds, and smells constitute a third feature of the hospital world so familiar to those who work there but not necessarily to those who are patients. Sights comprise more than the strange equipment that we have just described, and more than the variety of uniforms, mainly white. They include people in bathrobes, pajamas, nightgowns—the uniform that draws a sharp line between the patient and everybody else—or someone trying to walk down the hall on the arm of a nurse, taking tentative, halting steps, with a face marked by exertion and sometimes by pain. Sights also include people being wheeled by on stretchers. By and large the sights do not include rugs on the floor, frilly curtains, over-stuffed furniture, and so much of the familiar surroundings of home. There is every indication that this is an institution, not a home.[2]

—S.H. KING

I saw that one must oneself be a patient, a patient among patients, that one must enter into both the solitude and the community of patient-hood, to have any real idea of what "being a patient" means, to understand the immense complexity and depth of feelings, the resonance of the soul in every key—anguish, rage, courage, whatever—and the thoughts evoked, even in the simplest practical minds, because as a patient one's experience forces one to think.[3]

—OLIVER SACKS

Inpatient care and hospitals have changed drastically during the short history of the United States. At first, hospitals were relatively small, mostly charitable infirmaries where the ill, injured, and poor were given custodial care during long illnesses and before death. Starr clearly described the very drastic transformation of the health care industry within the past few decades.[4] Now, many health centers, especially academic institutions and for-profit conglomerates, are multimillion dollar operations that feature hospitals as their high-technology, high-visibility, high-rise, high-priced, high-cost showpieces. Physicians were once mostly independent entrepreneurs and practitioners who brought their patients to the hospital and dictated the care of the patients, the fee charged to the patient or payor, and the operation of the hospital. Now, governmental, industrial, and administrative rules, regulations, and operational hierarchies greatly compromise the independence of physicians, and their right and ability to manage patients according to their knowledge and instincts.

Patient care in the hospital in the modern era is very different from care in the doctor's office or outpatient clinic. Hospitals were previously regarded as major components of the health care system. Now insurance companies and governmental agencies see hospitals as cost centers to be avoided or limited. Diagnostic-Related Group (DRG)–based prospective payment systems or capitation systems attempt to control hospital payments. Hospitals, which are the only asset-based components of the health care system, must attempt to recoup their fixed costs from an increasingly hostile payor system. The lowest-cost provider may be sought for each task: licensed practical nurse (LPN) for registered nurse (RN), aide for LPN, pharmacy technician for pharmacist, physician assistant (PA) or nurse practitioner (NP) for physician. Another way for hospitals to reduce their overhead is to try to reduce lengths of stay, thereby allowing increased patient throughput and closure of nursing units to decrease staff costs. Payors may define patient days as "observation days" and then pay only outpatient rates for procedures done on those days. The net effect is to compress the patient's stay and force evaluation and treatment into less time and perhaps demand discharge before all results are in. The physician must either stay very close to the patient's evaluation or make some compromises in the logical sequence of the process, at a time when the hospital staff is increasingly stressed.

WHAT FEATURES OF THE HOSPITAL EXPERIENCE AFFECT THE DOCTOR-PATIENT INTERFACE

There are obvious advantages and disadvantages of inpatient care. Understanding both the positive and negative aspects should help guide physician behavior toward hospitalized patients. Let's examine the downside first. What's the bad news? Patients in the hospital are definitely, as a group, sicker than comparable outpatients. Utilization review committees and third-party payors now make it very difficult to admit patients to the hospital if they could possibly be evaluated and treated on an ambulatory basis. In a very basic and simplistic sense, people don't function as efficiently when they are sick as when they are well. When any of us has the flu or even a bad cold, our mental outlook, efficiency, spirits, and concentration suffer. Things that are ordinarily grasped quickly and readily when healthy take multiple exposures and repetitions to digest when we are under the weather. Sick patients are less effective historians and have more difficulty receiving information about their illnesses and treatment.

Hospitals are scary places to be in. The environment, the people, and the rules are very unfamiliar. Patients become depersonalized and lose their autonomy. When they first arrive, they are interviewed, usually in an office or the emergency ward, by a clerk who is charged with obtaining economic and billing information. Soon afterward, a hospital number and name tags are placed around the patients' wrists. Numbers are symbols of institutionalization that remind people of military "dog tags" or prisoner numbers. Jean Valjean in the musical *Les Miserables* sings about his imprisonment, "I am 24601." L.R.C. vividly recalls his thoughts during his own hospitalization while an intern at Boston City Hospital, when a name tag was slipped about his wrist. The tag made him remember a tour of duty as a pathologist when he was a medical student: The first reflex was always to check the wristband to make sure that the postmortem examination was performed on the correct patient. To this day, L.R.C. can never resist checking tags to ensure their accuracy. Gone are patients' own clothes; instead, they are given nondescript hospital "johnnies," which are usually quite different from any ordinary clothing, difficult to put on, and which expose patients' backsides, making them feel foolish and vulnerable. The food is not like at home. Patients are dependent on others to give them everything, including their own pills that they may have been taking themselves for years. Sometimes, they are not even allowed to go to the bathroom without permission or supervision. Unless patients have private rooms, there is absolutely no semblance of privacy. Other patients in the hospital are very sick, some are potentially contagious, and some are dying. Patients' belief in their own immortality vanishes very quickly, and every environmental cue reminds patients of their dependency and fragility.

Perhaps most frightening but also most powerful are hospital machines and personnel. Technology can heal and cure and yields incredible information about the mysteries of the human body, but everyone has heard or read of accidents and mistakes involving equipment. Machines have been known to collapse or deliver the wrong dose of irradiation. The workings of these machines are mysterious and frightening, especially to patients who are uneducated in their rationale and mechanism of operation (some, such as computed tomography [CT] and magnetic resonance imaging [MRI] scanners, are especially large and formidable). Many times, patients having a technical procedure do not see the physician in charge of the evaluation. They see only technicians who may or may not instill confidence that they know what they are doing.

In addition to machines, the hospital is full of people dressed in all manners of different uniforms. The patient literally needs a program to tell who does what with whom. Even when medical staff introduce themselves properly ("I am the neuromuscular disease fellow" or "I am the staff reproductive endocrinologist"), most patients still have little understanding of what function each caregiver has and how he or she relates to the overall schema of their care in the hospital. It is now very difficult to tell nurses from aides or technicians or house officers. Everyone may dress in similar garb and the identification tags may list only a first name and, in smaller print, an ambiguous title. Regarding the medical students and house officers, it is nearly impossible to tell who does what and their relative roles and power in the medical pecking order. Not only do the sheer numbers and heterogeneity of players confuse the patient, but there are two other concerns that patients have mentioned to us with increasing frequency. The first issue concerns coordination and integration of medical personnel. Do all these people talk to each other? When and how thoroughly? Who coordinates the data and is in charge? Patients are well aware that their doctors have other patients and other things to do and places to be such as their offices. If the attending physician (their doctor) sees the patient for only a brief visit each day, how can he or she really keep close tabs on what is happening to them in the hospital? Is there order in the seeming chaos? The second important concern relates to patient-perceived conflicts and clashing egos. Physicians are admittedly bright, ambitious, and often independent people. Patients are quick to pick up differences in style, variance in opinions, and competition among medical personnel. Open or implied criticism by one health provider of another fuels this sense of conflict. Patients may sense, especially if they are sensitive or naive about hospital dynamics, that they are in the middle and are the source of the dispute. Patients also recognize that some students, house officers, and staff lack polish, confidence, information, and power. Patients feel fragile in the hands of these individuals and hope and pray that the junior staff is being carefully and effectively supervised.

We have so far dwelled on the down side for the patient of being sick and in the hospital. What about the up side? For the doctor, there are definite advantages in having the patient hospitalized. Being confined to a bed in a specific locale in the hospital, the patient is nearly always available. The history and physical and neurologic examination findings can be checked and rechecked. Questions the physician forgot to ask initially can easily be pursued later. Prior answers can be elaborated on. Physical signs can be confirmed. Parts of the examination that are tedious and time consuming and require sustained patient cooperation, such as sensory testing and higher cortical function examination, can be done gradually and sequentially.

The availability of the patient also makes it possible to follow firsthand the course and progression of the illness. Health planners and utilization reviewers often naively consider hospitalization as a time for laboratory and procedural testing and treatment. Forgotten is the inestimable value in observing the acutely ill patient over a period of time. The development of new symptoms, new signs, and the course of resolution or progression of known abnormalities are often critical for accurate diagnosis. We have already mentioned but now reemphasize the great importance of repeatedly examining the patient with neurologic illness. The physician should not assume from the patient's report of no new symptoms and no change in ability to function that the admission findings are unaltered. After giving the hospitalized patient treatment that is expected to have acute effects, the physician can watch, document, and quantitate the results of that treatment by observing the patient and by sequential laboratory studies such as brain and vascular imaging, blood tests, and lumbar punctures. In regard to outpatients, all too often the physician must depend solely on the report of the patient as to whether the treatment helped the symptoms.

In the hospital, laboratory tests can be ordered and performed more efficiently, and rapid sequential decisions can be made. Let's use as an example a patient who describes unusual spells or episodic, poorly characterized central nervous system dysfunction. The physician might have great difficulty scheduling CT or MRI scans, electroencephalogram (EEG), ambulatory cardiac monitoring, noninvasive vascular ultrasound tests of the extracranial and intracranial arteries, and a five-hour glucose tolerance test all in the same or successive visits to an outpatient testing area. If they all could be scheduled, the results of one test, for example, an EEG with a definite seizure focus or an electrocardiogram (EKG) showing paroxysmal runs of ventricular tachycardia, might obviate the need or urgency for some of the other tests. There is little opportunity in outpatient facilities, with the exception of a very few efficiently run sites such as the Mayo Clinic, to review the results of previous tests sequentially before deciding on the next investigation. If the physician chooses sequential testing on an outpatient basis, this decision usually means multiple trips on multiple days to the outpatient testing facility, dragging out the time needed for diagnosis and making the patient more impatient and anxious. When the same patient is evaluated in the hospital, tests can be managed more easily, and results can be reviewed or called in before a decision is made on the need for the next test. Careful scheduling might allow an MRI, extracranial duplex, transcranial Doppler (TCD), and transesophageal echocardiogram to be completed in one or two days, allowing for a thoughtful decision on angiography to be made and discussed with the patient.

Consultations are also more easily and more quickly managed in the hospital. Many consultants are specialists and subspecialists whose major work is in the hospital. They live, so to speak, at least part of the time where the patients are housed. With the hospital record and house officers and other physicians readily available, physician intercommunication is theoretically easier in the hospital. It is rare that a complex patient evaluation can be performed in the office at a level of efficiency that can be achieved in an inpatient setting.

The presence of multiple and heterogeneous staff and of students and trainees at all levels has its positive as well as negative aspects. All these individuals want to help the patient. They provide ideas, some perhaps that the patient's own physician had not considered. They also provide an important checks and balances system. Americans love counterbalances and generally distrust monarchies and oligarchies; witness our complex and inefficient governmental system, with its many protections from autocracy. The responsible physician's behavior—diagnosis, testing, and treatment—is being carefully watched by others. Those low in the pecking order would love nothing better than to one-up their seniors or supervisors in the medical or academic hierarchy. The residents, fellows, and junior staff delight in outshining the professor. The community practitioners gloat at showing up the academics, and academics like to demonstrate the inferiority of the practitioners. This competition, usually friendly, innocent, and lighthearted (although it makes some patients uncomfortable), is also a protection and advantage as long as the different players and ideas are being coordinated. J.H. recalls evaluating a man with obvious acromegaly. Review of his hospital record of 5 years earlier showed a third-year clinical clerk note that listed possible acromegaly. On that occasion, no senior physician addressed the clerks findings or thoughts.

The constant presence of the patient can facilitate communication between physician and patient. Diagnosis, patient education, and all aspects of the communication interface described in Chapter 7, can potentially be facilitated in the hospital. Messages can be given piecemeal, a little bit at a time. Information can be given sequentially. We have already commented on the limitations of patients, especially when sick, in being able to handle a lot of complex information in one sitting. During a hospital stay, physicians have the opportunity to present information a little bit at a time, to repeat and review information, and to field questions. Individual patients often require time to digest and think about personal health information in order to ask questions. In the office, the interchange is so rapid that patients are often unable to grasp the significance of the information in time to be able to ask meaningful questions. Health planners see no problem in giving the patient the diagnosis, diet, medication instructions, activity limitations, plans for follow-up, and discharging the patient on the same day. To the extent that the information process can begin early and be repeated and developed during the hospital stay, some of the limitations of the "new health care" can be minimized.

Most ill patients who are not recluses or destitute have visitors. Family, friends, lovers, close associates, and even creditors may appear at some time during the hospital stay. Their absence says a great deal about patients and their plight. The patient's presence in the hospital affords the physician the opportunity to meet these significant others, obtain independent historical data, and communicate important information about the patient's illness, treatment, and prognosis. The same opportunity is less often available when the patient is seen as an outpatient.

For the clinician who is a student of the nervous system and of human responses, the patient can be the laboratory.[5] Concentrated exposure to an inpatient during a period of illness, whether that illness lasts three days, three weeks, or three months, allows the physician to ponder findings, test hypotheses, document ideas, and make advances in knowledge. Daily personal encounters with patients and the opportunity to discuss thoughts and findings with colleagues and consultants facilitates physician learning and discovery. As Osler said, "The important thing is to make the lesson of each case tell on your education. The value of experience is not in seeing much, but in seeing wisely."[6] There is also more opportunity to search the literature for help. All this can be done with outpatients but is more difficult during the short-term and decreased intensity of the single encounter. The hospital can and should be an excellent place for learning: for the physician, an opportunity to learn about patients and their diseases, and about medicine and neurology; and for the patient, a chance to learn about the illness.

THE INITIAL EVALUATION

The clinician should see the patient on the day or evening of admission. A full history and physical examination should be performed if the patient has not been seen before. If available time is limited that day, at least a partial symptom inquiry and examination should be performed and then completed the next day. If the patient has already been seen and examined as an outpatient, at the time of hospitalization the clinician should review the notes from the previous outpatient visits, then briefly review with the patient the salient historical points, and perform an interim examination to determine if the signs have changed.

Most patients are very naive about hospital rules and routine. Especially in an academic medical center, patients may be quite unprepared for trainees. It is always best to warn the patient, either before admission or during the initial inpatient visit, about what to expect during hospitalization. The patient should be told who will be likely to perform admission examinations. The roles of these individuals should be discussed, including the rationale behind these examinations and possible benefit for the patient and the trainees. We usually tell patients that we have purposely not shared data with the student and resident and have instructed them to start from scratch. The clinician should emphasize that he or she will personally take responsibility for supervising and coordinating the findings of all of these individuals. If investigations are planned, the procedures should be briefly described and explained.

If the patient will be cared for in an academic health center and trainees or students at any level will participate, it is best to allow them to face the patient without detailed preliminary knowledge of the neurologist's findings or thoughts and without the results of prior investigations. The chance for trainees to bring forth independent findings or ideas will often be lost if these impressionable individuals are biased by preliminary information. The admission history and physical examination should be a learning experience for the trainees and not just a routine pro forma procedure. At times, the seriousness of the patient's illness and the need for urgent diagnostic evaluation and treatment will obviate this leisurely approach. During the first 24 to 36 hours of hospitalization, the students and house officers should have taken careful and detailed histories, performed meticulous examinations, and recorded their findings, differential diagnoses, and plans of evaluation and treatment. The trainees should have an opportunity to review their findings and thoughts among each other. The responsible clinician should then review the trainees' findings, diagnoses, and plans and discuss any differences of thought with the group or the most senior resident. A modus operandi should be agreed upon. The shift in residency education to a more outpatient-based experience makes this critical aspect of patient care more demanding on both senior physician and house officer. After the initial evaluation period, the patient should be prepared for the upcoming procedures, tests, and treatments planned. The preliminary step of agreeing on a plan among the physicians should obviate embarrassment for all parties when gaps in communication become obvious to the patient. A responsible clinician feels foolish when a patient asks about a procedure that a resident has scheduled and discussed with the patient without the clinician's knowledge and acquiescence. Remember, also, that trainees look very inept if they do not know what is planned. All parties should work together as a team.

DAILY CARE AND SUPERVISION

During the hospitalization, the clinician should see the patient each day. Usually once a day suffices. If patients are very ill, changing rapidly, or unstable, they may need to be seen more frequently. When physicians are not on site, they should be able to be reached quickly by hospital staff. The senior clinician's visit is for many patients the high point of the day and is anticipated because of its importance. Don't treat the visit casually or turn it into a merely social occasion. Try to make the visit appear unhurried and yet efficient. During each visit, be sure to ask the patient whether his or her symptoms have changed and if new symptoms or problems have developed. After discussing the major illness, turn to other patient concerns. Little things or minor deviations from the norm seem to be magnified by the hospitalized patient. Patients focus on sleep, food, gas, bowel changes, annoying rules or interruptions or awakenings, noisy roommates, and so on. Perhaps these seemingly trivial concerns distract them from the painful anxiety that surrounds their neurologic problems. Give the patient a chance to tell you about these inconveniences and, when appropriate, prescribe symptomatic relief, such as minor sleeping sedatives, laxatives, or anxiolytics. Though these minor symptoms may seem very insignificant to the clinician in the context of serious disease, every detail is important to the patient.

On each visit, perform at least a brief physical examination or look at some physical sign. Hands-on contact—touching—is very important and therapeutic and reassures the patient of the closeness of the relationship.[7] The daily examination has three major functions: to monitor progression or improvement in signs, to look for complications of the illness or treatment, and to uncover new clues that might clarify or elaborate on the working diagnosis. In all cases, even when the examination is cursory, it should be hypothesis driven. In fact, we argue that, because of the brevity of the examination, it is even more essential that the clinician vigorously extract the utmost out of the short time spent. Before leaving the patient's bedside, restore to the patient's reach the nurse call button, phone, water pitcher, urinal, bedside table, eyeglasses, TV control, and whatever else was moved aside during the examination. This is especially critical when mobility is limited and the bedside table is the patient's total world. A colleague recovering from a serious illness commented on this and J.H. began to monitor his own behavior and discovered how often he was guilty of not paying attention to restoring the patient's bedside environment.[8]

Let's look at some case examples to illustrate the thought processes behind interim examinations. A middle-aged woman has been admitted because of confusion, somnolence, and low-grade fever. Your initial evaluation on day one showed a confused, inattentive patient with no focal signs and slight asterixis. CT and spinal fluid evaluations were normal, and no diagnosis has been established. You suspect a toxic-metabolic process and believe that the neurologic findings are caused by systemic illness. You concentrate on looking for evidence of organ failure such as kidney, liver, or pulmonary disease and occult infection such as endocarditis or an abscess. You listen for a murmur, look for signs of microembolism in the eye, fingers, and limbs, examine the abdomen for liver tenderness, splenic enlargement, and a local mass, and carefully listen to the lungs. You see if a flap is still present. You spend little if any time on looking for focal signs, but speak to the patient briefly to assess her present degree of confusion compared to that on admission.

Another patient is admitted with focal seizures affecting the left arm and is treated with a rapid intravenous infusion of phenytoin. You check for signs of right hemisphere dysfunction and quickly examine motor, sensory, and visual functions on the left and ask the patient to copy a diagram. You also look for signs that might correlate with a high phenytoin level, such as dysarthria, nystagmus, ataxia, somnolence, and a rash.

In some patients, the admission neurologic examination is suboptimal because of the patient's fatigue or confusion, decreased alertness, concentration, or cooperation. The patient may have received benzodiazepines for a seizure in the emergency department. When and if these initial problems improve, seize the opportunity to examine those functions that could not be evaluated properly on admission. Make a mental note to later assess functions that for any reason cannot be tested now. Unfortunately, many physicians, especially trainees, consider the clinical evaluation ("the admission H and P") to be the province of the first day or two in the hospital. Many patients leave the hospital without ever being fully examined. Laboratory tests, no matter how thorough, do not supplant or substitute for thorough analysis of the symptoms and signs.

Before or after seeing the patient, check the chart for the results of investigations, and notes and orders by other physicians, nurses, and health care workers. Seizures are rarely well described in the hospital chart. If time permits, check with the nurse responsible for your patient to see if he or she has anything to tell you about the patient's condition or behavior. Nurses are key individuals for sick patients. They are with the patient for much more time than any physician. Some patients confide to their nurses information and worries that they have not shared with their doctors. Nurses are often in a position to observe behavior during "spells" and to notice interpersonal problems during interactions with visitors. Patients ask nurses questions about their illnesses and tests that they are wary of asking their doctors or have asked and did not receive answers that satisfied them. Take a minute to talk to the nurse; provide a progress report, and answer any questions he or she has about the patient. Preserve good rapport and communication with the nursing staff; be sure they know that you appreciate their work and their professionalism.

On at least some of the daily visits, sit down in a chair or, with the patient's permission, on the patient's bed. Standing indicates that you are poised to move on. Use this time to discuss the diagnosis, provide the results of tests to date, describe upcoming tests, treatments, and procedures, and gradually educate patients about their illnesses. Answer questions. The visit should be a dialogue, not a monologue or a lecture.

If at all possible, try to visit patients on weekends. Saturday and Sunday are lonely days in the hospital. Activity abates and time seems to stand still. L.R.C. vividly recalls being very ill with hepatitis while a medical student. His physician, though not a hepatologist, faithfully came each day, including the weekends, to see and encourage him and let him know that he was fully aware of what was happening. Covering physicians can handle urgent decisions, but cannot really adequately substitute in patients' minds for "their doctor." Your appearance on a Sunday tells the patient that you care. If you cannot come in, a telephone call is next best.

REVIEWING RESULTS OF INVESTIGATIONS

The effective clinician anticipates circumstances in which errors and slip-ups are common and tries to prevent their occurrences. Check and double check. Misinterpretation, misreporting, and nonreporting or lost reports are common hospital problems that can lead to important errors in diagnosis and treatment and potential litigation. What should the clinician do to prevent these problems?

With respect to the clinician, tests can be simplistically divided into two types—those that are directly within the training and experience of the clinician and those that are not. This division does not relate merely to board qualification or certification. Neurologists have heterogeneous training and subspecialty interests. Many tests were and will continue to be introduced long after formal residency training. CT, MRI, noninvasive vascular extracranial ultrasound tests, TCD ultrasound, evoked potentials, and single fiber electromyogram (EMG) were all introduced after our formal neurologic training ended. Some of these investigations we feel quite competent in viewing and interpreting and others we do not. Even within one technological modality such as CT or MRI, there are great limitations in our own competence. We may feel well equipped to interpret cranial CT, but much less adept in analyzing images of the spine without help.

Few neurologists have any capability in interpreting the results from new technology far removed from their experience and training, such as ultrasound of the pelvis, echocardiography, and immunoassays, among many other tests. Competence is, of course, not always a black and white distinction; there are relative grades of competence. L.R.C. feels relatively confident when looking at chest X-rays, electrocardiograms (EKGs), upper gastrointestinal X-rays, and intravenous pyelograms, but completely at sea when shown a pelvic ultrasound or an electronystagmogram. J.H. is quite at home with imaging and much less so with electrophysiology.

When the responsible neurologist is competent with a particular test or technology, it is imperative that he or she reviews the raw data, whether it is images, tracings, or numbers. Knowing both the details of the clinical data in the patient and the technical aspects of the study gives the neurologist a great advantage in interpreting the meaning, clinical relevance, and importance of the investigations. A written report of a cranial CT, regardless of the capability of the reporter, never substitutes for looking at the films. The neurologist knows exactly what to look for. Important questions are not always answerable by a simple yes or no and often cannot be gleaned from reports.

Let's give two examples. You admit a 70-year-old man because of confusion, low-grade fever, and weight loss. You are not certain if the confusion is due to a systemic or toximetabolic process or to a degenerative cerebral process with atrophy. The resident tells you that the neuroradiologist, an expert in his field, has seen the CT scan and thinks it is normal; the brain substance is consistent with age. What can you conclude? It's probably safe to assume that your patient does not have multi-infarct dementia due to large artery or penetrating artery infarcts and does not have a large supratentorial tumor. You still wonder: How technically good were the films? Did this confused patient move and produce motion artifacts? Was the posterior fossa well seen? Exactly how large were the ventricles and the sulci? Was there any disproportion between the fourth and third ventricles and the lateral ventricles? Were the ventricles small, average, or a touch on the large side? All these size gradations might fit well within the bell-shaped curve of normality for age, but would have quite different clinical meanings. Small ventricles would effectively exclude chronic Alzheimer's or Pick's disease. Smaller-than-average ventricles, however, would be quite consistent with Creutzfeldt-Jakob disease and might even raise the possibility of bilateral subdural hematomas[9] and make you wonder if the study is technically sufficient to exclude this possibility. When you ordered the CT scan, neither you nor your residents had thought of this diagnosis and had not written "possible head injury" or "subdural" on the requisition or mentioned it in the initial discussion with the neuroradiologist. Many general radiologists do not distinguish between brain anatomy and vascular territory in a clinically meaningful fashion.

Another patient is hospitalized with a myelopathy of gradual onset and has spasticity, extensor plantar responses, numb hands, and loss of vibration sense in the feet. You are told that the neck X-rays show "neck arthritis." This interpretation is nearly useless. You want to know if the spondylitic changes affect the dural space enough to explain the myelopathy. Is there subluxation or impressive posterior osteophytes encroaching on the spinal cord space? What is the measurement of the space between the posterior border of the body of the vertebrae and the anterior aspect of the spine at the smallest diameter?[10] Perhaps one in a thousand reports by radiologists (nonneuroradiologists) contains this information, but we have not seen such an adequate report in the past 30 years.

Nothing quite replaces looking at the films yourself in these examples and in nearly all patients. In hospitalized patients, nearly all investigations are performed and are available on site, a distinct advantage over most outpatient circumstances. When tests are not done at the hospital, for example, an off-campus MRI or CT, copies of the films as well as the interpretation should always be sent to the hospital. The best of all circumstances is to look at the films with the neuroradiologist, with the opportunity to ask questions about any of the important points. Next best is to see the films yourself and read the radiologist's report. Less effective, but sometimes acceptable, is speaking to the neuroradiologist in person or by phone, with a chance to ask questions about the details and quantitative aspects of the films. Depending on written reports is seldom satisfactory. We have already commented in Chapter 6 on the value of tracing some films in the hospital record for easy later access.

When you are familiar with tests but not expert, try whenever possible to review the films or data with the test interpreter or an expert. We know of numerous instances of litigation surrounding the question of missed findings or erroneous or late reporting. Years ago, L.R.C. evaluated a middle-aged woman who was hospitalized because of the new onset of focal seizures. Careful clinical examinations, CT, angiography, and spinal fluid analysis all gave no clues as to the cause of the seizures and the patient was appropriately told that follow-up and repeat investigations would be needed. She later sought care elsewhere and died two years after admission with widespread cancer. The family initiated a lawsuit against L.R.C. and the hospital radiologist because in retrospect there was a suspicious finding on the chest X-ray taken in the hospital that had been reported as normal. L.R.C. had never personally seen these chest films.

A 63-year-old woman was admitted to the hospital with a severe cerebellar ataxia that worsened during the following weeks. She also had personality changes including memory loss and emotional lability. Plantar responses were extensor. Evaluation had included a normal contrast enhanced CT scan, MRI, and spinal fluid including cytology in addition to routine chest X-ray, complete blood count (CBC), erythrocyte sedimentation rate (ESR), chemistry profile, urinalysis, stool occult blood, and a vasculitic profile. Paraneoplastic cerebellar degeneration was considered. Anti-Hu antibodies were not then readily available. CT of the chest, abdominal CT, and gynecologic consultation were negative. A pelvic CT was then obtained that was reported as showing a benign ovarian cyst. Despite the fact that J.H. was not competent to evaluate ovarian pathology, he accepted this report without consulting the gynecologist again.

The patient was referred elsewhere for rehabilitation and was seen by a number of other neurologists. After a year, the patient returned with ascites and far advanced metastatic ovarian carcinoma. J.H. went back over the previous pelvic CT with the gynecologist who pointed out that he should have ordered a pelvic ultrasound and should have been suspicious of benign ovarian cysts in postmenopausal women. When J.H. informed the woman's sons, they did not sue for malpractice but expressed their anger in forceful terms. J.H. failed to utilize the readily available help in an area where he needed it.

In other instances, questionable or possible lesions on chest films or gastro-intestinal X-rays have been noted and described in radiology reports, but either the findings were not called to the attention of the responsible senior clinician, or the report was unavailable at the time of discharge and was later placed in the hospital record, or the report never reached the hospital chart or the clinician. For whatever reason, miscommunication or failure to communicate is common. Hopefully, new computer capabilities and quality review and systems personnel in the hospital will supervise and minimize these problems. The clinician must remain vigilant and develop a system for handing test results unavailable on discharge.

The preceding discussion and examples have emphasized radiographs and imaging procedures. The same problems and rules apply to other investigations except that the interpreter is more often a specialist in a different field. Let's briefly look at two examples. You hospitalize a young patient with the sudden onset of a left hemiparesis and hemianopia. CT shows a possible right cerebral infarct. An echocardiogram is interpreted as normal. We are totally incompetent in looking at echocardiograms. We would need to discuss with the cardiologist whether the study was adequate in excluding an inter-atrial septal defect or patent foramen ovale or a cardiomyopathy. Was a bubble contrast Doppler study done? What was the ejection fraction? Seeing the study would not give us the answers to those questions, and, unfortunately, many formal reports do not satisfactorily include this data.

Another older patient is admitted with confusion, cough, asterixis, and a high serum CO_2 level. There is muscle atrophy; the limbs are weak, and reflexes are diminished. The patient smokes and has chronic lung disease. You order pulmonary function tests and the report of the pulmonary consultant who interpreted the results and the raw data is available in the hospital chart. You wonder if the findings are due solely to the patient's chronic bronchitis and emphysema or is there hypoventilation due to a neuromuscular disorder? Only discussions with the pulmonary consultant will suffice to answer this question, and more testing may be necessary.

COMMUNICATION BETWEEN DOCTOR AND PATIENT IN THE HOSPITAL

We have already commented in the first part of this chapter on the advantages of inpatient status for doctor-patient communication. Judgment is required to decide when to begin serious discussions about diagnosis, prognosis, and treatment. How much information should be shared? Should the family and significant others be included and, if so, when?

By the time the patient leaves the hospital, diagnosis should be discussed. In some, the diagnosis may have been made before admission and already discussed on an outpatient basis. In some patients, the diagnosis may still remain unsettled at discharge; if so, this status should also be communicated. Harm can be done by premature sharing of differential diagnostic possibilities or preliminary diagnostic opinions that later prove wrong. What would your response be if you as the patient were told by your doctor that you "probably" had a brain tumor and later your condition was diagnosed as a stroke or a medicinal side effect? What would these shifts in opinion do to your confidence in your doctor? Who is to say that the latest diagnosis is correct or if it will be changed later to something else? Suppose that your car repairman tells you it is the motor that is responsible for your car failing to start and replacing it or fixing it will be expensive. He later calls you to say that he erred and it is only the spark plugs. How much confidence would you have in your car repairman?

When there is diagnostic uncertainty, don't be afraid to share this fact with the patient and family. If the diagnosis is uncertain, however, you as the responsible physician must be prepared to demonstrate to the family that you are taking all appropriate steps to clarify the diagnosis or at a minimum are excluding those conditions that are reversible or remediable.

Wait for the "right time" to discuss diagnosis. The major determinants that guide timing are the nature and certainty of the diagnosis and the patient's wish to know the diagnosis and receptivity to discussion. Definite good news should be shared as early as possible. Some patients do not want to be told the bad news by their doctors right away. They have gleaned from clues, facial expressions, indirect allusions, and by the nature of their treatment that they have a serious problem with a bad outlook. Hearing the words "you have a malignant brain tumor" or "you have motor neuron (Lou Gehrig's) disease" might give a finality to their lives that they are presently unprepared to handle. Do not shove the diagnosis down the patient's throat. Seek clues from your daily interchanges with patients. Do they ask direct questions about their diagnoses? Do they press you or other doctors about information regarding their condition? Or do they seem to change the topic every time you begin to talk about their diagnosis or condition? By the time of discharge, the patient, the family, or the caregivers should know the nature of the illness and the certainty of the diagnosis. At the bare minimum, the physician who will assume follow-up care should be contacted directly and brought up to date on the diagnostic data and what the patient has been told.

Discussions with and about patients who are reaching end-of-life care are particularly sensitive and can be problematic. Von Gunten and colleagues describe a systematic approach to communicating with terminally ill patients and their families that is well worth reading and rereading.[11]

Daily or periodic discussions should involve the nature and risks of upcoming tests and the results of prior investigations. Again, we emphasize that some patients do not want to know about bad results; the clinician will have to seek clues as to patients' desire and receptivity for information, and also the appropriate amount and technical complexity of the information given. At a minimum, the patient must know about significant risks of procedures and tests. A good strategy is usually to share a minimum of data and be prepared to answer questions with the degree of detail the patient desires and you feel comfortable with and able to share. The same basic rules apply to discussions of treatment.

Discuss important risks and be prepared to answer questions about the rationale, length, expected utility, monitoring, and minor effects of treatments recommended or being considered. The length of the individual communication sessions and the pace of discussion will depend on how sick the patient is, the projected length of the hospital stay, and whether you will have an opportunity after discharge for discussion.

What if the patient is not competent or able to discuss diagnosis, prognosis, and treatment? Especially in hospitalized neurologic patients, decreased level of consciousness, memory loss, aphasia, and cognitive abnormalities make some patients unable to understand or digest the material in a meaningful way. In these patients, the family or other intimates or caregivers should be communicated with, depending on their interest and availability and the severity of the illness. There is a major difference between the patient who is incapable of asking and the person who chooses not to ask. The clinician should be able to tell the difference. In any event, in the patient who doesn't ask despite being given multiple opportunities and adequate time, engaging in lengthy detailed discussions is probably a waste of time, if not counterproductive. Ability to gauge the amount, complexity, and timing of doctor-patient communication is both an innate and acquired skill, which the effective clinician should strive to cultivate.

DISCHARGE

Release from the hospital provides a clear and definite finale or terminus to the inpatient evaluation. The termination of outpatient care is seldom as clear-cut, unless for some reason your involvement in the patient's care will be definitely terminated. The responsible clinician should sit down with the patient and significant others at or shortly before discharge. In some patients, this will be your last opportunity to bring up to date discussions about diagnosis, prognosis, and treatment because other doctors will be assuming later responsibility. In other patients, you will, hopefully, have ample opportunity during outpatient follow-up visits. Again, the details of the nature of the dismissal discussion will depend to a great extent on how much has already been said, how receptive the patient is, and the opportunity for later discussions. In all cases, be honest, be sensitive, and make the patient and family feel that there has been ample chance for questions and discussion.

Death in the hospital is one circumstance that is often poorly handled by physicians. Remember that the family lives on and they will need to understand the death and come to terms with it and with the patient's care. Make yourself available to discuss family members' issues and questions. This should not be a hurried discussion. There is no urgency for this discussion and, in fact, dispassionate exchange is usually easier with the passage of time. Lack of discussion with the family after a patient's death, especially if death was unexpected, or after a bad treatment outcome is often an important factor that fosters litigation. If the patient has been referred by another physician, failure to quickly communicate the outcome may prove a source of great embarrassment for that individual.

At discharge, be sure that the patient and responsible others know what they are to do. Should the patient be seen after discharge? By whom? When? Where? If you tell them to see or contact you in three weeks, are there foreseeable circumstances that should trigger an earlier call? Does the patient know what drugs and treatment have been prescribed? When should pills be taken and with or without food or other pills? Are there side effects or complications to watch for? Would any of us know how to take fifteen pills at specific times without confusion? Don't assume the patient will know these details. We would love to have a nickel for every patient who mistakenly takes antihyperglycemic therapy at bedtime or incorrectly takes all of their pills at once during the day. Be as specific in your directions as possible. Write down the key points of treatment, appointments, key physician names and phone numbers. Invite a phone call if patients are confused about directions once they are home. When the patient is going to another health care facility, be sure the written summary and instructions for treatment and follow-up are clear.

For doctors who spend much of their time working in hospitals, the hospital environment is often intellectually stimulating and the camaraderie with professionals and personnel is usually pleasant. Doctors often forget that for patients, hospitals are almost always unpleasant, frightening, and difficult places to be. Doctors who have been hospitalized can readily recall their own experience as inpatients. As physicians we must identify with the patient in the hospital bed. There but for the grace of God go we. Hospitalized patients find that they are completely in the hands of their physicians and they anxiously await any interchange. Any extra time, kindness, or empathy that the physician can tender to the patient is appreciated and helpful.

Often in neurologic patients, hospitalization is merely a phase in the care of the patient. Patients are herded in and out quickly, often without resolution of symptoms. Physicians must help their patients understand that the function of the hospitalization is to settle certain diagnostic questions and sometimes to render specific treatments. Other diagnostic tests and treatment can be pursued on an ambulatory basis. Physician explanations can reduce the anxieties and unpleasantness of the hospital experience.

REFERENCES

1. Kobler J. *The Reluctant Surgeon: John Hunter.* New York: Doubleday, 1960.
2. King SH. *Perceptions of Illness and Medical Practice.* New York: Russell Sage Foundation, 1962;353.

3. Sacks O. *A Leg to Stand On.* London: Picador, 1991;132.
4. Starr P. *The Social Transformation of American Medicine.* New York: Basic Books, 1982.
5. Caplan LR. Fisher's rules. *Arch Neurol* 1982;39:389–390.
6. Bean RB, Bean WB. *Sir William Osler: Aphorism from his Bedside Teachings and Writings.* Springfield, IL: Charles C Thomas, 1961.
7. Benjamin WW. Healing by fundamentals. *N Engl J Med* 1984;311:595–597.
8. Joynt RJ. Personal communication, 1997.
9. Greenhouse AH, Barr JW. The bilateral isodense subdural hematoma on computed tomographic scan. *Arch Neurol* 1979;36:305–307.
10. Ferguson KL, Caplan LR. Spondylitic myelopathy. In L Kranzler, R Penn, G Dohrman (eds), *Neurologic Clinics.* Vol. 3, No. 2. Philadelphia: W.B. Saunders Co., 1985;373–382.
11. Von Gunten, CF, Ferris F, Emanuel LL. Ensuring competency in end-of-life care. Communication and relational skills. *JAMA* 2000;284:3051–3057.

11

Outpatient Care

In the waiting room, the floor paint was peeling, the high paneled walls were a dirty olive color, and the large slatted benches did not provide enough space for all the patients who had come from far off. Many sat on the floor—Uzbeks in quilted cotton gowns, old Uzbek women wearing white kerchiefs, young ones wearing lilacs or red or green kerchiefs, and all in boots and galoshes.[1]

—A. SOLZHENITSYN

The people who came to him or called him out were far too poor to dream of troubling the doctor unless they were really ill. Thus, he met diphtheria in queer stuffy rooms above converted stables, rheumatic fever in damp servants' basements, pneumonia in the attics of lodging houses. He fought disease in that most tragic room of all: the single apartment where some elderly man or woman lived alone, forgotten by friends and relatives, cooking poor meals on a gas ring, neglected, unkempt, forsaken.[2]

—A.J. CRONIN

Outpatient care, whether delivered in a doctor's office away from the hospital or in an office on hospital grounds or affiliated with the hospital, or even in an outpatient clinic, is vastly different from care on an inpatient basis. There are also vast differences in the care delivered at each of these outpatient sites. The identity of the individual patient in the hospital is merged with a vast milieu of other people. All the trappings of individuality and home environment, including clothing, are left at the front door when the patient is admitted to the hospital. It is as if patients were suddenly yanked away from their own beds by a lift and deposited in some strange, complex, and frightening environment. The patient's doctor, no matter how eminent an individual, is just one of hordes of people in the hospital. In contrast, visiting an outpatient facility is more like a trip to a shop. Patients choose their clothing, their transportation, and their companions. The major focus of the visit is close, personal contact with one person, the doctor, who may have some assistants; the major actors in the outpatient drama will return to their usual environment before retiring that night. Inpatient experiences are largely institutional, whereas outpatient office visits are, or should be, personal.

Another major difference between the inpatient and outpatient sites of care relates to the issue of time. In the hospital, very little seems to take place on schedule. Tests and physician and trainee visits can happen any time, even when patients are fast asleep or sitting on the toilet or in a bathtub. Only meals, change of nurses' shifts, daily rounds, and clocks give any clue as to the time. As an outpatient, there is a designated time for the office appointment. Even though patients are well aware that the physician, like an airline flight, may be and, in fact, frequently will be late, still there is some approximation of the visit time and its likely length. There is a finite quality to the encounter, a beginning and an end, and then a return to usual routine.

The contrast between hospitalization and a visit to a hospital outpatient clinic is less stark because, in clinics, depersonalization and vague time constraints are also prevalent. In this chapter, we will not consider neurologists' function in clinics because few neurologists spend much time in outpatient clinics after their training.

The term "clinic" conjures up a picture of house officers and trainees treating impoverished patients who sit on benches or chairs in a large, barren, chaotic waiting area. All too many clinics book morning or afternoon patients who all share an appointment time. The physician may be a transitory figure who may go off rotation or complete training. We firmly believe that clinics are very impersonal and ineffective and should be discontinued. Individual physicians, not clinics, should take care of patients. The only possible benefit of a clinic is the presence of other physicians and ancillary allied health providers (therapists, psychologists, social workers) who are knowledgeable and interested in a particular disease or problem. This advantage can be retained by having the physician, or group of physicians, schedule their individual patients with a particular problem on specific days when other health personnel will be available. Although patients perceive that clinics are much cheaper, in fact, for those who can pay, the difference in charges is very small. The main distinction between a clinic and a doctor's office (regardless of site) is that at an office patients have specific appointments with a certain physician who forms with them a physician-patient relationship. The physician and assistants (nurse, secretary, and others) are identifiable and available to the patients when they become ill or have pressing questions or problems. Clinics do not promote good doctor-patient relationships. The introduction of teams or firms, that include a senior physician as well as trainees, allows for some constancy in care that mitigates some of the problems of the clinics.

In most patients' and physicians' minds, clinics are a symbol of second-class care, a remnant of the charity hospital where the poor come because they cannot afford anything else and have no alternative. If given a choice, what physician would seek medical care at an outpatient clinic? How can we as physicians continue to set up, run, or work in a health care setting in which we, ourselves, would feel uncomfortable as consumers? Unfortunately, in many urban hospital outpatient settings, the number of patients requiring attention is so great, and physicians available to care for them so few, that there seems to be no alternative to the clinic system. In this chapter, however, we will confine our remarks to outpatient offices of individual physicians or groups of physicians.

HOW DO PATIENTS FORM IMPRESSIONS OF THEIR OUTPATIENT EXPERIENCES?

Doctors would like to think that patients judge their office visits solely by the quality of the doctor-patient interaction. If the doctor's performance was personal, thorough, sensitive, and effective, and the technical aspects were exemplary, doctors assume that the visit will garner high marks in the patient's mind. After all, the essence of the physician-patient interaction is the quality of the personal contact no matter where it takes place. James Garfield said about another similar relationship, the teacher-student interface, that the best college in the world is "Mark Hopkins on one end of the log and a student at the other."[3] The very best health experience should consist of an excellent physician ministering to a needy patient in private. Unfortunately, this often is not the case, and the environment does make a difference.

Patients choose physicians by the three A's: availability, affability, and ability—in that order. The outpatient's experience with the doctor is somehow submerged in and dwarfed by the totality of the visit. How far did the patient have to travel? Is the office accessible by public transportation? By taxi? If a car is necessary, can parking be found, and how conveniently, and at what expense? Will there be heavy traffic on the way? Is the office hard to find? Is there a great deal of walking? Is access a straight path or a complex maze the patient has to traverse? Are there facilities for the handicapped? To reach the office, are there long waits in overcrowded elevators that stop at each floor?

What is the waiting room like? Is the reading material ancient and worn? L.R.C. recalls vividly sitting with a sick son about to get an inoculation in a pediatric waiting room littered with toys and coughing and crying children amid a sea of chairs and infectious organisms. He also recalls visiting a dermatologist's office with another son. We were packed into a small anteroom with patients with acne and great weeping rashes. Such waiting room experiences, though they may be unavoidable, create an unpleasant impression.

What is the office staff like? Does the secretary snap at patients officiously when they approach the desk or is she warm, friendly, and helpful? Does she recognize patients as people and inquire about their families or health, or tell them that she is glad to see them?

Are the furniture and decorations attractive, bright, and in good taste, or does the office look and feel sterile, institutional, medicinal, and poorly planned? Are the chairs arranged so that all patients face each other as though in a train station? What about the temperature: Is it boiling hot in the waiting room and freezing in the examining room where patients are undressed? Is there a smell? Is the place clean? What about toilet facilities: Are they adequate, easy to reach, and clean?

How long must patients wait for the doctor? Are they hurried in and out, or is the pace leisurely or geared to the nature and seriousness of the medical problem? How much does the visit cost? Too much or too little can each leave negative impressions. J.H. remembers referring a patient with a difficult diagnostic problem to Dr. Robert Joynt, a renowned senior neurologic consultant. The patient returned with a diagnostic and therapeutic plan. He was grateful to J.H. for recognizing his limitations and for his choice of consultant. He was somewhat puzzled as to why Dr. Joynt's consultation fee was less than that of J.H. when Dr. Joynt's opinion was more helpful. Who will pay: the patient, a third-party payor, or the government? Are copayments needed? Must patients pay cash at the time of the visit, or are they sent a bill? Are there large signs "reminding" patients that payment is expected with service? Are Medicare, Medicaid, and insurance forms handled conveniently for patients, or does the secretary treat them as if they contained plague bacilli?

All these factors, some very minor, some seemingly trivial and inconsequential, add up to the sum of the patient's impression of the visit. Was it a warm, pleasant experience or a big hassle? L.R.C. recalls, years ago, asking his wife how a doctor's visit had gone. He had arranged an appointment for her with a very competent and fine internist. She said she wouldn't go back because "the office is cramped and cheaply furnished, the secretary is a witch, and there are uncapped, smelly urine sample bottles left in the john." She liked the doctor, but would never return.

It behooves doctors who would like to succeed and service the needs of patients to pay close attention to these seemingly small details. The location, organization, and decoration of the office and its atmosphere, maintenance, and cleanliness are very important.

Most important in our minds are the attitudes of personnel. Secretaries and office managers play key roles. Most patients view these individuals and nurses as extensions and reflections of the doctor. Nurses by nature and training should know how to nurture the sick and not so sick. Secretaries and office managers often do not. The best-run, most efficient business office would be a disaster as a doctor's office. Secretaries are often seen by patients as barriers they must hurdle or evade to get to the doctor. We all know the character of the loyal, efficient administrative secretary to the corporate executive or lawyer whose perceived major function is to protect the boss from needless intrusions, especially by "lesser individuals." Only very important people (VIPs) get through the secretary's net. Unfortunately, many office personnel seem to act either like watchdogs at the gate, warding off intrusion, or like very efficient administrators who are quite impatient at being interrupted from their paperwork. Medical office personnel must operate very differently.

Secretary-patient interchange is not limited to the office visit. Secretaries or answering machines are on the other end of the line when the patient makes the first contact with the doctor's office. What is the initial response? Icy and impersonal ("Please wait while I put you permanently on hold")? Or is it: "Mary Jones, how good to hear from you. The doctor was worried. How did the test go?" Is it easy to make an appointment? Is the timing of the appointment appropriate to the nature and urgency of the problem? How are messages handled? Can patients leave a single message indicating the medical problem and urgency of the call and expect to be called back by the doctor? Instead, do patients have to tell the secretary the intimate details of their personal and medical history, recognizing that the message will probably not be passed on unedited to the doctor? Are there certain hours for calls? Is the line always busy?

Choose your office personnel very carefully. Tailor their jobs to their abilities, experience, and personalities. Warm, cheerful people belong out front and on the phone. Cold, efficient business types belong in the back office with the typewriters, computers, and files. Educate personnel about your expectations.

Whenever possible, service should be both efficient and friendly. The doctor and other personnel are there to provide a service to patients, not vice versa. Patients, like customers, should be catered to. They are the core, the raison d'être, of the system, not its victims. Interchange should be personal. A good mnemonic for medical office staff is FEST: friendly, efficient, skilled, and timely. Patients are people, not names, diseases, or test results. Wonders are done for rapport when office personnel greet patients by name, ask about their families and health, seem glad to see them, and are warm and solicitous. Once again, medical personnel should apply the Golden Rule, remembering that they themselves will one day be patients.

THE INITIAL OUTPATIENT VISIT

The physician should spend some time thinking about how best to schedule first visits. Will the doctor see all comers or just patients referred by other physicians or other health care providers? There are advantages and disadvantages to both open door and selective policies. It would be wonderful if all patients had capable and available general practitioners who knew them well and cared for them when problems arose. But many people don't. Insisting that patients who call a neurologist see a general practitioner first for referral often adds an unnecessary step and considerable time to their care. Some people cannot easily arrange an appointment with a good generalist because there are too few in the system. Some generalists are not very good, especially with neurologic problems, and will mismanage patients before or instead of referral to the appropriate specialist. Many managed care systems view specialists only as generators of cost by ordering expensive tests and performing costly procedures. Health care economists and managers, more concerned with the "bottom line" of cost than with the quality of care, have tried to institute and enforce obligatory "gatekeeper" systems, which mandate that a triage person must screen all patients before referral to specialists. Moreover, in most managed care systems, the triage specialist would have economic and other incentives for not referring patients to specialists. Which is more expensive: multiple visits to a generalist, whose ill-conceived efforts result in inappropriate neurologic investigations delaying the diagnosis, occasionally precipitating litigation, or a single visit to an experienced clinical neurologist who may arrive at a diagnosis more quickly, obviating some unnecessary, expensive tests? Few, if any, neurologists' charges for an initial visit rival the cost of one computed tomography (CT), magnetic resonance imaging (MRI), electroencephalogram (EEG), electromyogram (EMG), or angiogram. A neurologist's consultation is the best bargain in town.

There is no easy answer to the medical gatekeeper issue. Much depends on the people involved, who the gatekeeper and the specialist are and how they function. Clearly, a neurologist would rather not be confronted in the office by a patient for whom a full hour has been scheduled who says she is there because she is nervous ("Aren't you a 'nerve doctor?'"). Can you visualize an older gentleman who begins his initial visit by telling the neurologist that he gets up often at night and has difficulty peeing? After a brief history and the doctor's explanation, he replies, "Oh, you are a neurologist. I asked for a urologist!" The problem concerns not only which patients will be scheduled for visits, but also who will be allowed to make the appointment. Sometimes clinics, emergency wards, other physician's secretaries, and well-intentioned relatives or friends try to make arrangements for patients who have absolutely no intention of keeping their appointments.

The *when* of the first appointment is probably as important as the *who*. In some neurologists' offices, patients who call are given "the next available appointment," in 4 months. Patients who can wait 4 months for a visit probably don't need to be seen. By the time of their scheduled visit, a significant number would have worsened and gone to a hospital or another doctor. Others would have had a remission or great improvement in their symptoms so that motivation for the consultation is no longer present. Some patients, especially those with intellectual loss, will have forgotten their appointment in 4 months. Long delays in obtaining an appointment means many no-shows. The doctor must institute a system for contacting and reminding patients about their upcoming visits in order to avoid a no-show and wasting of an hour of scheduled time. We believe that neurologists should be flexible about scheduling new patients. If the doctor is to be useful, sick people and acute problems must be seen quickly. If a young woman were to develop Bell's palsy today, it would be foolish for her to wait 3 months to be seen. Because of the difficulty that patients with acute, but not serious, neurologic problems have in arranging appointments, most wind up in emergency wards. Entrapment or pressure neuropathies, recurrent headache, back or neck pain with root radiation, Bell's palsy, and local regions of numbness or paresthesia are extremely common problems that are poorly dealt with in emergency rooms and only serve to distract personnel there from life-threatening emergencies.

Does each new patient need a full hour for the first visit? Again, triage is a useful concept. We think it is better to reserve some time for brief, almost triage, visits for patients with acute problems. These patients can be screened quickly and investigations or treatment begun. Later, they can be scheduled for a more complete visit. Some patients will be seriously ill and can be admitted directly to the hospital where they can be examined at a more leisurely pace later.

A triage system can determine what patients are scheduled and when. A well-trained nurse, a physician's assistant, or a competent secretary can be trained to triage according to preset guidelines. In difficult or unfamiliar circumstances, the doctor can be contacted to help make a decision. An alternate approach is to have the secretary simply record the referral and data given by the patient, and the doctor will decide later on the details and timing of the appointment.

If the initial appointment is scheduled more than a few days in advance, the doctor should consider mailing the patient some written information. The American Academy of Neurology has made available a short booklet describing neurologists. For patients who will be seen in an outpatient area of a hospital facility, the mechanics of the initial visit can be quite confusing, especially if the hospital is unfamiliar territory. Some hospitals have booklets describing the location of the hospital, directions for reaching the facility by car and public transportation, parking availability and cost, registration procedures, and a diagram of the locations of various buildings. The doctor may also want to send the patient a cover letter describing how to reach the specific location of the appointment and reiterating the scheduled time of visit. Some doctors have also written short booklets that answer frequently asked questions about the mechanics of the practice. (What does a neurologist do? How should appointments be arranged? How are telephone calls handled? How will bills and payments be managed?)

The first visit is often a trying experience for the patient. For this reason and to start the doctor-patient interaction off on the right foot, it is very important that the neurologist spend sufficient personal "quality" time with the patient during this encounter. Most often, this involves a warm-up, get-acquainted period, followed by a thorough and meticulous history and examination. Some physicians watch the clock closely; in patients with a long and complex history that occupies nearly the full hour, they will call a halt to the encounter after the history and postpone the examination for the next visit. In our opinion, this tactic is not wise. Some examination, even if abbreviated, should occur at each visit.

In academic medical centers, there is a strong trend for relocation of more resident and medical student education and training to the outpatient arena for very cogent reasons. It is best to have beginning, inexperienced trainees observe an experienced clinician carry out an initial patient visit before allowing trainees to see patients alone. When ready, trainees will learn more by seeing new patients under the close supervision of a clinician than by struggling on their own. After introducing the trainee to the patient, the clinician should emphasize that he or she will return shortly to review and discuss the problem. Some patients will refuse to see trainees. That is their prerogative. When trainees have completed the history and examination, they should present the information while the clinician, the patient, and appropriate family members are together in the examining room. As parts of the history are covered, the neurologist can ask the patient to elaborate on certain features. The trainee should present the results of the examination, while the neurologist checks key signs and performs parts of the examination that were omitted or inadequately performed by the trainee. While the patient is dressing, the clinician and trainee can discuss the problem and formulate a plan of action in an adjacent room. When everyone has recongregated, the clinician should deliver the summary and dismissal interview while the trainee observes how it is done. Most important, the neurologist must spend sufficient time in the room and must perform some parts of the examination personally. Even when the trainee is a senior resident in whom the neurologist has considerable confidence, it is imperative that the neurologist make physical contact with the patient.

If the patient encounter is a single-visit consultation, the clinician must decide how much to tell the patient directly and how much should be left to the discretion and judgment of the referring doctor to convey to the patient. After the visit, the physician should dictate a note about the patient that later will be typed, or generate a report directly using a word processor and a personal or office computer. The note serves as a record of the visit and can be sent to referring doctors for their information, records, and action. Make the length of the report manageable, preferably less than two full typed pages. There should be two parts to the report. The first should include the data—the history and the examination described concisely in simple English. The second part should begin with a summary of the clinician's thoughts on the major findings and problems and the diagnosis or principle differential diagnosis. Close with a paragraph that enumerates suggested diagnostic investigations and treatments. Make clear what tests have been scheduled and what treatments prescribed and which are to be left to the referring doctor to carry out. Sometimes it is useful to send a copy of the note to the patient. The neurologist should call the referring doctor when the diagnosis is serious and unanticipated by the referring doctor and when quick action should be taken.

FOLLOW-UP VISITS

Scheduling for previously seen patients must also be flexible. Attacks of demyelination, breakthrough in seizure control, anticonvulsant intoxication, and recurrent brain ischemia are just a few examples of acute problems that need urgent management. When the physician knows the patient and the problem well, treatment can often be rendered quickly. Time must be reserved in the schedule to fit in past patients with acute follow-up problems. If those patients cannot be seen during regular hours, they must be handled outside the usual schedule. Once physicians have assumed responsibility for patients' care, they must not desert them in time of need. These patients should not be referred to emergency wards unless treatment is not feasible in another ambulatory setting.

The ratio of time spent in diagnosis to that spent in discussion should decrease the longer the doctor knows the patient. An interim history and focused physical and/or neurologic examination usually suffices to clarify the nature of new problems and the progression of the illness and treatment. Let us repeat once again that we always do some physical examination, even if it is to look at just a few signs, because the simple laying on of hands can be therapeutic. The remainder of the visit can be profitably spent in discussing prognosis and progress, treatment alternatives and prescriptions, and answering questions that relate back to prior discussions. This is a chance to improve rapport and cement the relationship. If things are going very well, the session can be abbreviated; there is no point in belaboring long discussions when the situation is satisfactory and the patient has no desire to rehash past issues. When a new problem arises that is quite separate from old diagnoses, more time will be necessary to retake the history and perform necessary parts of the physical and neurologic examinations. Allotted time should be proportional to the extent of the problem, not limited by the schedule.

Effective neurologists develop rapport with their regular patients. Many of these patients, who have chronic neurologic diseases such as multiple sclerosis, epilepsy, stroke, or myasthenia gravis, come to rely on the neurologist as the principal care provider ("their doctor"). While this might be appropriate since the neurologic problem is often the major health concern, few neurologists deliver truly comprehensive medical care. Neurologists should beware of what we call the "specialist's syndrome."

While serving as a medical officer in the army, L.R.C. recalls seeing a 65-year-old man in the emergency room with shortness of breath and difficulty urinating. Though discouraged and ill, he gave an account of his care. He praised the army system. Since discharge from the service at age 45, he had regularly attended various clinics supervised by topflight specialists. At a hypertensive clinic where he was referred because his military discharge blood pressure was 145/85, he was asked about headache, ankle swelling, and chest pain. His blood pressure was always described as "borderline but not high." At an arthritis clinic where he was referred because of a single attack of gout 15 years before while taking hydrochlorothiazide, medical personnel asked about his joints and measured his serum uric acid, which was always "a little high." At a neurology clinic that he attended because of an old, stable, slight alcoholic neuropathy, the staff inquired about tingling, burning, and weakness of his feet, tapped his ankle reflexes, and tested sensation in the hands and feet. On examination, L.R.C. had no difficulty diagnosing his chronic obstructive lung disease, acute upper respiratory infection, prostatic hypertrophy, and obvious depression. During the past 20 years, he had attended specialty clinics, regularly going to each at least three to four times each year. During that time, no one had performed a full physical examination, taken a complete history, ordered a chest X-ray, or done a rectal examination. None of the problems for which he was obtaining care were of any consequence, and none of his important medical problems had been addressed at all. Yet, he was more than happy with his care. This patient may be an extreme example, but we don't think so.

Many patients, especially those in the upper economic strata, consult many specialists who look after specific problems, but no one coordinates their medical care or looks after their entire soma or psyche. Optimally, patients should have a generalist (family practitioner, internist, or pediatrician, not an obstetrician) who delivers concurrent medical care. Neurologists should insist that their patients also acquire a competent generalist. Some chronic neurologic problems can be managed well by generalists, with the neurologist in the wings available for consultation. Alternatively, regular care by the generalist, plus regular but infrequent visits with the neurologist, is satisfactory. The neurologist should recognize that capability as a generalist fades with time in specialty care. With this reservation in mind, the neurologist should make every effort to deliver complete health care within his or her capability when the patient will not follow advice to consult an internist or family practitioner, or none can be found that prove satisfactory. This may include periodic rectal examinations, chest X-rays, electrocardiograms (EKGs), general blood tests, and so on.

Telephone contact is a very important part of follow-up care. Patients can report changes in symptoms and response to treatment by phone; doctors can use the phone to provide some results of laboratory tests, make minor changes in therapy, discontinue drugs with toxicity or intolerable side effects, and call in prescription renewals. Physicians should develop their own rules for telephone follow-ups. Is there a system for differentiating urgent from routine calls? Is the doctor to be interrupted for calls? If so, under what circumstances? Which calls can be handled by the secretary or the nurse? Are routine calls to be taken by the doctor at specified times in the day, for example, only morning, lunchtime, or later in the afternoon when the physician is usually in the office, but not with patients? When and how are routine, nonurgent calls handled: Will the physician return those calls that day or evening or at the next leisurely time? Should the secretary write down some information extracted from the caller about the problem? If so, how much? What should be done about problem callers? Each doctor has certain patients who call often, ask redundant questions, and use up a great deal of time with very little obvious benefit. No matter what rules and systems are put in place, the demeanor and timeliness of the person answering the phone is important. Friendliness and a desire to help are essential. The secretary's kind words, recalling the patient, and asking about his or her well-being are therapeutic.

Though telephone contact is often adequate, convenient, and efficient because it saves office time for more pressing physician activities, there are potential problems. No doctor can recall all the details of all patients' illnesses and care. A message to call Mrs. P. may be enough to evoke vivid recall of a very familiar patient and her care, but sometimes recollections are vague and the doctor draws a blank. With unfamiliar patients, the chart should be available for reference before or during the return phone call. Also, it is helpful to be able to add to the chart the transmitted information or changes in treatment or progress. A brief dictation or a note written in the chart can do this. Some physicians prefer to always have the chart for all calls, but this requires valuable secretarial time to pull the charts and return them to the file. Again, a system is needed and will depend on the individual physician.

Some physicians may prefer to have patients use e-mail for follow-up contacts, especially for reporting results of tests back to the patient. E-mail contact has the advantage of allowing the physician to review the chart and look up laboratory and imaging results before responding. For some physicians who regularly access e-mail while out of town, it provides a means of contact even when they are away from their practice. E-mail also provides a convenient way of printing out the contact and attaching it to the patient's chart. Patients should be instructed to include contact phone numbers with their e-mail messages so that the physician can call them if the message or response requires explanation or if the response is personal or may be emotionally charged. There has recently been a marked increase in e-mail prevalence. Patient surveys suggest that a higher proportion of patients than physicians are comfortable using electronic communication.

USE OF NURSES AND PHYSICIAN'S ASSISTANTS

Paramedical personnel can be of great help in the outpatient setting if they are properly trained and supervised. Unfortunately, all too often, especially in the outpatient clinics of hospitals, paramedical personnel serve either as managers or perform routine tasks that do not take full advantage of their professional training or skill. Placing patients in examination rooms, weighing, taking routine pulses and blood pressures, assisting patients in disrobing, and chaperoning are commonplace tasks that can easily be carried out by personnel with less formal education. Nurses and physician's assistants require on-the-job training to fulfill various other professional functions that we will discuss in the following paragraphs. This training is best done on site since the styles and activities of neurologists differ widely, as do the interests, training, and abilities of nurses and assistants. Possible functions include the following.

Triage

Telephone contact and triage are crucial to running a successful office. We have already commented on the critical importance of optimal timing of visits and being able to accommodate patients who should be seen quickly. Nurses and physician assistants often have sufficient medical and technical training to be able to function quite well as triage officers who make decisions about how soon the patient should be scheduled. They may also be able to intercept inappropriate appointment requests. A secretary can answer the phone, obtain the data, and, except for routine follow-up visits, seek clearance and guidance from the nurse or physician assistant for new appointments and urgent follow-ups.

Answer Some Phone Messages

Prescriptions require physician signatures or quick approval, but a nurse or physician assistant can mail the prescription or call it into the pharmacy. The nurse can serve as a very useful go-between, extracting the key questions and data from the patient, answering the patient's questions directly when able, or if not, obtaining the answer from the physician and then responding to the patient. Telephone calls can be the bugaboo of practicing and academic neurologists because they take up so much time that there is insufficient time for work. The telephone is probably the most abused substance in the doctor's practice, far exceeding overuse of drugs and alcohol. A small number of patients, perhaps less than 10 percent of the total, occupy over 50 percent of the telephone time and become very well known to office personnel. If a nurse or physician assistant can absorb some of this time, a large service is rendered.

Following Some Patients with Chronic Diseases

Interpersonal skills and practicality are assets traditionally associated with nurses. They often do a superb job of following patients with chronic illnesses such as seizures, headaches, muscular dystrophy, and mental retardation, and obtaining good rapport and compliance. Nurses and physician assistants can supervise the scheduling of visits, especially when new problems arise or treatment is changed. Nurses and assistants can also supervise the dosage of medicines such as Coumadin anticoagulation, adjusting the dosage to the results of the prothrombin time. In many offices and clinics, the patients who are followed for years occupy much of the schedule and leave little time for the physician to see new patients and for consultations. The majority of these chronic patients are stable; many could be handled equally well, if not better, by generalists. If the nurse or physician assistants can assume direct responsibility for these patients, the physician's load will be appreciably lightened.

Seeing and Examining "Walk-In" Patients

Nurses and physician assistants can be trained by the neurologist to take a pertinent history and to perform a reasonable screening examination of patients squeezed into the schedule due to acute problems. They then can present the patient to the physician much as a medical student or house officer would. This will allow the physician to spend less actual time with the patient but still be confident about the thoroughness of the encounter.

Coordinating Various Clinical Activities and Studies

As medical and neurologic practice becomes increasingly centered in outpatient areas, clinical research will, of necessity, also involve more ambulatory patients. Practicing physicians, as well as traditional academicians, will need to be recruited to participate in these studies; many community-based physicians are ready and able to participate in research trials. Nurses and physician assistants can become excellent study coordinators, ensuring that patients are scheduled at the correct times, records are kept, and forms are filled out. In our experience, nurses and physician assistants enjoy and appreciate being part of a research endeavor. Their rapport with colleagues is enhanced and they feel more professional.

Nurses and patients are usually able to meet scheduled appointments, but emergencies or other responsibilities sometimes interfere with visits to the physician. Physicians must be aware that they are legally responsible for the actions of their assistants.

FILING SYSTEMS FOR CATEGORIZING AND RETRIEVING PATIENT DATA

Neurology patients are a rich resource for research and case reports if the material can be retrieved. Unfortunately, if no system is created prospectively, retrospective retrieval becomes very difficult. Let us cite an example from our own experience. In the early 1970s, L.R.C. saw two individuals with very similar problems within a span of 3 months. Both were young male homosexuals who had urinary retention, impotence, perineal paresthesiae, and a slight cerebrospinal fluid pleocytosis. Despite cultures and serologic tests, a specific diagnosis of the condition could not be made. Their symptoms and findings gradually resolved and some unusual sexually transmitted disease seemed at fault. About 5 years later, L.R.C. saw a patient, also a male homosexual, who had a primary herpetic vesicle on his penis and inguinal lymphadenopathy who was hospitalized with herpes simplex virus type II (HSV II) meningitis. During the recovery phase, he developed urinary retention, impotence, and paresthesiae in his perineum and legs. L.R.C. then saw several patients, male and female, with genital herpes who also developed urinary retention and sexual dysfunction.[4] He naturally wondered if the two original patients seen 5 years earlier might have had unrecognized herpes. In the early 1970s, genital herpes was not as widely known and he did not recall inquiring about it or testing for it. He wanted desperately to review the old records and to contact the patients, but had absolutely no office system for retrieving their names, outpatient records, or hospital numbers. L.R.C. had to review all hospital admissions to the neurology service at the Beth Israel Hospital during 2 years to find the patients; even after limiting the chart search to men born after 1945, the retrieval process still took many hours of work. Finally, he did find the records and was able to find the patients' phone numbers and call them. Lo and behold, each recalled a "blister" on the penis and swollen inguinal nodes just before the onset of urinary retention. One had told him of the eruption but it had not rung a bell at the time. This experience taught him a lesson. If charts are filed by diseases, problems, international classification of disease (ICD) codes, or any other system, they can be coded (by color or some other system) for easy retrieval. Neurologists may also, at some point, want to review their experience with all patients with multiple sclerosis, epilepsy, head injury, dizziness, and so on. The advent of office computers, with their great capability for storing data, can potentially solve the retrieval problem. Neurologists must decide how much to put in the classification database. Should it include only diagnosis, name, date of birth and record number, and a brief synopsis of the problem, or answers to a long checklist data bank? Neurologists must fit the system to their own needs. The larger the database, the more likely it is that the required information will be available for later review. No matter what length and complexity is in the database, it is unreasonable to assume that information desired at some future time will be coded for retrieval. Time and energy are required to enter the data. A relatively simple database with a small group of categories relevant to an individual physician's practice seems more helpful. Many years ago J.H. designed a detailed data storage system that not only was impossible to maintain but also did not include the fields that he later wanted to retrieve.

MANAGED CARE

Thirty years ago the dominant health care format was that of independent practitioners or group practices reimbursed predominantly by an indemnity health care insurance system covered through employers. Individuals without insurance might manage to pay the costs of health care, albeit slowly. When Medicare developed in the mid-1960s, hospital reimbursement was cost-based with physician reimbursement on a fee-for-service basis. With federal support of Medicaid, states developed a similar reimbursement scheme. Physician fees were generally set well below clinics' fees and private practitioners found participation burdensome. Rising health care costs led to the development of the Medicare Prospective Payment System (PPS) and fixed reimbursement for Diagnosis-Related Groups (DRG). While hospitals were now given incentive to contain costs and shrink length of stay, physicians were reimbursed primarily by fixed fee for service. This was perceived to be a misalignment of incentives and a host of programs and plans were developed to reduce payer cost. Health Maintenance Organizations (HMOs) receive premiums and are responsible for the financial cost of an enrollee's health care.[5] Physicians are now faced with a myriad of plans or organizations imposing diverse restrictive testing policies and conflicting formularies. A detailed discussion of managed care is inappropriate here. A summary of the rationale and goals of these organizations can be found in the book by DeMuro.[6] The Practice Committee of the American Academy of Neurology has created a variety of documents and programs to assist with the business aspects of coding and contractual relations with providers. These are updated regularly and should be consulted as needed.

HMOs that only used employed physicians at a designated HMO center accomplished limited penetration and so many managed care organizations sought to increase their panel by contracting with other physicians. This could be in the form of a Preferred Provider Organization (PPO) or through a panel without walls in the form of an Individual Practice Association (IPA). Physicians in an IPA are not truly practicing in an integrated manner but participate as a means of contracting with an HMO. At first, the goal of managed care organizations in relation to their physician panels was only to discount fees for service. This progressed to preauthorization of procedures, hospitalizations, and consultations. Continued hospital stay reviews were based on perceived medical necessity without concern for personal patient issues. Retrospective reviews resulted in rejection of claims for services already delivered. Increasing costs of specialized services, increasingly expensive technology, rising costs of newer medications, and the need to support corporate bureaucracies and profit margins led to the development of capitation schemes. Capitation offers the insurer an ability to define cost and shifts risk to the providers (physicians or hospitals). The physician is paid a fixed amount per member per month (PMPM). Primary Care Physicians (PCPs) were perceived as gatekeepers whose incentives were to be brought in line with the managed care organization through capitation and through withholds or other means to punish excessive consultation, testing, and hospitalization. Resource Based Relative Value Scale (RBRVS) was introduced by Medicare in 1992 to enhance compensation for cognitive skills but served to reduce physician payments. In "mature" managed care communities HMOs will probably attempt to manage care through protocols, controlled utilization, and pharmaceutical management systems. Despite increasing interference in physician judgment, HMOs are protected from malpractice liability.

Hospitals perceive that they are the target of HMOs and IPAs. Cost reductions are sought through reduction in hospital utilization. Twenty-three–hour admissions may be all that is authorized to avoid payment of DRGs. This may leave hospitals with the costs of their infrastructure while their occupancy and incomes fall. Some hospitals have looked to Physician Hospital Organizations (PHO) to allow them to capture some of the risk savings. The PCP is now considered desirable. The specialist who attracts complex patients requiring expensive procedures is less desirable when the hospital is capitated. Subcapitation of specialist providers is desirable from the perspective of PCPs and HMOs but will clearly be quite risky for the specialist, as the pool of capitated individuals is relatively small.

Quality is frequently established by measuring only items captured by computer programs such as frequency of routine immunizations or scheduled mammography. Costs are kept under control by having services provided by the lowest level provider or location for each service. Proprietary programs, such as that of Milliman and Robertson, are widely employed to set standards for patient care. The proprietary nature of these programs does not allow for review of the decision-making processes involved in these idealized guidelines that seem primarily addressed to minimizing cost. The specialist may feel a need to participate in multiple arrangements.

Neurology is a specialty that is increasingly under attack by HMOs that accept the types of guidelines that assign care of most neurologic disease to PCPs. The PCP may be urged to avoid consultation or to authorize only one visit. At the same time, much neurologic training for primary care residents may be provided by PCPs poorly educated in neurologic disease. A limited time is provided for neurology with no attention to the neurologic method or localization. The studies a neurologist uses are increasingly expensive but the neurologist's fee is a small part of the cost of neurologic disease. Some HMOs have come to realize that allowing a specialist to see a "bleeder" (a participant whose care and testing is generating excessive cost to the HMO) may save considerable money in the long run. Capitated PCPs may prefer to have a chronic daily headache patient out of the office.

Patient care is quite different in a closed panel HMO from that provided in the office of a single practitioner. Though perhaps less expensive, HMO care is also less personal and more "institutional." Generalizing from L.R.C.'s own experience regarding closed panel HMOs:

1. There is a higher generalist/specialist ratio than in the community.
2. Referral to specialists is discouraged unless absolutely necessary; the HMO usually uses a gatekeeper who is given incentives for limiting referral to "expensive" specialists like neurologists.
3. Patients are usually scheduled for brief neurologic visits.
4. Hospitalization is aggressively discouraged and, when hospitalization is allowed, patients are pushed out "sicker and quicker" unless the hospital is trapped in a DRG contract. Other health care providers such as nurses and assistants, who are perceived as less expensive than physicians, are used more heavily than in most private doctors' offices. Other than surgery, eye problems may be handled entirely by optometrists. Some allied health providers work under protocols to screen which individuals will be allowed to see the doctor. These nonphysicians, following the protocol rules handle minor problems.
5. Doctors spend most of their time with new patients and regularly scheduled follow-up visits and are not as available for past patients who become acutely ill. Acute problems are usually managed in a walk-in clinic by some other physician (rarely, if ever, a neurologist).
6. On-call schedules are such that physicians are not on call many evenings or weekends. This makes it easy for doctors to schedule a golf game in the afternoon off or a social event in the evening, but makes it unlikely that neurologists will be available when one of their patients becomes ill.
7. The press of physician responsibilities leaves little time for communicating with and getting to know patients and developing a personal physician-patient relationship.
8. Administrative HMO personnel urge physicians to dictate shorter notes into the computer record for the purposes of economy and efficiency.

All of these HMO characteristics make it harder for neurologists to deliver high-quality personalized care. Neurologists working in an HMO system have to be extremely careful in training allied health personnel in an adequate system of care delivery.

L.R.C. worked part-time in an HMO for about 6 years. Patients were herded in and out quickly, and there was always pressure to see more patients in less detail during a shorter time interval for the same remuneration. A patient with Bell's palsy can be seen quickly and the medical issues sorted out correctly: The neurologist asks about mastoid and ear pain and checks cranial nerves V through VIII, scratches the toe contralateral to the facial palsy looking for a Babinski response, and watches the patient walk. The patient is then shunted out the door. Next case. After many such patients, the physician feels like an automaton on an assembly line. Try to handle a complex patient with dementia or a child with learning disabilities in the same way! Little time is available to get to know patients and communicate with them. Patients become a blur of faces and diagnoses, not real people. When patients call on the telephone when the physician is not at the HMO, record review is difficult. A treating physician with just the bare bones included in the HMO charts is helpless when testifying in court. L.R.C. found himself more and more dissatisfied and frustrated with the system.

J.H. worked for 3 years as a preferred provider for a closed panel HMO. The laboratory studies often did not come back to his office. Imaging studies were contracted to a radiology group and were frequently read by nonneuroradiologists. Considerable resistance was offered to having the films made available to J.H. in a timely manner. When he requested ophthalmology assistance it was usually arranged through an optometrist. The office at the HMO was not very helpful in providing information from the records. He belonged to a number of IPAs and was able to see considerable variability in policy. Unless there is a dominant HMO-IPA in a community, specialist physicians will find themselves pressured into joining multiple provider organizations to maintain an adequate referral base. When there are choices available, the neurologist may wish to consider the policies of the HMO-IPA carefully. Is the IPA truly representing its physician members or is it a creature of the HMO to which it is linked? What is the control of the IPA? Is it primarily PCP or more balanced? A referral limited to a single evaluation visit does not allow the patient to return for an exit interview after the test results are known. An IPA in Rochester, New York, is utilizing a policy that automatically downgrades payment if the neurologist makes a diagnosis that is perceived by their administrators to be manageable in a briefer visit (e.g., migraine). A PCP designed a program to reduce imaging studies by creating a list of allowable diagnoses for imaging. If the clerk detected an inappropriate diagnosis, the ordering physician would be fined and the radiologist would not be paid. Only considerable rebellion led the IPA to accept that there was neither validity to the list nor any physician consensus. The new version retains sufficient hassle factor that physicians will hesitate to order needed studies. One can sympathize with the IPA officers who have to confront an HMO raising its charges to cover increasing pharmaceutical costs while not allowing increasing payments to the IPA despite increasing imaging costs. The possibility that the wisdom of the gatekeeper concept may be flawed has been considered but does not seem to have much penetrance. The worst HMO abuses have been paraded in Congress and the press and reform may well be in the offing. Neurologists continue to need to battle in order to be able to deliver quality care.

We suspect that only a minority of neurologists find themselves happy and comfortable in closed panel HMOs because of the high hassle factor and the difficulty of caring for patients in a thorough and sensitive manner and the lack of incentive for high-quality care. The issues that we have described should be carefully weighed before neurologists explore practice in an HMO setting. If they do choose an HMO, they should attempt to maintain a high standard of care despite administrative and economic pressures.

Group practices are extremely variable and depend greatly on their size and the individuals in the group. Is the major goal of the group to make money, perform lots of procedures, or to practice and deliver high-quality care? Is time designated for education, conferences, and rounds? Are there discussions within the group about patients with difficult diagnostic problems? Is there a pleasant atmosphere in the office and good rapport within the group? All these factors relate to the quality of a group practice.

This chapter has emphasized the importance of the totality of the outpatient experience to the patient and the need for systems and rules in managing ambulatory care. Though the physician visualizes the ambulatory visit with the patient as consisting of his or her contact with the patient, for the patient the visit includes a multitude of experiences and contacts. Reaching the facility, parking, secretaries, phone contacts, ancillary personnel, billings, elevators, decor, bathroom facilities, phlebotomists, waiting rooms, and other patients all entwine to form a symphony of images and sounds of people, places, and things. It is this symphony, plus the doctor, that comprise the totality of the patient's experience. To be successful the physician must heed the details of the full environment. By success, we are not referring only to economics but also having the patient return and comply with advice and treatment.

There are lots of outpatients with many different problems and lots of phone calls and lots of records. No single physician can possibly keep track of it all in his or her head nor is time available to do so. Rules and systems are needed for triaging, scheduling, billing, record retrieval, call-back of patients with abnormal test results and patients who should be seen, but have not returned. Also important is communication with other physicians involved in the patients' care. The physician should try to ensure that personnel, rules, and systems are in place to meet and anticipate problems.

REFERENCES

1. Solzhenitsyn A. *The Cancer Ward.* New York: Dial Press, 1968;2.
2. Cronin AJ. *The Citadel.* New York: Bantam Books, 1962;191.
3. Rudolph F. *Mark Hopkins and the Log: Williams College, 1836–1872.* New Haven: Yale University Press, 1956.
4. Caplan LR, Leeman E, Berg S. Urinary retention probably secondary to herpes genitalis. *N Engl J Med* 1977;297:920–921.
5. Tarlov AR. HMO enrollment, growth, and physicians: the third compartment. *Health Aff* 1986;5:23–35.
6. DeMuro PR. *The Fundamentals of Managed Care and Network Development: A Business Guide for Healthcare Professionals and Providers.* New York: McGraw-Hill, 1999.

12

Consultations

The consultant should be ever mindful of the difficult problems encountered in the everyday practice of medicine, and he should therefore make
a deliberate effort to buttress the position of the primary physician. If the
consultant concludes that the primary physician is in error, the matter
should be discussed with him directly. It is exceedingly wrong to sacrifice
the equanimity of the sick person and his worried family because of bun-
gled relationships between the consultant and the primary physician.[1]

—P. Tumulty

The consultant reacts to a situation with his or her whole being and
with a behavior that is determined less by a process of deliberate decision making than by a complex of trained reactions and experiential
responses.[2]

—G. Lippitt and R. Lippitt

SEPARATION OF NEUROLOGY AND
MEDICINE AND SUBSPECIALIZATION LED
TO INCREASED CONSULTATION

The complexity of all aspects of medicine has increased almost exponen-
tially during the past two decades. Thirty or more years ago, when we were
finishing our neurology residency training, there were not many neurologists.
Neurologists that were trained in the few accredited programs were clustered
in a few large urban centers—New York, Boston, Philadelphia, Minneapolis,
Chicago, and Los Angeles—almost entirely practicing neurology within academic programs.[3] Clinical neurologists practicing in the community were a
rarity. Few were able to earn a living without practicing psychiatry. The neurologic clinician of that era was capable of managing nearly all problems that
might present to neurologists. As diagnostic technology grew dramatically and
the number of neurologists multiplied, subspecialization became the norm.
Many neurology trainees began to take a fourth year of neurology training (a
fellowship) in a subspecialty area such as epilepsy, stroke, electrophysiology,
neuromuscular disease, behavioral neurology, or neuropathology. The same

pattern of specialization was also occurring in surgery and internal medicine. General surgeons and internists became endangered species and subspecialty physicians and surgeons predominated. Today, most academic neurology departments are staffed by subspecialists with separate divisions devoted to child neurology, neuropathology, neuromuscular disease, and so on. Even in practice, some clinician neurologists who had subspecialty fellowships continue to specialize and seek referrals for consultation in their areas of special expertise. Specialization undoubtedly has led to an acceleration of research advances in each subspecialty, but, at the same time, has made it very difficult for any physician to become proficient in all areas of neurology. Consultations among subspecialty neurologists have become increasingly prevalent in this era of subspecialization.

Neurologists of thirty years ago had more training in internal medicine than those trained today. Most neurology training programs were divisions under umbrella departments of medicine. An internship and junior residency year in medicine were prerequisites for neurology residency training. Following the divorce between academic neurology and medicine departments, medical sophistication among neurology trainees declined dramatically. Medicine, with all of its subspecialization in hematology, cardiology, endocrinology, rheumatology, and so on became much more complex and technologically and procedurally oriented. The neurologist's ability to keep up with internal medical advances in knowledge diminished. Neurologists by necessity work very closely with general internists and medical subspecialists in caring for patients with complex illnesses. Conversely, when neurology left medicine, the neurologic training and sophistication of medical house officers also suffered greatly. Today's graduating medical residents, in general, know very little neurology and feel obliged to consult neurologists about patients with the most simple and routine neurologic problems. (This trend is not as prevalent in some countries such as Great Britain and Australia where internists and general practitioners are much better schooled in nervous system problems.)

Despite the great increase in consultations among subspecialty neurologists and between neurologists and other specialists, few trainees are given guidelines in asking for or delivering consultations.

INDICATIONS FOR SEEKING CONSULTATION

When the Outcome Will Likely Be Bad

When should neurologists seek out consultation with colleagues? One important indication for consultation is when a patient that the neurologist is treating will have a very bad outcome. Motor neuron disease, malignant brain tumor, progressive dementia, and paralyzing neuropathy with little prospect of effective treatment are examples of conditions in which the neurologist knows the prognosis is poor. Especially if neurologists are junior or specialize in another branch of neurology, they should anticipate subsequent criticism by family members and associates. As the patient's condition declines, the family is certain to question, "Has everything possible been done?" or "Could the diagnosis be wrong?" "Have all the treatment options been explored?" "Why is this happening?" Consultation with another neurologic colleague goes a long way toward allaying these potential criticisms. The consulting neurologist should be well known or specialize in the area of the patient's illness. Whenever possible, the consultant should meet with the family and patient so that they hear the consultant's prognosis and opinions about management firsthand.

When the Disease Is Outside the Neurologist's Area of Expertise

Another important reason for seeking consultations or transfer of responsibility for care is a disease or problem outside the neurologist's area of expertise. This indication for consultation is relative. Some neurologists specializing in stroke, epilepsy, or another field are well qualified to care for patients in other categories. This varies with the neurologic specialist, the subspecialty area of the patient's disease, and the complexity and specific nature of the patient's illness and its treatability. As a stroke specialist who now spends a considerable portion of time seeing patients with cerebrovascular disease, L.R.C. still feels reasonably comfortable in caring for patients with behavioral and neuro-ophthalmological problems and diseases of the spinal cord. He is less confident of his ability to care for patients with myopathies, but feels competent to manage patients with uncomplicated myasthenia gravis and polymyositis, disorders in which he has had ample past experience. J.H. and L.R.C. always agree to a consultation when this is suggested by the patient or a family member. We tell the patient that we are willing to suggest a consultant, or to provide the names of a number of capable consultants. We accept any consultant they suggest who is knowledgeable in the area of concern. Decision to consult or transfer the patient will depend on the neurologist's competence to handle the problem and the availability of a neurologist who is more able to manage the specific problem in question. The strength of the rapport that the neurologist has established with the patient and general physician and the treatability of the patient's illness are other factors to consider. If the patient has a familial neuropathy for which there is no available effective therapy, then the factors favoring consultation would be lower than if the patient had a potentially remediable, immunologically mediated peripheral neuropathy with which the neurologist has had little personal experience. If the patient has a long-standing relationship with a neurologist, the patient may feel that even discussing the possibility of consulting another physician will be seen as betrayal. In this circumstance, it is wise for the neurologist to initiate the discussion about a possible consultation, affirming that he or she would welcome any input that might benefit the patient. The patient and family should be assured that a consultant is selected because of his or her expertise and may offer some help in the patient's care and that the patient's well-being is your goal. In the final reckoning, the deciding criterion should be the Golden Rule: If you had the patient's problem and were confronted with the same circumstances, or the patient were your parent, spouse, or child, whom would you choose to care for you? Would you ask for a consultation? If so, with whom?

When the Neurologist Lacks Confidence in Management

Another important consideration is the neurologist's confidence in his or her present management. Does the neurologist know what is wrong with the patient and what should be done? Clearly, the less that the neurologist knows, the greater the need for consultation with others who may be able to clarify aspects of diagnosis, prognosis, and treatment. We have commented already that "scattershot" evaluation or treatment is expensive and ineffective. Better to consult than to take a "whole body biopsy" approach or deliver potentially harmful treatment.

Surgery, radiotherapy, chemotherapy, and even immunotherapy (if available) are all plausible treatments for patients with nervous system neoplasms. The neurologist should anticipate the requests of the family. They will surely hear somewhere that "Aunt Jane's neighbor with a brain tumor did well with BCNU or X-ray treatment" and will ask why their relative did not receive these treatments. Better that the neurologist seek and suggest consultation before the family's or patient's request. Patients and their families should be confident that the neurologist has touched all the bases and thought seriously about the problem. Furthermore, the neurologist is the team leader and should guide the management rather than being led passively by the recipients of care.

When Treatment Is Controversial

Consultation is also wise when the neurologist has chosen an unusual, novel, controversial, or nonstandard plan of management. Though the neurologist's judgment may be absolutely correct, the chosen approach may leave the neurologist vulnerable to criticism by the patient and family if things go wrong, and may even later lead to legal retribution and litigation. Ethical considerations could also be involved.

Let's consider two case examples that illustrate this point. You have been referred an 82-year-old demented woman from a nursing home who has the recent onset of weakness of the right arm. When you examine her on the first hospital day, she has a slight conduction aphasia, right arm and leg paresis, and a low-pitched loud focal left carotid bruit. Conversations with the nursing home staff and the patient's two daughters document that the patient has been severely demented for 4 years, does not recognize her daughters or grandchildren, is incontinent, and has been chronically unhappy. Her right-sided weakness clears, computed tomography (CT) shows considerable atrophy and no infarction, and noninvasive testing demonstrates severe (greater than 95 percent) stenosis of the left internal carotid artery origin. The daughters call to say they want "everything done for poor mother." Guilt feelings about their own perceived maternal neglect seem evident from your conversations with them. You do not think that aggressive treatment (carotid artery surgery) is warranted in this patient, despite the daughters' request. Consultation is important in this setting to support your approach.

A young woman with a several-month history of diplopia, dysphagia, and intermittent dyspnea is brought by her protective mother to see you. You diagnose myasthenia gravis and are worried because of her decreased vital capacity. You believe that an aggressive approach is indicated, including thymectomy and vigorous immunosuppression. The patient does not appear to be very ill or disabled now, but you anticipate that serious problems will surely develop. You realize that the earlier immunosuppressive therapy is begun, the greater the opportunity for a cure. You are aware that some other neurologists, given the present circumstances, would probably suggest more conservative treatment and that the therapeutic course you have chosen does have potential risks and serious complications, including death. Given these circumstances, it would be wise to consult another physician, preferably someone with considerable experience in the treatment of patients with myasthenia. The consultant chosen should be a physician who is open-minded and not biased against an aggressive treatment viewpoint.

When Patients and Families Are Hostile

Another stimulus for consultation with another neurologist is the perception that the environment in which care is being delivered is potentially hostile. Is the patient angry, contentious, aggressive, dissatisfied, or previously litigious? Have family members or friends of the patient called with criticisms or aggressive queries? Have there been past medical disasters involving this patient, whose antiphysician attitude may already be very high? Is a lawyer involved? Has the neurologist been contacted by another physician at the instigation of the family to question management decisions? Consultation with a well-respected physician who will review the case and management and give approbation or help may allay potential criticism. It is tough to fight battles alone.

Consultation with Nonneurologists

The previous discussions concerned circumstances that should lead neurologists to consult other neurologists. Let's turn now to consultation with internists, generalists, and other nonneurologists. We have already shared our view in previous chapters that most patients should optimally have a generalist involved in their care. If a hospitalized patient has no general physician and the neurologist has identified a physician who is willing and able to accept the patient after discharge from the hospital, it is wise to have that physician consult while the patient is still in the hospital and preferably as early as is feasible. After discharge, it may be very difficult for the generalist to catch up with data generated during the hospitalization. Also, the generalist should be given the opportunity to be involved in important diagnostic and therapeutic decisions. If the patient already has a generalist, he or she should be included in the patient's hospital care. Needless to say, if a medical or surgical problem arises that the neurologist is not equipped to handle, a consultation should be arranged.

The neurologist should be careful, especially when a number of consultants have been called in, to retain control of the patient's care. Medical care by committee is invariably poor medicine. One individual must assume the responsibility for coordinating care, weighing various opinions, and making decisions. When the neurologist is the senior clinician responsible for the patient's principal problem he or she must take the role of coordinator and director. If the patient's problem is such that others are better qualified to take charge of the care, then the patient should be transferred to their care.

SELECTING A CONSULTANT

A number of factors will influence your choice of consultants. If you have a strong opinion about the nature of the treatment you feel is indicated for the patient, you should consult a specialist who is likely to concur with your approach. Suppose that you have a patient with severe lumbar pain and radiculopathy who has not responded to conservative treatment. Radiography documents a large herniated disk compressing the root appropriate to the patient's clinical symptoms and signs. You are convinced that surgical therapy is now indicated. You should consult a neurosurgeon who is likely to agree. Suppose, instead, that you have a patient with back pain who has been injured on the job. There are no definite localizing root signs. You are reticent to suggest surgery at this time because of the real uncertainty of the relationship of the disk to the clinical picture. In that situation, the consultant you choose should be a more cautious surgeon who is likely to suggest a conservative approach, or another neurologist. Of course, if you are uncertain about the best course of action, then you should select one or more consultants who are open-minded and likely to render a balanced opinion. These consultants should not have reputations for being wedded to either overly aggressive or conservative viewpoints.

The age and sex of the chosen consultant are also important. If you are relatively young and might be perceived as inexperienced by the family, choose an older "graybeard" as the consultant. On the other hand, if you are aging and might be perceived as being outdated or stodgy, choose a young consultant who will be viewed by the family as injecting fresh, up-to-date ideas into the case. Similarly, depending on the patient, the sex of the consultant might be important. If you are a woman and the patient is a "traditional" middle-aged or older man, you are probably wise to choose a male consultant. If the patient is a woman or girl and you are a man, a female consultant might be preferred. When in doubt, discuss the issue of the age and sex of the consultant openly with patients, asking if they have a preference.

The specialty of the consultant is obviously important. Especially with patients with a poor prognosis, for whom you want to provide a balanced approach, involve consultants from different specialties so that all plausible angles are considered. If the patient has a brain or spinal cord tumor, consult a neurosurgeon, radiotherapist, and oncologist. Be sure all of the bases are covered.

At times, especially in difficult situations, you will want to choose a "professorial" consultant to calm the waters. Some patients who view themselves as VIPs are satisfied with nothing else. If the environment is potentially hostile or critical, the prognosis is grim, or there are serious diagnostic and therapeutic dilemmas, an eminent opinion may be very useful. Seek an individual well known and well respected in the community who has impeccable credentials and will treat the patient with consideration and humanity. This consultant can be a person with a high academic position or be a well-recognized senior practitioner in the community.

In difficult situations, you may want to involve a consultant with whom you clearly have no relationship. Avoidance of any appearance of "collusion" or "conspiracy" is sometimes crucial. By suggesting consultants from different medical centers with whom you are not affiliated or even consultants from different cities or regions, you may appeal to the patient's and family's sense of thoroughness and fairness. We have found it a very useful tactic to give the patient and family a list of suggested consultants, any of whom would be quite acceptable to you and helpful to them. You should offer to rank the list if desired. Patients should be given the option of contacting the consultant themselves. Some patients do not want a new consultant to be biased in any way by what you may have told them. When a consultant is chosen, offer to facilitate the consultation as much as possible by making records and films readily available and smoothing the interchange. If the patient and family agree, make a call to the chosen consultant describing the data, the circumstances that led to the request for consultation, and the role that you would like the consultant to play. Are there specific questions that you would like the consultant to address? Are there controversial issues? Is there a hidden agenda?

Referring patients to doctors and medical facilities in distant cities has advantages and disadvantages. By geographically widening the available choices, the referring physician can direct the patient to consultants and centers that have special expertise in the patient's problem. The distant super specialist also commands respect in court cases that come to litigation. There are also definite disadvantages of distant consultations in addition to inconvenience and expense. A visit to a distant specialist is beneficial when there is a pressing question that can be answered by a brief hospitalization or outpatient evaluation. Questions concerning diagnosis and diagnostic or therapeutic procedures may be answered by such a visit. In other patients, there is no focused question, merely discontent on the part of the patient, family, or referring physician with regard to the course of the illness and its present management. Some chronic illnesses are best managed by day-to-day, week-by-week contact. Parkinson's disease, movement disorders, multiple sclerosis, and pharmacological control of seizures are examples of problems that require sustained contact. Treatment is empiric and is "played by ear," depending on the patient's progress and response to the latest treatment and dosage of medicine. A good coach can construct a wise game plan but must be prepared to revise and modify it, depending on the success of the early action. Chronic problems do not readily lend themselves to solutions during single consultations. However, in some instances of chronic disease, distant consultations might serve as a valuable starting point; the consultant can be contacted later by phone or letter for follow-up advice.

For some patients, the referring physician seeks a single consultant with special expertise. In other patients with very complex or multisystem diseases, it may be more appropriate to refer the patient to another medical facility where there is a team of specialists who could work together to solve the patient's problems. This requires not only the presence of multiple capable consultants, but some coordination and efficient cooperation. Some institutions such as the Mayo Clinic and Lahey Clinic have achieved renown for their facility because of their efficiency in coordinating care. This approach has great advantages.

TIMING OF CONSULTATIONS

Be as considerate of the consultant as possible. Since most neurologists frequently function as consultants themselves, this advice hits very close to home and needs little emphasis. Call consultants early enough to involve them in the decision-making process, but if significant information is likely to be generated from early investigations and the patient is stable, wait to call the consultant until sufficient baseline data are available. Consultants are placed in a very awkward position if they are called in after key decisions have already been made.

L.R.C. vividly recalls being asked to see a patient with a gradually progressing right hemiparesis thought to be explained by a mass lesion in the left hemisphere that was detected by brain imaging. On examination, he found a left visual field defect in addition to the already described right hemiparesis, which suggested the presence of multiple metastases. He examined the patient in the early evening. He spoke to the patient's worried husband, who said that his wife was scheduled for brain surgery early the next morning. When L.R.C. suggested to him that in his opinion it might be better to wait and evaluate the problem further before deciding on an operation, the husband responded that he had been told by the neurosurgeon that she might die if surgery were delayed. L.R.C. had been placed in an untenable position. If he stopped the surgery, he would be blamed for the subsequent bad outcome that was more likely than not. If he did not protest the proposed plan of action, the family (and courts) could justifiably take his silence as tacit approval. This situation could have been avoided by requesting a consultation before the decision to operate had been made and shared with the patient and family. In this case, L.R.C. told the patient and family that he thought that surgery could and should be safely delayed. He discussed the poor timing of the consultation with the referring surgeon in an attempt to prevent the recurrence of this problem.

Similarly, stroke neurologists are frequently called in as "courtesy consultants" by vascular surgeons after the patient has had angiography and the patient is scheduled for surgery. Families and courts often assume that all doctors involved in a case at a particular time of critical intervention have participated in the decisions made. The consultant's involvement in a case will be taken as evidence that he or she agreed with decisions made by the referring physician, and the consultant will be culpable if things go wrong. Do not place your consultants in this awkward position; consult them before decisions are made!

FUNCTIONS OF A CONSULTANT

The consultant should see the patient as early as possible after the consultation request is received. If the consultant wants to be involved in the case before irrevocable decisions are made, the diagnostic and treatment process should not be delayed. In a hospitalized patient, consultations should occur, at the latest, within 48 hours of the request.

Consultations take time. They should not be performed casually or in a cursory fashion. The patient and the family must gain the impression that the consultant's opinion has been based on a careful and thorough review of the case. Almost always this means adequate time spent with the patient and not just with the hospital or outpatient record. Doctors care for people, not charts.

The most important single rule, in our opinion, is that the consultant must acquire the primary data directly (or with the aid of the resident or fellow). The consultant should take the history from the patient, examine the patient, and examine any radiographic or imaging films. Reports are insufficient. A rehash of previously acquired data is not likely to be productive. A consultation has been requested because the accumulated data have not been sufficient to provide answers to the patient's problems. Tumulty put it quite well when he described the function of the consultant: "His should be a fresh and brand-new look and not simply an overview of old material already assembled. He should trust no one's judgment but his own and rely only upon that clinical data that he has evaluated himself."[1] To perform a thorough consultation, two things must be done: the data must be acquired from primary sources, and the chart must be reviewed to find clinical and laboratory information that has been missed and to understand the questions that have been asked. Consultants use different styles. Most review the chart before seeing the patient. L.R.C. prefers seeing the patient first before looking at the chart so that he approaches the case unbiased by prior opinion and analysis. After seeing the patient, he then reviews the chart to be sure he has not missed some data or questions. When necessary, he then returns to the bedside to clarify remaining issues. J.H. prefers to review whatever data is available, and then meet the patient in the office. In the hospital he prefers to take the chart in with him so that the patient is aware that he has seen the data, but he elicits the history from the patient and family, unless the patient is incapable of providing a history.

After seeing the patient, the consultant should write a brief, concise summary note in the hospital chart outlining major findings, diagnosis, and suggested evaluation and management. If the patient was also seen by a student or trainee, it is insufficient for the consultant to simply initial their notes. Trainees can provide a listing of the data and findings, but their discussions and suggestions are seldom focused enough. If a student's or resident's assessment of a case is judged by a consultant to be complete, either that trainee is extraordinary or, much more likely, the consultant is inadequate. A more complete dictated note can later be sent to the referring physician. This note should be added to the chart to meet the requirements of management and payers. If the patient is seen on an ambulatory basis, the note should arrive within a week. Some communication should be made with the referring physicians at the time of the consultation. Optimally, this should be a phone call discussing findings and suggestions. At times an e-mail containing the key points will suffice. In the bustle of hospital life, phone contact is not always feasible and physicians are sometimes hard to reach; in routine cases, a note in the chart will usually suffice. There are circumstances when a call is essential:

1. The patient is critically ill and the consultant has diagnostic or therapeutic suggestions.
2. When quick action is imperative.
3. When unexpected findings are discovered.
4. When the consultant disagrees with present management.
5. When the consultant's opinions are likely to be controversial and need explanation.
6. When the consultant is uncertain of the referring physician's expectations, questions or preferences regarding who should talk directly to the patient and the family.

Consultants are called by referring physicians for a variety of different purposes. In different situations, a consultant's role might involve:

1. Confirmation of a serious neurologic disease or prognosis.
2. Provision of a diagnosis or cogent differential diagnosis in a heretofore puzzling case.
3. Guidance in investigating the patient's problem.
4. Assistance in ordering tests such as CT, magnetic resonance imaging (MRI), angiography, or myelography. In some institutions, these neurologic procedures cannot be ordered unless the patient has been seen by a neurologist or neurosurgeon. Invasive procedures should always require specialty input. Although specialty input would probably enhance the appropriateness of imaging studies, the pressure on modern hospital facilities is such that the neurologist is not able to function as a gatekeeper in most facilities.
5. Help in deciding on the best treatment.
6. Introduction to a patient whom the referring physician would like the consultant to follow as an outpatient after discharge.

7. Help in discussions with the family. The consultant's opinion may lend weight and credence to the family's confidence in the patient's care.
8. Arbitration of differences in medical opinion.
9. Informational or courtesy consultation, furnishing access to a disorder of special interest to the consultant or one in which he or she is conducting research.
10. Access to a patient who has a disorder with which the consultant is involved in a clinical trial.
11. A teaching function for the trainees of the referring physician or the consultant.
12. A pro forma consultation to meet the expectation that neurologic problems will be seen by a neurologist, since to do otherwise would be against form.

Consultants should always ask themselves immediately after performing a consultation why this referring physician has asked them (instead of another neurologist) to see this patient at this time. If the answers to these questions are still obscure after seeing the patient and reviewing the record, the consultant should call the physician and ask. The questions must be known in order to provide useful answers. Dr. John Kelly and L.R.C. have written a book on neurologic consultations that discusses the differential diagnosis and evaluation of common neurologic problems that the neurology consultant faces.[4] We also urge neurologists to review a brief article by Goldman, Lee, and Rudd that guides internists in answering consultations.[5] We summarize their ten commandments for effective consultation here:

1. Determine the question.
2. Establish the urgency of consultation.
3. Look for yourself. Acquire the primary data; don't rely solely on the chart.
4. Be as brief as appropriate in your note.
5. Be specific in your recommendations.
6. Provide contingency plans.
7. Honor thy referring physician's turf. Do not covet thy neighbor's patient.
8. Teach, but with tact.
9. Talk is cheap and effective. Use direct personal and phone contact often.
10. Follow-up is important.

When requested by the patient or family, and after obtaining clearance from the referring physician responsible for the patient's care, consultants should make themselves available for discussions with the family. The best arrangement is to have the principal physician and the consultant meet with the patient and family, but this is sometimes difficult to manage. The consultant must be very careful during discussion with the patient to avoid criticizing or demeaning the primary physician, including casual comments that could be taken as critical ("You mean you are still taking steroids?" "You actually had that procedure?" "I can't imagine why your doctor told you that." "That's an interesting theory."). These statements can be quite damning in the patient's mind and are best omitted. The patient should never be specifically told that, in the consultant's opinion, the physician did wrong. Whenever possible, the primary physician should be supported and buttressed, enhancing the patient's and family's confidence in his or her care. Consultants should not under any circumstances steal the patient away from the primary physician unless that physician has specifically requested them to assume responsibility. Patients and families often prefer being directly under the care of consultants, but this should be resisted. Ships have only one captain. The impression should be of a team effort, with the principal physician guiding and coordinating the team.

DISAGREEMENT OVER MANAGEMENT AND CARE BETWEEN THE REFERRING PHYSICIAN AND THE CONSULTANT

Understandably, there will be differences of opinion between consultants and referring physicians and between consultants. Consultation is requested to provide fresh insight. As an honest, independent thinker with special knowledge in a field at times mysterious to nonneurologists, the consultant's point of view may seem novel or frankly off-base to the referring physician. Disagreements often arise concerning the facts of the case, their interpretation and meaning, or translation into management of the problem and the patient. Disputes sometimes entail differences in philosophy, style, and ethics, despite general agreement about the medical facts of the case.

How should consultants respond when their advice has gone unheeded or a different plan of action has been adopted? They should call or meet with the referring physicians to discuss the issues. Sometimes ideas and suggestions have been misinterpreted, misunderstood, or poorly communicated rather than ignored or disputed, and the problem can easily be rectified. At times, the referring physician will be correct. Though the consultant may have analyzed the neurologic components of the problem well, his or her suggestions may not fit in well with the overall care of the patient as seen from the broader perspective of the generalist. Remember, consultants have no monopoly on truth and wisdom. They should acknowledge when they have erred and compromise when the health of the patient is not at stake. At other times, even after discussion with the principal physician, consultants still feel that their view is right and the referring physician is wrong. If the differences are minor, academic, or trivial in relation to the patient's care, consultants should continue to follow the patient and avoid making a mountain out of a molehill. When the differences of opinion and management are more serious and the consultant feels that the health and well-being of the patient will likely be compromised by following the present management plan or not pursuing suggestions offerred by the consultant, then he or she is obliged to make the disagreement known to the patient and family. This should be done only after repeated attempts to settle the issues between the consultant and the referring physician. Consultants have a grave responsibility to the patient as well as to the referring doctor and so they must communicate their views to patients. This should be accomplished calmly and dispassionately, avoiding any comments that might demean other doctors' views. Angry or arrogant notes should never be written in the chart. A meeting should be arranged with the patient after the consultant has informed the referring physician. The consultant should explain to the patient and family that there is a basic disagreement about the patient's care. If possible, the differences may be explained in simple terms ("Dr. X favors an operation on your carotid artery, while I feel the best course at present is to wait and treat you with aspirin."). It should be stressed that medical problems are like other issues of judgment—that there is room for disagreement and no individual is always right. There are many ways to skin a rabbit. If a consultant feels that because of differences of opinion he or she can no longer be helpful and plans to withdraw from the case, the consultant should suggest that another consultant be brought in to help settle the differences of opinion and make a brief note in the record to that effect. If, after the additional consultation, the patient and responsible physician would like the original consultant to stay involved, the consultant should do so if they will agree to heed his or her advice.

At times, the issue is informed consent. The consultant has a difference of opinion about what should be done but feels strongly that ultimately the patient and family must decide. It is the patient's body and destiny. In our opinion, it is mandatory for the consultant to be sure that the patient has been informed about the risk and benefit considerations of the various diagnostic and treatment alternatives. Whenever it is possible to arrange, we have found it useful as consultants to meet with the patient and the referring physician together to discuss the issues. The commonest dispute is between a surgical and a medical approach. The surgeon and the medical or neurologic consultant can usually generally agree about the advantages and disadvantages of each approach and the risks involved. Quantitative estimate differences are common and should be shared openly ("Dr. X estimates that your risk of stroke without surgery is about 10 percent per year, while I think it is closer to 5 percent a year."). After learning the facts and opinions, the patient should decide. The consultant has done the responsible thing by informing the patient of the alternatives. If the patient or family wants another consultant to help with the decision, this should be encouraged and they should be provided with the names of different capable experienced consultants.

REFERENCES

1. Tumulty P. *The Effective Clinician.* Philadelphia: W.B. Saunders Co., 1973.
2. Lippitt G, Lippitt R. *The Consulting Process in Action.* La Jolla, CA: University Associates, Inc., 1978;41.
3. Denny-Brown D, Rose AS, Sachs AL. *Centennial Anniversary Volume of the American Neurological Association.* New York: Springer Publishing, 1975.
4. Caplan LR, Kelly JJ. *Consultation in Neurology.* Toronto: B.C. Decker, Inc., 1988.
5. Goldman L, Lee T, Rudd P. Ten commandments for effective consultation. *Arch Int Med* 1983;143:1753–1755.

13

Medical Students, House Officers, Trainees, and Academia

It will therefore be proper to investigate the matter more closely, to study the movement of the heart and arteries not only in man but in all animals possessing a heart and to search out and find the truth by frequent experiments in living animals and by constant observation.[1]

—WILLIAM HARVEY

No physician can be all things to all patients. Each physician tries to be as much of a humanist as he can, but the physician and the patient both demand that he never depart from his role as a scientist. Balancing the two is difficult. Juggling a third role, that of teacher, adds another complication. If I err in balancing these three demands, I undoubtedly err in the direction of teacher.[2]

—HAROLD L. KLAWANS

Diagnosis of disease may be compared to the recognition of birds. The student of ornithology will learn to recognize a rook or crow in an aviary. He will see a large black bird with a white beak. If he finds a dead rook he can name it from a textbook picture. If, however, the student goes out into the field with an ornithologist he will find that the problems of recognition depend upon a different set of circumstances. The field-worker will indicate a small black dot flying in the distance and will identify it as a rook. His reasons for his apparently arbitrary statement would be: (a) it is one of a flock and he knows that rooks are gregarious; (b) it is sunset and rooks always fly home to roost at this time; (c) there is a rookery in the nearby trees.[3]

—THOMAS HODGKIN

The successful teacher is no longer on a height, pumping knowledge at high pressure into passive receptacles . . . he is a senior student anxious to help his juniors.

—WILLIAM OSLER[4]

243

Clearly, space will not permit a long essay here on various aspects of academia. In this chapter, we will limit our comments to academic issues that impact on patient care, especially patient care in an academic medical center.

THE NECESSITY FOR TRAINEE SUPERVISION IN PATIENT CARE

In our opinion, the raison d'être of hospitals and physicians is patient care. In academic medical centers there is an oft-cited triad of responsibilities: patient care, education, and research. But they are not of equal importance. In clinical departments, patient care must come first.

Patient care is best delivered by knowledgeable, experienced neurologists who like to take care of people. Certainly, students, interns, residents, and fellows are absolutely essential for creating a vibrant learning and teaching environment. Their presence promotes further learning for academic clinicians. Regardless of the age and experience of clinicians, they will always be students. When physicians stop learning, they lose the ability to provide up-to-date patient care and become ineffective teachers. The very best teachers are eternal students who share their enthusiasm and methods of learning. "What a great teacher does that is most important is to make it possible for a student to share with him his own enthusiasm and happiness in the pursuit of knowledge."[5]

But education and research cannot be at the expense of the patient. Inpatient and ambulatory services must have as their goal optimum patient care and service. Trainees, no matter how smart or proficient, are not experienced enough to assume full responsibility for the care of neurologic patients. All patients, rich and poor, private or charity, black or white, complex or simple, in the hospital or ambulatory service should be under the direct responsibility of experienced clinicians. This does not mean that all care must be delivered directly by staff physicians. It does mean direct supervision of all aspects of care. Would physicians choose otherwise for themselves or their families? Is it morally justified to do otherwise for our patients?

The Distinction between Clinician and "Bench" Researchers

Supervision should be by physicians who are clinicians. Medical advances in clinical and scientific sophistication now dictate a clear separation between physicians engaging in productive basic "bench" research and physicians who care for patients and perform clinical research (herein referred to as clinicians). Basic research is difficult and competitive and is essential if medical science is to advance. Many M.D.s and Ph.D.s compete for a shrinking supply of research dollars. In order to compete, the physician scientist must be productive in the laboratory. Few physicians will be able to compete successfully for research funds unless they put their full effort into research. Significant periods of time spent away from the laboratory detract from research productivity. Furthermore, clinical neurology has also become more complex, and clinicians must work very hard to keep up with current technology, information, and literature relating to care of the patient. Part-time clinicians cannot deliver the same quality of patient care as full-time clinicians who devote all their energy and time to the clinic, just as part-time researchers cannot compete with equally qualified full-time basic researchers. Doctors who divide their time evenly between bench research and the clinic become mediocre researchers and mediocre clinicians. It is still possible for bench researchers to remain clinically active in an area relevant to their research such as dementia, multiple sclerosis, or epilepsy, and to work in a regular outpatient clinic in a subspecialty, but it is not reasonable to expect them to remain competent as general neurologists. We also feel it is counterproductive to insist that all academic neurologists spend some time in basic research. Clinical neurology is difficult and is not a part-time job. We believe that the time has passed when neurologists could do both jobs well. Even the National Football League years ago categorized individuals as offensive or defensive players or other specialists like kickers. We believe, in the future, academic neurology departments will and should be made up of two different groups of people: those interested in and able to deliver clinical patient care and do clinical research and those scientists who will work at the bench. These two groups need to communicate, collaborate, and share goals, vision, achievements, and ideas.

The academic clinician group might be composed of full-time and visiting physicians in practice or, in some full-time institutions, might be comprised entirely of full-time staff neurologists. Units in epilepsy, stroke, neuro-oncology, neuromuscular disease, neuro-ophthalmology, neuro-immunology, child neurology, and behavior are important for research, teaching, and patient referral. In order to make advances in their subspecialty areas and to continue research and teaching, subspecialists must have access to patients with illnesses in their domain. This should take place in the hospital both on the inpatient and consultative services and in ambulatory settings. A stroke neurologist must be continuously exposed to stroke patients; an epileptologist will be stymied without a steady source of patients with seizures. Also helpful in clinical departments is a cadre of general neurologists competent to handle most neurologic problems.

In small centers, it would be difficult to support all these divisions. In large cities, it is probably unnecessary to cover all the bases at each hospital since different medical centers can cross-refer patients that they are not fully equipped to manage. Cooperation and collaboration should be the watchwords of the future, not unnecessary competition and duplicated resources.

The assignment of a trainee to a general outpatient team (or firm) that includes one or two senior clinicians allows for both long-term continuity of patient care and promotes development of an ongoing mentoring relationship between trainee and faculty. When the number of trainees permits, residents may have clinical periods assigned to subspecialty firms.

INPATIENT "WARD" SERVICE AT A TEACHING HOSPITAL

Composition of the Team and Its Direction and Approach

The inpatient neurology service of a teaching hospital is directed by a staff neurologist. The trainee members of the team vary considerably and might include a senior (second- or third-year) neurology resident, junior (first- and/or second-year) neurology residents, interns, and third- or fourth-year medical students. The nursing staff are especially important members of the team and are usually the most stable. The head nurse and chief assistants are really the only "permanent" residents of the ward, often occupying it year after year, while patients, staff neurologists, and trainees come and go. The senior nurses should assume key administrative roles and be prominent in orienting medical personnel to the way the ward runs. English hospitals for generations have recognized the supremacy of the "ward sisters," the senior nurses who run their domain with an iron hand. Nursing leaders, now both male and female, should be granted authority and responsibility if they are capable of assuming leadership roles. In some large hospitals and neurology departments, there may be more than one ward team, each led by a different staff neurologist and composed of different groups of trainees.

The staff neurologist, also traditionally referred to in some centers as the "attending" or "visit," has the principal role in patient care and trainee education during the time "on service," usually a month. There are two basic systems in general usage. In one, the supervising neurologist assumes care for all patients, and in the other system the supervising neurologist is responsible for teaching but patient care is divided among staff members.

Single Atending Physician System

Let's first discuss and analyze the system in which a single attending neurologist takes full responsibility for the ward. The term "ward" originally referred to charity patients housed in a single, large room or multiple four- to eight-bed rooms. We were trained in such units, typified by the old Peabody ward at the Boston City Hospital, F Main at the old Peter Bent Brigham Hospital, the Bullfinch and White 11 wards at the Massachusetts General Hospital, and 9 Center at Columbia-Presbyterian Medical Center. These units, and we suspect all similar wards, have long ago been replaced by hospital floors with one- and two-bed rooms (occasionally four beds). Most present trainees and junior staff have never personally experienced the old ward system.

These "charity" patients were individuals who had no doctor of their own and were referred to the inpatient unit from a clinic or emergency ward. Now, mainly for remuneration purposes, it has become customary to assign these patients to a staff physician who theoretically supervises their care and bills for services. The staff physician in the unitary system takes responsibility for all patients and supposedly sees all patients daily, as well as presiding over a daily teaching round in which all new patients are presented and examined and treatment plans generated. Another duty involves being in charge of the charts. Full admitting notes on each new patient are required. Regular progress notes on all patients are also mandated by nearly all reimbursing parties. Most often, the staff physician in this system has a one-month duty rotation, beginning on the first of the month and ending on the last day of the month. This month is very busy, and the responsible staff physician's time is taken up fully with the ward duties, leaving little opportunity for most other academic activities. On the first of the next month, a new attending physician appears and the old one returns to the laboratory, clinic, or administrative office. Discharged patients are usually referred to the outpatient clinic of one of the residents active in the patient's inpatient care.

There are advantages of the single attending physician system. The residents, trainees, and nurses have only one individual to serve. Direction of patient care is simplified, and teaching is more easily organized. Communication is much easier than in the system of multiple attending physicians. After the month is over, the physician is "free" to return to the research laboratory and need not be "bothered" with patient care responsibility on the inpatient unit or with follow-up care. Scheduling activities is much easier for individual staff members who know when they are on and off duty.

There are also great disadvantages in this system. We firmly believe that the disadvantages far outweigh any advantages. No single staff neurologist in this modern era is competent in all fields of expertise. If your mother or wife had a stroke, would you be content with an attending physician who is a peripheral nerve specialist? Should a complex seizure patient be managed by a myologist? Most neurology departments are staffed by subspecialty neurologists. They achieve their reputations by seeing patients with diseases predominantly within their chosen area of specialization and performing research in this area. Over the years, competence in areas distant from their field of specialization dwindles. Though able to discuss a case in general terms, they are not well equipped in the recent advances and nuances of care of patients with diseases outside their special area of expertise.

There is also a "numbers problem." Most wards have fifteen to thirty sick patients. Neurologic care consists of much more than making an erudite diagnosis and leading a discussion of the problem with trainees. The true physician must have knowledge of the social and personal backgrounds of the individual patients, be available and able to lend emotional and intellectual support to the patients and trainees, and be willing and able to communicate with families and significant others. No single staff physician can perform these complex functions, which are very time consuming, for all ward patients. In practice, most of these functions are delegated to the trainees, and their performance of these duties is not monitored or well supervised. Staff physicians usually make one- to two-hour teaching rounds in which new patients are discussed. They should also be available for urgent patients who are admitted during off hours. They may make walking rounds with the trainees to note progress of old patients.

Many disappear when teaching rounds are over. Very few submerge themselves in the daily tribulations of caring for sick patients and their families, but they are available to help trainees with the "science" of medical care.

We believe that this system shortchanges the patient. Trainees do not have the experience or sophistication to care for the patient in the same way as experienced clinicians. The trainees are deprived as they are expected to carry out functions for which they have had little if any training and experience, virtually without supervision. They desperately need models to show them how to do it.

Another disadvantage of this system is the regular changing of the guard depending on the lunar calendar. When physicians first come on service, they inherit many patients. It is seldom possible to become very familiar with these old patients who were "worked up" under the supervision of the previous attending physician. The tactic is usually to continue the present modus operandi as gleaned from the chart and residents. The staff physician usually leaves the in-patient ward at the end of the month when the tour of duty is completed. Follow-up is relegated to someone else. This change of care at month's end allows the physician to return to the lab, but is inconsistent with good patient care. The sudden abandonment of the patient at month's end is, in our opinion, very destructive to optimal patient care. Patients want to feel that their doctor has gotten to know and care for them and does not just think of them as cases with disease X.

The system of a monthly full responsibility visiting system is good for taking research physicians out of the labs and exposing them to trainees. These physicians are in the labs usually because they like that type of activity and are competing successfully. Many bench researchers are less fond of patient care. Many are less proficient at patient care and less able to instruct students and trainees in the details of the care of sick people than are full-time clinicians. Fully trained and intelligent, they can readily present the tenets of diagnosis that they learned during their training; they can also lecture on activities in their own lab and the research world. But is it fair for patients to be managed by individuals with these propensities? In practice, due to the staff physician's lack of concern, daily care details are completely delegated to trainees.

The single physician system is also a problem for clinician-researchers. A specialist in movement disorders needs to continue to see and treat the bulk of patients with Parkinson's disease to enable his or her research. A specialist in posterior circulation vascular disease would like to see, follow, and study all patients who enter the hospital with strokes in the vertebro-basilar system. What do these clinicians do on their months off service? Research in various subspecialty areas suffers unless the ward team consistently consults the various subspecialty services regarding patients with conditions that fall within their chosen domain of interest.

Single Teaching Physician Aided by Clinicians for Patient Care

We strongly favor the alternative system of having a single teaching neurologist but spreading care responsibilities among full-time clinicians. Patients are assigned to particular staff physicians in one of three ways:

1. Patients with a subspecialty problem should be cared for by a specialist in that area. Stroke patients will be managed by stroke service staff, seizure patients by epileptologists, and so on.
2. Private patients or patients already being cared for by staff doctors ordinarily should be assigned those doctors when admitted to the hospital. Familiarity with the patient should override specialty considerations since subspecialty consultations can always be arranged.
3. Patients may be referred specifically to certain staff clinicians at the medical center. Though these referrals are often "political" and may involve mostly VIPs, there are important reasons to maintain and promote referral services.

When patients do not fit into one of these categories, they are referred to the staff teaching physician or to any other capable available member of the staff, sometimes on a rotation basis. The physician assigned to the patient manages the patient while the patient remains in the hospital and maintains care on an ambulatory basis or refers the patient back to a physician in the community. The patient's staff doctor is responsible for calling or writing to the physician who will assume responsibility after discharge and, of course, to the referring physician, if a different individual. If a staff physician has to be away or otherwise is unable to sustain responsibility for his or her patients, they should be transferred to another staff physician. Before leaving, the physician should perform patient rounds with the new physician, introducing patients and discussing their cases.

We believe that the system of multiple staff physicians and one teaching physician has many advantages. Each staff physician usually has a smaller, more manageable complement of patients. Personal care can be delivered to 3–8 patients, but not to 15–30 patients. Personal care is better delivered by staff physicians than by unsupervised trainees. Patients benefit by being taken care of by doctors who like and are interested in patient care, and who are knowledgeable in their field of illness.

Trainees also benefit. Trainees can learn the art of patient care by apprenticeship and modeling their behavior after senior clinicians whom they watch dealing with patients and their families in sensitive, difficult situations. Also, trainees are to some extent freed up for medical management and reading. For each of the patients that they evaluate, trainees receive tutelage from two staff neurologists, the patient's staff physician and the teaching physician. Exchange of ideas and variance of staff physicians' styles is helpful in the education of trainees.

The input of two senior physicians is useful for quality control. There is greater opportunity for detection of errors or omissions in diagnosis and treatment and introduction of fresh opinions and cross discussion.

Continuity of care is facilitated. Hospitalization for acute illness is just one phase of patient care. Exposure to patients during this acute period is essential, but only by long-term observation and management can the longitudinal aspects of illnesses be clarified. Many patients discharged as "wrecks" from the hospital return to seemingly normal function months later; patients who look like "roses" on discharge often dwindle badly afterward. Prognostic lessons learned only from the acute hospitalization often prove to be false.

Clinical research is facilitated. Frequent exposure to patients in their own subspecialty allows staff to study the illnesses more fully and facilitates research and trial protocols. Trials begun during hospitalization can be continued in ambulatory settings.

The education and maturation of subspecialists are enhanced by constant exposure to material within their realm of interest and study. They can learn from their experience. What would myologists do if they were not exposed to patients with muscle disease? Perhaps work in a laboratory on related basic research? Perhaps massage and analyze old trials and the data of others? Perhaps work in a general neurology clinic? But knowledge of the clinical findings and nuances of inclusion body myositis will come only from careful study of groups of patients with this disorder.

This system does make communication more difficult because residents, students, and nurses must contact different staff physicians for different patients. This disadvantage, in our estimation, is more than compensated for by improved patient care, trainee teaching, and clinical research. The system should not have an adverse effect on basic research, since bench researchers would either remain where they are most productive (in the lab) or take an occasional turn as a teaching physician with little patient responsibility.

Daily Rounds

Morning activity and rounds on an inpatient, teaching ward should be consistent and routinized. Timing and integration with nursing activities and schedules may vary between hospitals and neurology services. The head nurse should enforce a daily routine that is consistent and independent of the changing rotation of the resident and attending staff. The workings of the ward cannot change each time a new physician comes on board. The nurses' rules about morning and afternoon ward activities should be discussed with the senior neurology staff and written down. New residents rotating on service should be indoctrinated by the head nurse. The chief of service must back up the authority of the head nurse who runs the ward.

There must be three separate morning rounds. During the earliest round, individual house officers (or teams if an intern and resident or student work together) see each of their individual patients. At the minimum, this should include an interim account of new symptoms and changes in old symptoms, getting a sense of how the patient is doing compared to the previous day, listening to any complaints or problems, at least a brief examination, and a review of the latest laboratory data and imaging reports. Time should also be spent on emotional support. A nod, a smile, a pat on the shoulder or hand, a few seconds or minutes to "shoot the breeze" are appreciated by the patient. If the patient is feeling frightened or depressed, clearly more time will be needed. The early round should take about thirty to sixty minutes, depending on the number of patients, the acuteness and severity of their illnesses, and the house officer's efficiency.

The next round includes all resident staff and students and available members of the nursing staff. These should be walking rounds and must not take place in a room away from the patients. The head nurse should accompany rounds and as each bedside is approached, the staff nurse caring for that patient should be available to join the discussion. This nurse should be made to feel like an active and important part of the professional team. Ordinarily, the responsible house officer will present an interim report and the nurse should comment on his or her observations. Patients should be greeted warmly and asked if they have anything to add or dispute related to the house officer's and nurse's accounts. If there is any question about progress, the senior resident in charge of the round may want to ask questions and do a brief examination. Before leaving the bedside, the team should decide on the day's tests, activities, and treatment, and orders should be written in the chart. All concerned with the patient's care should be informed, so that the nurse will be able to answer the patient's or family's questions about activities when queries are forthcoming later. If there are major questions or uncertainties, final plans should await discussion with the patient's attending staff physician. All patients should be seen at least briefly. Obviously, more time will need to be spent with acutely ill patients and those who remain diagnostic or therapeutic dilemmas. Patients who are stable and have been on the unit for a long time can be seen briefly.

After the resident's rounds, some time should be devoted to patient care activities, looking at radiographic films, and urgent diagnostic or therapeutic procedures. This is the best time for various attending physicians to make their own daily rounds. They can make note of the day's planned activities and can discuss any discrepancies or problems with the resident staff.

The key event of the morning should be the visit of the teaching attending physician or monthly visit. The teaching physician should be presented all new patients who will come under his or her responsibility. If time permits, interesting or instructive patients under the care of other physicians should also be presented.

We feel very strongly that patient presentations must be at the bedside or the patient should be brought into the conference room during the presentation. Rounds in a closed room without the patient are sterile, academic exercises, not patient care. The experienced clinician gains much insight from seeing the patient and interacting directly. The trainees must observe the attending physician in action, focusing not only on the patient's illness, but also on the patient as a person.

There are many reasons for the patient being present during the presentation. This is such an important issue and so central to patient care and trainee teaching that we want to elaborate on the reasons for the rule and the suggested method of the presentation. We suggest the following general procedure. The individuals present, particularly those involved in the patient's care, should be introduced to the patient by name and description ("Drs. A, B, and C are neurology residents who need to know about your care because they often cover for each other; Susan P. and Tom X. are medical students, and Dr. O is a medical intern rotating through our service."). The patient should then be told that the details of his or her illness are going to be presented to the attending physician, preferably in simple terms that the patient can understand. The patient should be encouraged to interrupt to correct any points or elaborate when there is additional important information. Then the student or house officer who has "worked up" the patient should begin the presentation, telling the history the patient has related, adding information related by others that adds to or questions the patient's account. Whenever possible, the patient's words should be used, and translations or substitutions of "medical lingo" should be avoided. Simple English should be used. Sensitive personal facts can be omitted. If there is potentially emotionally charged medical data that may not be fully known to the patient, it should also be omitted. Rather than saying that the patient had "a highly malignant small-cell cancer of the lung removed two years ago," if the patient has not been told the diagnosis in those terms, the house officer can merely say that "a shadow on a chest X-ray led to chest surgery and removal of a part of the lung. This was followed by radiation." This conveys the information that the patient related. Medical data, lab results, and sensitive items can be added later in the privacy of the conference room. After or during the history presentation, the attending may and, in fact, should interrupt to elicit more detail or explore other areas not mentioned. After the history presentation is over, others present should be invited to ask the patient questions that they feel are important and have not been fully explored. The patient should also be invited to add information.

The examination findings can be handled in a number of different ways. The presenter can describe the examination, with the attending checking key findings during or after the presentation. Alternatively, the attending might perform the examination while the others observe. Sometimes it is useful for teaching purposes to have one of the residents do the examination while the attending and others watch. If the examination findings are presented, the presenter should avoid comments that might be interpreted by the patient or family as pejorative. The presenter should not say that the patient is demented. Instead, the data can merely be stated ("The patient said she was in the Boston Common, and the date was February 31, 1381, and George Washington was president" or "serial 7s were reported as 100, 93, 81, 70," etc.). After the attending physician's examination, others present should be asked if there are other parts of the examination that they would like performed. Before leaving the patient, the attending physician should ask the patient again if there is any other information to add. The patient and family members, if present, should also be invited to ask questions that concern them. The group should then retire to a conference room or, if the patient has been presented in the conference room, he or she should be ushered back to bed.

The procedure outlined answers many of the following complaints and criticisms often made by patients and doctors.

1. The "players" are identified. Patients often comment that they do not know the various individuals involved in their care and have no idea of their roles.
2. Information is shared and described fully and fairly. The staff involved in the patient's care functions as a team led by the attending physician. Some patients are annoyed or puzzled by the need for examinations by multiple individuals. They wonder if the information is transmitted to the attending physician or is extensively edited. They wonder if the team members talk to each other and relate the details to the attending physician. The method described lets the patient hear what has been said and to whom.
3. Patients get their "day in court." They are allowed to hear, edit, and elaborate on the data. This should confirm the patient's impression that information is complete and fairly described.
4. The patient feels that adequate time has been spent. When patients are presented in a conference room out of earshot and sight of the patient, the actual bedside time spent may be very brief, sometimes only 5–10 minutes. Patients have no idea what has been said in the conference room; they observe only the time spent with them. When a short time is spent, patients naturally worry that information is incomplete and that decisions are hastily made without adequate time or deliberation.
5. The attending has more time with the patient to make direct observations. There is no substitute for watching the patient.
6. The attending physician need not repeat all parts of the history and examination. The presentation allows the attending to be eclectic and explore key parts of the history and physical findings, and yet the patient knows that the attending has been told the remainder of the data. When attending physicians come to a patient's bedside after a conference room presentation, they are faced with two unsatisfactory choices. They can either be very selective in performing parts of the history and examination and take the risk of the patient noting the incompleteness, or they can tediously review the full history and examination, boring all those present, dragging out rounds, and unnecessarily decreasing time for discussion and teaching. How much the attending physician reviews depends on the experience of the clinician, the perceived reliability and experience of the presenter, the complexity or straightforwardness of the problem, and the time available.
7. Social and psychological factors can be explored. The attending should be alert to cues that the patient feels uncomfortable with the turn of the inquiry. These issues and other sensitive matters can be explored later when the attending returns to the bedside without the full team. The attending's interest in the social environment and psychological factors shows trainees that these matters are of utmost importance and relevance to patient care. Trainees use experienced

clinicians as role models. Despite staff protestations about the importance of psychological factors, if trainees see that all patient encounters with the staff involve only strictly biomedical aspects, the actions will belie the words.

After the patient has left, or the team has returned to the conference room, sensitive data and prior laboratory results can be reviewed. At this point, before introducing the results of any laboratory or imaging results done during the current hospital stay, discussion should focus on the clinical problem. We believe that trainees learn more when they are led through the thinking process concerning diagnosis than when the attending didactically discusses and expounds on the case. Students and house staff should tell the attending what they feel are the major problems. They should work out the differential diagnosis of the disease mechanism and lesion anatomy. Trainees must be guided through the process of planning evaluation and investigations. Then the attending should summarize and clearly state his or her own diagnosis and how their own approach differs. Then the laboratory results, X-rays, or imaging tests performed to date should be discussed or reviewed.

After the patient's problems have been fully explored, the case should be viewed in broader terms. This may involve a discussion of the disease, for example, the usual physical findings, clinical features, course, and laboratory results in series of patients with progressive supranuclear palsy and how this patient with that disease fits into the spectrum of the illness. Discussion could relate to a clinical or laboratory phenomenon such as loss of vertical eye movement, tremor, partial complex seizures, high CSF protein, or oligoclonal banding. Alternatively, treatment might be emphasized, with a review of past therapy in the particular disease. Adaptation, communication with the patient, psychosocial and environmental influence, or coping strategies could be emphasized. Each patient's case offers many lessons.

If the attending is the patient's doctor, at some point after rounds or the next day, he or she should communicate with the patient either alone at the bedside or with the trainees who are also responsible for that patient. Attendings or staff physicians responsible for patients should round individually on patients under their care who have already been discussed at rounds. Problems and progress in these "old patients" can be mentioned and reviewed at the beginning or end of daily attending rounds. Walking rounds each day, with the attending and the house staff seeing each patient together, is wasted time. Too little time is spent with each patient, and psychosocial factors and minor daily problems are ignored because of the lack of privacy and press for time. Furthermore, the house staff has already walked around, and their time is wasted in the repetition. Attendings should see their own patients alone each day. These daily private visits transmit to the patient the attending's personal involvement and concern. Patients must look on the attending physician as their doctor, not only as the leader of the pack.

If the teaching attending has opinions that differ from the patient's physician, these should be discussed between the two staff physicians. The patient's physician has the last word and the major responsibility, not the teaching attending, no matter what his or her academic rank or seniority. The buck must stop with the patient's staff physician, not with the residents or the teaching attending.

Ordinarily, when patients are discharged, they should be sent back to the care of the referring doctor, with an appropriate call from the attending, followed by a letter and discharge summary. Some patients will be followed on an ambulatory basis by the attending or by an involved resident with staff supervision.

Inpatient Consultation Service

In most teaching hospitals, the large number of consultations and inpatients under the care of staff neurologists mandates that there be two separate services, one dedicated only to consultations. In smaller institutions, or in hospitals where few patients are directly under the primary responsibility of neurologists, the two services might be combined or all patients might be consultations. Some neurology departments in the United States, for example, the University of Rochester, use a system loosely modeled on the English system of "firms" in which house officers and students are assigned to individual physicians or groups of physicians. These firms or teams care for inpatients, answer consultations, and attend ambulatory sessions together.

Let's consider here the more traditional neurology consult service, which is usually headed by one staff neurologist for a 1-month rotation and staffed by one or more neurology residents and sometimes medical and psychiatric residents and medical students. The staff neurologist usually serves from the first to the last day of the month and then is replaced by a different staff physician.

Consultations are called or requested in writing or through computer communications. When there are multiple trainees, the service should be coordinated by the most senior neurology resident, who assigns patients to individual trainees. Depending on the experience and capability of that trainee, the neurology resident may need to review the case with the trainee before presentation to the staff consultant. During daily consultation rounds, new consultations are presented to the staff consultant. We strongly favor presenting all patients at the bedside for the same reasons explained in the previous section on inpatient care.

After the patient has been seen, and the case discussed among the team, it is the staff consultant's responsibility to communicate the findings and suggestions to the staff physician or the responsible resident who requested the consultation. If the patient is acutely ill or urgent action is recommended, the communication should be immediate and by phone. If the consultant's findings are unexpected or if the suggestions are controversial or problematic, it is also best to call to discuss the case. For routine cases, a brief, concise, clear note in the chart will usually suffice. Trainees should write more complete notes, recording the pertinent historical and examination findings. It is not enough for the consultant to simply countersign the trainee's note; there should be at a minimum a few short sentences written by the consultant capturing the essence of the case and recommendations.

Consultations must be answered quickly, within 48 hours of submission and preferably the same or the very next day. During the weekend, this might be done by the resident and staff neurologist on call, but during the work week it should be done by the consult team. Urgent cases should be seen by the staff neurologist soon after the neurology consult resident and should not wait for the next day's rounds.

Follow-up of consultations is very important. The staff consultant who sees the patient should follow the case whenever possible until discharge from the hospital or resolution of the neurologic problem. Judgment will be required to decide which patients need to be seen only once, which can be seen occasionally, and which require frequent visits and close supervision. As a senior neurology resident at the Boston City Hospital in the late 1960s, L.R.C. recalls being literally swamped by new requests for consultations. He saw 8 new patients a day, 40 a week, and nearly 500 during a 3-month consultation rotation. He had time to see only new cases, no follow-ups. L.R.C. saw the patient, pontificated in the chart on the diagnosis and treatment, and never returned. At that time, he thought he was the world's best consultant, unerringly pinpointing difficult neurologic diagnoses in each case. When L.R.C. became a staff neurologist at a teaching hospital used by private patients, he was then able to follow up on his initial opinions. He was quickly humbled to find that, more often than not, the initial assessment was wrong or at least found wanting when all the data later became available and the course of illness became clear. Even now, there are few cases in which even experienced neurologic consultants don't learn something by following the course of events and the results of investigations and treatment.

Trainees should follow the patients they have seen and presented. If trainees become aware of a problem that needs the staff consultant's input or learn data that would modify the original opinion, they should contact the consultant. Nevertheless, we feel it is very important for staff neurologists to follow patients themselves. Ordinarily, follow-up rounds should be made separately by the staff neurologist and the trainees for the same reasons discussed under inpatient service rounds. Long walk rounds in which the entire team, staff and trainees, visit each patient are tedious, time consuming, and not very effective for either patient care or teaching. The staff neurologist who initially examines the patient should follow that patient throughout the hospitalization even if the calendar month of duty has passed. Continuity of care is essential. When this practice is not followed, the new consultant cannot effectively pick up all the old cases, and patient care suffers.

In many neurology departments, a single assigned attending neurologist answers all consultations directed to the service, no matter whether they are ward patients or the private patients of other physicians. This system of one consultant simplifies communications and coordination of team activities, but it does not always meet the needs of the patients and the other medical and surgical departments optimally. We favor allowing staff physicians from other services to, at times, request an attending neurologist other than the monthly designated consultant to see their patient. These requests are made for a variety of reasons, the most valid ones being that the requested physician had previously cared for that patient, has appropriate subspecialty expertise, or is known personally or by reputation by the patient or family, who initiated the consultation. When willing and available, the requested neurologist should answer the consultation. Continuity of care is very important; whenever possible, the neurology staff consultant who had seen the patient before should be involved again if the patient is readmitted. Even when this request for continuity is not made by the service initiating the consultation, the neurology resident should recognize the situation and contact the previous consultant. The neurology resident should examine the patient first and present the case to the attending alone or with the consultation team. The case is then not lost to the trainees. Patients with stroke and brain tumor, two potentially serious and mortal diseases, may need the subspecialty expertise of neurologists specializing in these disorders, especially if the monthly designated consultant is an epileptologist, peripheral nerve expert, or myologist.

We have attempted to deal with the problem of subspecialization by having subspecialty services function in addition to the ordinary consultation service. The regular consult team should see the patient first. When appropriate, they will also call in the stroke service, oncology service, and so on, after clearing this with the physician or service requesting the original consultation. In this way, the subspecialty services gain constant exposure to most patients in the hospital in their field of interest and expertise, and the patients and trainees are well served from a teaching viewpoint.

AMBULATORY CARE

The wealth of clinical neurologic material now seen in ambulatory settings makes the outpatient arena potentially the most productive resource for teaching trainees. The scheduling of trainees in ambulatory settings must, however, be carefully planned to optimize patient care and satisfaction and resident and student training. Patients will be very unhappy if they must stay at the clinic for hours, with long delays between being examined and prodded by multiple trainees.

For very inexperienced trainees, the best first step is observing a trained clinician take a history, perform an examination, and communicate with the patient. The encounter can then be discussed with the trainee after the patient leaves. Later, trainees should interact alone with patients, under supervision.

"Resident clinics" are not very worthwhile for training. Usually, these clinics are attended by "unwashed" long-term patients either left over from the last resident (or even generations of past residents) or collected by the resident during the years of training. The charts are lengthy records of housekeeping chores, with the significant material hard to glean. Most of the more interesting, compliant patients get weeded out. Little room is left on the schedule for new patients. Those new patients who are referred to the residents are often the "dregs" of the material seen in the ambulatory area. Patients with difficult or "interesting" neurologic problems are referred directly to more senior neurologists attending the clinic. Private paying patients request staff clinicians. Patients who have little income or health insurance coverage, do not have their own doctor, come from other resident clinics, or have what seem like relatively mundane or "psychological" problems to the triage person are usually directed to the residents. The chaff is delivered to the residents after the wheat is removed. The pace of the resident clinic and the type and number of patients seen usually makes staff supervision difficult and mostly pro forma.

We favor instead a system that integrates trainees into the outpatient schedule of staff physicians. The trainees are assigned to a specific staff physician for a period of time such as 6 months. They are scheduled to see two or three new patients each session. The patients are individually referred to the consulting staff physicians; the types of problems seen usually reflect the subspecialty interest and expertise of the staff preceptor. If L.R.C. were to work with a designated trainee, that resident would see mostly stroke patients during their tenure with him. If the resident were then to rotate to the tutelage of a peripheral nerve specialist an epileptologist, or a myologist, the patient exposure would be quite different. After appropriate introduction and explanation, the trainee examines the patient first. Soon after finishing the history and examination and thinking about the case, the trainee presents the patient to the staff physician in the examining room with the patient present. In most cases, family members are invited in if their presence will be helpful. The consultant should review the history and examination in the fashion similar to that described in the section of this chapter on inpatient attending rounds. After the examination, the trainee and preceptor should move to another office or private area to discuss the case and plan management. They then both return to the patient room, and the staff physician talks with the patient about the findings and plan, while the trainee observes the communication. Later in the rotation, the resident should, in selected cases, be asked to deliver the dismissal interview while the preceptor supervises.

Whenever possible, a period of time could be set aside for a conference for all those attending the outpatients that day, presenting interesting, puzzling, or instructive cases seen during that session. Charcot derived many of his leçons du Mardi from outpatients attending the clinic at the Salpêtrière,[6] and demonstrations at the National Hospital Queens Square, London, England, often concern ambulatory patients. This preceptor system is usually applied to trainees and is scheduled for regular sessions, for example, once or twice a week in the ambulatory care facility. Also useful are ambulatory rotations during which the resident has a different preceptor for each clinic session and follows some patients with short-term problems under supervision.

This system does not allow the trainee much follow-up exposure. Trainees do see patients that they have examined with their preceptor when the patient returns to the ambulatory care facility during the resident's tenure with that preceptor or during the ambulatory rotation. They do not, however, develop a cadre of their own patients to follow longitudinally. L.R.C. believes they will readily get longitudinal experience as soon as they begin practice or become staff clinicians after their training period. In his opinion, the increased exposure to new patient material and increased tutelage and observation of potential role models in action more than compensates for the paucity of clinic longitudinal care. J.H. feels that the outlined plan offers great educational (and patient care) value but finds the "firm" concept offers the opportunity to see new patients while maintaining long-term continuity. He suggests that residents begin their first year in a generalist firm one half-day per week. In the second year a second half-day is added that includes subspecialty supervision.

TEACHING STYLES AND METHODS

The medical trainees of a bygone era learned their trade by apprenticeship. Rather than classroom teaching, the essence of their training was observing their masters performing the daily acts of physicians of that period. After a long period of observation, masters allowed apprentices to do some procedures, while carefully supervising their technique. Eventually, apprentices were allowed to practice on their own, after variable periods of training, when the master recognized that apprentices had achieved competence. Medical students, during the third and fourth years, are taught by a mix of didactic instruction and observation. Intern and resident training is fashioned after the apprentice system, but, in contrast to the apprentice of days of yore, today's trainees are given too much responsibility too soon and with too little direct supervision. Good patient care training of house staff requires (1) exposure to an adequate number of patients with diverse medical problems, (2) role models and mentors to observe in day-to-day patient care activities, (3) consistent questioning and inquiry of the staff by the trainees and of the trainees by the staff, (4) exposure to adequate reference material and guidance by staff on how and where to find key information, (5) close supervision of trainee activities, especially early in training, and (6) increased responsibility commensurate with increased competence.

We cannot overemphasize the importance of role models and mentors. Quoting Penfield again, "No man goes alone on his eventful journey through medical school. He makes his own little images of those whom he chooses to be his heroes, setting them up in his personal shrine as he progresses."[5] Trainees should be exposed as much as possible to senior clinicians "doing their thing." If senior clinicians are taken away from the bedside or clinic, away from direct patient care responsibilities, they will not be available for trainees to emulate. Emulation does not come from attending lectures!

The method of teaching is also important. Most young teachers have a great urge to tell the student the material. This is often done didactically by lecturing, distributing handouts of written information, or writing journal articles. By sharing their accumulated wisdom, these teachers hope to spare students the arduousness and pain of acquiring the information themselves. But unfortunately, this method does not work. Parents learn this lesson when they try to spare their children the pain of lessons the parents have learned with time. "If youth but knew and age but could," the old saying goes. But sons and daughters don't listen to their parents' words; they need to acquire the lessons themselves. Similarly, trainees learn more by being pressed to think for themselves. Recent scrutiny of present medical school education policies led to a forceful statement urging a diminution in the amount of data and didactic instruction given to medical students.[7]

During his stroke fellowship year, L.R.C. was blessed by having an apprenticeship with an unparalleled master clinician and teacher, Dr. C. Miller Fisher. For the first 6 months of his fellowship, Dr. Fisher never told L.R.C. anything directly. He taught by questioning and by example. Each evening, Dr. Fisher and L.R.C. would meet for about 4 hours, during which time L.R.C. would present two patients seen that day or a preceding day. While Dr. Fisher listened carefully, L.R.C. would begin by presenting the details of the history and exam. Dr. Fisher would often interrupt and ask L.R.C. to elaborate on or clarify a point ("What was the patient doing at that time?" "Did the left eye move laterally as quickly as the right eye moved medially?" "Was sensation as impaired in the thumb as in the face?"). Then he would ask L.R.C. how he would put the case together. After listening, he would continue to question ("I see, but how did you explain this finding?" "Weren't you bothered that there was no nystagmus?" "Why did he have a headache?"). Gradually, he would paint L.R.C. into a corner. L.R.C. had to state his opinions and reasons clearly. Then they would go and see the patient together. Dr. Fisher would review parts of the history, always eliciting new key information. He would then go over some of the aspects of the examination, again always uncovering some new findings and raising questions about others. Dr. Fisher showed L.R.C. that the data aquired by L.R.C. during the history and exam were good but not quite good enough. L.R.C. had missed key information that helped answer some of the questions raised in the preliminary discussion. At the beginning of the year, L.R.C. would naively ask Dr. Fisher what he thought after seeing the patient. He usually responded, "Difficult, eh?" or "I just don't know what to make of it," or "I am anxious to know how you finally solve this one." Often, when L.R.C. had been painted into a corner by repeated questioning and quoted a source in defense, Dr. Fisher would say, "You might take a look at . . ." citing three or four sources that usually either ran counter to L.R.C.'s interpretation or added important considerations.

Residents should not be spoon-fed. Attendings should avoid giving them a lecture or a didactic exposition after seeing each case. They should be made to clarify, organize, and synthesize their thoughts and venture their own opinions. Then they will learn. There is a useful little book on how to teach evidence-based medicine.[8] It is not written as a bedside paradigm, but can be adapted to a patient-centered approach. We are increasingly impressed that students and trainees ask for more lectures, more handouts, and more didactic sessions. Unfortunately, didactic sessions teach little except what is important to be learned. In our opinion, grand rounds, which in many teaching hospitals are composed of "canned" talks by experts, are usually sterile experiences. The person who learns most is the individual who prepares the talk. But watching a teaching physician examine a patient and review the details of a case helps trainees to clarify their own thoughts. Grand rounds should include mostly case presentations and discussions.

Periodically, during the house officer training period, it is useful for trainees and staff clinicians to administer an oral practical examination. Emulation of the neurology board examinations patient session is an excellent way to monitor trainee progress as well as to prepare the house officer for the board exam. Senior faculty watch while the trainee takes a history and examines the patient (25 to 30 minutes). The faculty preceptor then asks the trainee to summarize the data concisely. What is the differential diagnosis and the most likely diagnosis? How should the patient be investigated and treated? Then the resident can be interrogated about issues raised during the patient encounter and related subjects. The session should last about 1–1½ hours. Each trainee should be examined by at least two faculty members. Patient vignettes or videotapes can also be used but do not substitute for live patients. There is no substitute for watching the resident in action with the patient. Trainees appreciate constructive feedback on their techniques, their progress, and any critiques. We have used this approach at Strong Memorial Hospital and the New England Medical Center. As examiners, we have learned a great deal about residents' skills as well as their ability to synthesize their fund of information and the clinical findings. It is helpful to then offer constructive criticism to the residents. These examinations should occur regularly beginning in the first year. In this way both the examiners and the trainees can gauge progress.

Another very useful teaching device used frequently by psychiatric training programs is taping a clinical encounter between a resident and a patient. Optimally, this would be by videotape, but audio tape recording of the history and information transmittal sessions is also useful. Trainees can watch or listen to their performance, and the tapes can also be reviewed by staff preceptors. This technique is used very effectively by swimming, tennis, and golf instructors. Why not bring it into the more serious business of training clinicians?

CLINICAL RESEARCH AND WRITING

During the training years, faculty hope that house officers and students will catch the "writing bug." Preparing a manuscript for publication is an excellent way for trainees to learn about the subject reported and to learn about submitting material to the medical literature. Case reports and literature reviews are both good ways to get the house officer started. But house officers are usually just as naive about writing as they are about the nuances of patient care, often even more so. They need prodding, supervision, and help.

When a patient is presented with very instructive features, students should be encouraged to write it up or at least explore the finding further in a prospective group of patients. They should conduct a literature review on the subject. Trainees should be encouraged and later reminded to discuss their preliminary findings with the teaching physician. If the material will add to the medical literature, the trainee should start the process of preparing the manuscript. They need guidance in finding key references and sources of information about the subject. After discussing the general outline of the report, they should then write a rough draft, combining the clinical data and the literature review. The staff preceptor then reviews and critiques the draft. The manuscript should develop through successive reviews of the drafts. When the paper is in reasonable form, the staff physician should revise and add to the paper. It is essential for the preceptor to go to the literature to be sure that the source and citations are complete and the descriptions accurate. The trainee's name deserves to go first on the paper.

A similar process of literature review can be stimulated by discussion of a particular conundrum such as "What is known about the toxic effects of Amicar?" or "What has been the experience with thrombolytic agents in forms of vascular disease other than stroke?" The student should be encouraged to write and publish when the information would, in the preceptor's opinion, make a useful addendum to the literature.

Trainees should also be exposed to the rigor and systematic logic of research during their training. Research and patient care should go hand in glove. They should be encouraged to participate in clinical research projects or be given some time at the bench to explore that discipline. However, trainees and students should never be used to do the research work of the staff. They should be encouraged to start projects of their own with staff input, supervision, subsidization (if available), and help.

The other chapters in Part III deal with issues of central concern to all neurologists and physicians. Ambulatory care, hospitalization, consultations, and unfortunately, medicolegal issues are an integral part of physicians' everyday activities and concerns, no matter where they practice. Academic issues are different. To some physicians the academic world is a distant recollection. Any close connections were severed as soon as residency training ended. To others, like L.R.C., whose entire careers took place in academic medical centers, the teaching environment is absolutely central to all medical activities. J.H. has spent much time at an affiliated teaching hospital with extensive time spent in resident and medical student teaching. There are many physicians between these two extremes who have some academic activities but who work predominantly in a nonacademic environment.

Both academic and nonacademic hospitals and medical centers exist primarily to care for ill patients and to promote public health and well-being. Research and teaching are very important but should not take precedence over patient care. Clinicians actively engaged in taking care of patients and clinical research are best able to teach medical students and trainees how to care for patients. Students learn by emulating these clinicians. Academic physicians teach best by stimulating trainees to learn with them.

REFERENCES

1. Harvey W. *Exercitatio Anatomica De Motu Cordis et Sanguinis in Animalibus.* Springfield, IL: Charles C Thomas, 1968.
2. Klawans HL. *Toscanini's Fumble and Other Tales of Clinical Neurology.* Chicago: Contemporary Books, 1988.
3. Hodgkin T. *Towards Earlier Diagnosis.* 5th ed. Edinburgh: Churchill Livingstone, 1985.
4. Bean RB, Bean WB. *Sir William Osler: Aphorisms from His Bedside Teachings and Writings.* Springfield, IL: Charles C Thomas, 1961.
5. Penfield W. *No Man Alone, A Neurosurgeon's Life.* Boston: Little, Brown, 1977.
6. Goetz G. *Charcot. The Clinician: The Tuesday Lessons.* New York: Raven Press, 1987.
7. Muller S and the General Professional Education of the Physician Committee. *Physicians for the Twenty-first Century.* Washington, DC: Association of American Medical Colleges, 1984.
8. Sackett DL, Straus SE, Richardson WS, Rosenberg W, Haynes RB. *Evidence-Based Medicine: How to Practice and Teach EBM.* London: Churchill Livingstone, 2000.

14

Medicolegal Aspects of Neurologic Care

The laws of evidence seem to me the strangest thing about the whole legal system, and I never got used to them. A witness is in the stand, doing his best to give a clear, connected statement of the facts as he knows them, but the laws of evidence require that the simplest story be interrupted, parts of it prohibited, the telling of it so cabin'd, cribb'd, confined that both witness and jury are confused.[1]

—ALICE HAMILTON

A disproportionate number of state and federal legislators are lawyers. As lawyers, they believe that the common law tort of negligence has been a useful method of disciplining the medical profession. The lawyer's belief is that the threat of a malpractice suit keeps a physician practicing high quality medicine, and that the jury award of damages punishes the "bad doctor." This trust is badly misplaced. As a method of assuring competence among physicians, the tort of medical negligence is erratic at best. It is far more likely to punish the bad result, and it is not effective in flagrant cases of negligence that do not cause injury sufficient to make the compensating damages worth a lawyer's time. Furthermore, the punishment for a malpractice judgment, even if accurate, comes far too late to help those patients who are treated by the negligent physician in the subsequent five to ten years before the suit comes to trial. Since the determination of standards of care and of the physician's deviation from the standard is left in the hands of persons carefully selected for their ignorance of the subject—a jury rather than panel of experts—the result is at least as likely to be due to emotional reaction to the attorney's plea as it is to any evaluation of physician incompetence.[2]

—RICHARD S. WILBUR, M.D.

What hung in the balance, I painfully realize was S.'s whole sense of herself as physician, her identification with the profession at which she worked so conscientiously. I knew better than anyone her intense concern for her patients, her untiring efforts to place their welfare ahead of everything else. Found negligent, she would never be the same again—

265

and maybe we wouldn't, either—for charges of professional malpractice aim finally at the soul and spirit.[3]

—Eugene Kennedy

Legal issues, disability problems, and malpractice suits are unfortunately becoming more and more of an issue for doctors, patients, and society in general. Though neurologists are involved in a small fraction of malpractice allegations and suits, legal issues have nevertheless insidiously infiltrated all aspects of neurologic clinicians' activities. Defensive medicine, defined by a federal commission as "the alteration of modes of medical practice, induced by the threat of liability, for the principal purposes of forestalling the possibility of lawsuits by patients as well as providing a good legal defense in the event such lawsuits are instituted,"[4] permeates the care of patients with nervous system diseases. If polled, most if not all physicians might compare the legal invasion of medical practice to a glioma whose cells invade brain tissue, gradually and insidiously but relentlessly impairing brain function. But bewailing the presence of the uninvited guests (lawyers and courts), name-calling, or throwing stones will do little good and will probably disaffect the general public. We must try to extract some good from the bad. Though AIDS is probably the worst plague of our century, rivaled only by the second World War, it has undoubtedly taught physicians and scientists a great deal about viruses, immune function, interaction between viruses and cells in the nervous system and the usual findings in unusual infections of the nervous system rarely seen in any numbers before the AIDS epidemic. Lawsuits may have been the only way patients could seek redress and compensation for undeniably bad medical care. The medical profession must find ways to police itself without the necessity of court interventions using more effective peer review.

There are a number of reasons for our present medicolegal crisis, including litigious patients; an overabundance of lawyers, some of whom are greedy and less than completely ethical; a slow, inept, costly legal system; and a process (the advocacy system, with cases decided by scientifically and medically unsophisticated jurors) unsuited for fair and equitable solution of complex medical issues. Other important causes, which physicians often lose sight of, are bad medicine and poor medical practices. We must do all we can to improve the care of patients. Only as patient advocates will we gain support for meaningful change; after all, aren't we practicing medicine and neurology to help patients? In recognition of concern about patient care, the medicolegal committee of the Council of Medical Specialty Societies, representing over 290,000 physicians, has chosen to call itself the Patient Safety Committee, and its major education project the Patient Injury Prevention Program.

An in-depth analysis of the medicolegal problems that neurologists face is beyond the scope of this chapter. Interested readers are referred to a monograph by Beresford that includes detailed descriptions of the legal process, as it involves neurologists[5] and a guide to medical malpractice issues from Illinois.[6] Here, we will begin by briefly touching on disability concerns, a common problem that patients, lawyers, and various governmental agencies bring to neurologists. Turning then to the malpractice problem, L.R.C. will present some suggestions to neurologists for prevention of allegations and lawsuits and describe the neurologist-lawyer-court interfaces, with advice to neurologists about their involvement. L.R.C.'s experience in "legal" neurology has come mostly from testifying in court on behalf of defendant physicians (especially neurologists), testifying as an expert witness for some legitimately injured patients, and preparing reports about his own patients at lawyers' requests. J.H. has had some experience reviewing the records and testifying primarily in defense of physicians and hospitals and concurs in the comments.

DISABILITY, CIVIL SUITS, AND NONMALPRACTICE CLAIMS

Two different situations, civil suits for injury other than malpractice and disability assessment for worker's compensation or social security disability, present similar problems for neurologists. In civil injury suits and worker's compensation cases, the patient claims an injury, usually physical, but occasionally there are also alleged emotional and economic consequences. Physicians evaluating these patients may benefit by consulting an American Medical Association monograph on disability evaluation.[7] Compensation under worker's compensation or social security disability may be awarded in the absence of proof of fault or wrongdoing, in contrast to civil suit cases.

In all of these circumstances, the physician is asked to determine if the injury is real or fancied, the relation of the alleged event or injury to any disability found, and the degree and nature of any disability. Almost always, the physician will be asked to furnish a report, sometimes followed by testimony, to a lawyer, insurance or governmental agency, or court. Neurologists and other physicians have no obligation to perform this type of evaluation. If it is not "your cup of tea," we urge you to avoid these injury and disability assessments. If, however, a patient seeks your help to diagnose and treat an injury, your position is more difficult. We believe it is important at the outset to clarify with patients whether they are seeking legal retribution for an injury. If you take the case, be sure that your notes are complete and that they do not conflict with the report that you later write. The report is intended for the review of an insurance agent, lawyer, or a governmental agent, rather than a physician. Use simple terms and avoid medical jargon when possible.

The report should include:

1. *The facts of the case.* If there is an alleged injury, begin by recording the description of the injury as reported by the patient and any witness accompanying the patient to your office. Specify the source of your account. What are the patient's symptoms? What are your find-

ings? You need not include in the report the full description of your physical and neurologic examinations, but should keep detailed notes on the extent of the examinations and findings. Are there significant positive or negative laboratory findings? Are there important pre-existing illnesses, past injuries, or other medical problems that might affect assessment of disability or the causality of the alleged injury to the symptoms?

The bulk of disability assessment patients come to neurologists because of back, neck, and head injuries. Chronic headache, backache, neckache, whiplash, and postconcussive symptoms are the bane of many neurologists because the symptoms and complaints usually far outweigh any objective physical or laboratory findings. There is "more smoke than fire." If there are findings that make you believe that the patient is greatly exaggerating or feigning the injury, you should record that. Remember, however, that you are the patient's advocate, not the judge. Record any positive findings, even if they are nonneurologic, such as muscle contractions, increased lordosis, or straightening of the vertebral column. Many musculoskeletal and head injuries produce severe symptoms and disability despite few objective findings. Give patients the benefit of the doubt. Treat them kindly and sympathetically. The patient's response to therapies and to the passage of time often gives an indication of the cause of the complaints.

2. *The diagnosis.* State the working diagnosis and its basis simply and briefly. What findings led to this diagnosis? In disability assessments, the extent of the disability is usually more important to the assessor than is the actual medical diagnosis.

3. *The presence of any temporary or persistent disability.* The extent and nature of the disability are the important considerations. Some disabilities might affect certain activities or occupations but not others. For example, seizures disqualify patients from being airplane pilots or bus drivers, but not from most other jobs. You should include in the report the patient's description of the handicap and your assessment from objective testing.

4. *The presence of any causal relationship between the alleged injury and any symptoms, findings, or disability.* Courts often use two general rules for assessing causality, which are identical to those used in malpractice concerns. The "but for" rule asks if the doctor can state that but for the act or event the patient would not have sustained the injury or disability. The substantial factor rule asks if the action or event proximately and substantially contributed to the injury.[5] Lawyers want the physician to accompany the statement of causation disability with the legal lingo "with reasonable medical certainty." "With reasonable medical certainty" is used by some to mean "more likely than not" and others to mean "beyond a reasonable doubt."

5. *The long-term prognosis for the injury and disability.* If this is quite uncertain, say so. Remember, however that waffling on this issue may delay settling of the claim and consequently the therapeutic "green poultice" (monetary compensation) effect that often follows settlement.
6. *Treatment.* What treatment is reasonably anticipated? For how long? We think that it is very important for neurologists not to pursue procedures or treatments that they would not customarily use if there were no alleged injury. We almost never suggest myelography or surgery in patients with low back pain unless there are definite root symptoms or signs since asymptomatic disc protrusions and degenerative changes are so common in the population. Lumbar spine films, computed tomography (CT) scans, and magnetic resonance imaging, when indicated, are noninvasive tests that are often helpful in defining abnormal anatomy. Some patients have peripheral nerve or muscle injuries, and these can be well assessed by neurologic examination and electrophysiological testing.

Recall that your notes, your report, and your testimony may be requested. Do not record any statements that could embarrass or discredit you later. Make sure that your recorded database is sufficient to answer questions that may be posed later. The case could be delayed for months or years, by which time your personal recollection of the patient and the case may be dim or nonexistent.

MALPRACTICE

General Rules

Most physicians and neurologists have vigorous opinions about the malpractice issue. We suggest the following general rules or principles:

1. *Improve patient care and communication.* Satisfied patients who have been well taken care of rarely sue, and even more rarely are their suits successful.
2. *Work to reform the system.* Physicians' best allies are patients and businesses or municipalities that also face product or personal liability claims. The problem is not strictly a doctor problem but a very expensive, ineffective, often unfair and inefficient system for determining liability and recompensing damages. The whole legal system for dealing with liability issues needs reform. Airlines faced with huge damage suits, schools that can't field football or hockey teams for fear of suit because of uninsurable helmets, and towns unable to maintain skating rinks or swimming pools because of insurance considerations and possible suits are potential allies in modifying the system. The legal profession lacks motivation for reform due to fears that they may be adversely affected. Reforms are likely to hit lawyers in their pocketbooks.

3. *Discourage, discipline, and weed out poor or hazardous medical practice and practitioners who threaten patient safely.* Unfortunately, the present laws do not always protect well-intentioned physicians who act honestly in this endeavor.

4. *Work to revise qualifications for medical expert witnesses.* There are physicians who repeatedly act as "hired guns" stretching truth to advocate one side in courts of law. These individuals will testify for money on either side of the issue with low regard for truth or their own competency to testify.[8] The rules for the qualifications of medical expert witnesses allowed to testify in medical malpractice cases must be revised so that those testifying are truly experts in the issues under consideration in the case. Medical societies or the courts must find a way to eliminate from the courts so-called medical experts whose testimony is inconsistent, not based on evidence, clearly erroneous, or fabricated. Testimony in court is a matter of public record and is potentially available for independent peer review.

5. *Be a truthful witness.* The advocacy system is a poor way to settle medicolegal issues. Yet legitimate arguments can also be made against other proposed alternative systems. If you are called as an expert or treating witness, you should advocate the truth. The truth usually lies somewhere between the disputing parties' versions. Don't appear partisan to anything but the truth. Discuss the case as you see it, irrespective of which side you are testifying for.

6. *Help patients get recompense by testifying for them.* Patients deserve recompense if they are injured through no fault of their own. If legitimate medical experts don't defend patients, less capable individuals may testify and the legal process will suffer as a result.

Causes and Prevention of Suits

The best way to prevent initiation of malpractice actions is to practice careful and thorough clinical neurology. Diagnosis cannot be handled casually or hurriedly. Sufficient evaluation time must be spent with the patient, and the diagnosis should be pursued in a rigorous, systematic fashion (as described in Part I). Take time to establish a personal and solid doctor-patient relationship. There are four other key behaviors:

1. Communicate with the patient and family often and honestly, especially about risks, limitations of treatment, and the seriousness of the prognosis. Convey the impression that you care! Be sure to obtain informed consent for any diagnostic or therapeutic procedure with potential risk.

2. Keep complete notes and records documenting the completeness of your evaluation and communication with the patient.

3. Use consultants liberally, especially in situations in which the outcome is likely to be bad or the patient is potentially hostile or litigious.

4. Some suits are unwittingly precipitated by doctors' comments. Avoid adverse comments or inferences about the care provided by other physicians, while seeking the best care for patients. (This is discussed in the chapter on consultations.)

Failure to Diagnose or Delay in Diagnosis

Analysis of malpractice claims shows that the most frequent reason given by patients suing neurologists is failure to diagnose or delay in diagnosis. Spinal cord lesions that are potentially reversible are especially problematic. Juries are very sympathetic to paraplegic and quadriplegic patients in wheelchairs, especially when subsequent testing uncovers a compressive lesion that was missed. Brain tumors not detected early can also lead to legal action. We know of instances in which neurologists and other physicians have been sued because of lung tumors not described on radiologists' reports of chest X-rays. In these cases, subsequent films have shown obvious tumors and review of the old films with the retrospectoscope allowed recognition of the lesion originally missed. The lesson should be clear: review films yourself with the radiologist if there is any suspicion of a neoplasm and liberally order chest CTs in tumor suspects. We are aware of a number of suits brought against neurologists for alleged failure to diagnose carotid artery stenosis or occlusion. Invariably, the suit was precipitated by a surgeon's remarks after a stroke to the effect that earlier detection of the vascular lesion would have prevented the stroke. Juries are also understandably partial to disabled stroke patients. It has been said that neurologic patients wear their disorders on the outside where it is easy for even laymen to appreciate their plight. Another circumstance that can lead to litigation is failure to recognize traumatic brain lesions, especially subdural and epidural hematomas. Stupor may have been falsely attributed to alcohol and only belatedly or at necropsy were traumatic lesions appreciated.

Neurologists cannot be held liable for missing a diagnosis as long as they practice up to the standard of care of "average neurologists." Usually, they are sued when a diagnostic procedure that would have detected the lesion was omitted. Especially difficult to explain to juries and courts are diagnoses missed because of failure to perform noninvasive, innocuous tests, such as CT, neck ultrasound, echocardiography, or electroencephalogram (EEG). Was the omission an error in judgment or was it a cost-saving decision? Consideration of expense is not a valid excuse in court. The saving of a few dollars pales in importance when serious neurologic diagnoses are missed. Omission of myelography or angiography has also led to suits. If, ordinarily, a given test would be performed, but there are cogent reasons to omit the test, describe your reasons fully in the chart for later protection.

Complications of Diagnostic Procedures

Just as neurologists can be sued for failure to perform diagnostic procedures, they are also sued for complications of diagnostic procedures such as angiography and myelography. Neurologists are often put in a catch-22 position of potential litigation if they don't pursue an investigation that might diagnose a remediable disorder and also if the procedure is ordered and is followed by a complication. We know of two suits that illustrate this situation. One physician was sued for not ordering angiography for a patient with a carotid bruit and possible transient ischemic attacks; the patient subsequently had an ischemic stroke ipsilateral to the bruit. A surgeon later ordered angiography that showed occlusion of the involved carotid artery and contralateral carotid stenosis. The surgeon told the family that angiography before the stroke probably would have prevented the stroke. A suit was brought and decided for the plaintiff, even though doctors testified in court that noninvasive tests at the time of the patient's admission were not readily available or reliable. In another case, a neurologist was sued successfully because he ordered angiography. The patient had a slight fluctuating neurologic deficit with some progression since admission, and digital subtraction angiography suggested critical ipsilateral carotid artery stenosis. Carotid angiography was followed by a disabling stroke.

Suits have been brought because of alleged side effects or complications of procedures. Some of these alleged complications are merely progression of the illness, to be expected whether or not the procedure is performed. It is the neurologist's good fortune that improvements in noninvasive testing have reduced the frequency of potentially hazardous studies. There remain times (e.g., subarachnoid hemorrhage) when such procedures remain necessary and it behooves us to proceed after alerting patient and family to the potential risks and documenting the discussion in the record.

Doctors have no absolute protection from these suits. Adverse outcomes and litigious patients and lawyers can lead to suits irrespective of the presence of negligence on the part of the physician. In the circumstance of complications of procedures, the best protection the physician has is maintaining detailed notes in the hospital chart or office record. These should document: (1) The indications for the procedure. The fact that the physician has considered alternative diagnostic procedures, but has decided that the procedure to be performed is necessary. The relative risks and benefits of the procedure have been carefully considered in the decision. (2) The expected outcome if the procedure is not done. (3) Informed consent obtained by a full disclosure to the patient of the risks and benefits of performing or not performing the procedure and potential alternatives. With this type of documentation, it is very unlikely that a legal suit can be brought successfully unless the procedure was not indicated or was performed negligently. When the procedure scheduled is potentially risky, and indications are questionable or dubious, it is best to obtain consultation before proceeding.

Side Effects of Treatment

The third large category of suits are brought because of side effects of medical or surgical treatment. An important reference that considers the neurologic complications of medical care is the recent collection of Biller.[9] Even when injury arises after surgery, the neurologist who had referred the patient for surgical opinion or surgery is potentially liable, as well as the surgeon. If you are involved in a case at the time of surgery, you should be sure to document that you also obtained informed consent from the patient and discussed your reasons for referring the patient for surgical opinion and that you concur with the planned surgery.

If the physician does not agree with the planned surgery, this must be discussed with the surgeon (see discussion in Chapter 12 on consultations). Suits are brought in relation to medical therapy for a number of reasons:

1. *Using a drug that is not indicated.* Government approval for use of a drug in a given circumstance lags far behind knowledge that the medicine is potentially useful. Among neurologists, the utility of propranolol for prophylaxis or treatment of migraine preceded approval by many years. Physicians are not prohibited from using an approved drug for a nonapproved indication, but, when they do, it is necessary to explain the circumstances to the patient and record this in the chart. If the use of a medicine is experimental or investigational, it is important to obtain informed consent.

2. *Failure to elicit a history of prior drug reaction or allergy.* Severe anaphylactic or systemic reactions to medicines can lead to lawsuits if physicians have not taken reasonable care in eliciting a detailed history of past exposure and reactions. A different problem occurs when the physician knows about past reactions and records them in the record but the patient is negligently given that substance.

3. *Failure to consider drug interactions or adverse effects of a drug on a preexisting medical or psychiatric condition.* We now know that drug interactions are common. The combined use of some drugs, such as aspirin and warfarin, can cause bleeding. The addition of some drugs affects blood levels of other drugs, such as phenytoin. Sedative or hypnotic drugs can potentiate each other. Drugs useful for a neurologic disorder could potentially be problematic for other diseases. Atropine may worsen glaucoma, leading to decreased vision; propranolol may adversely affect asthma and can diminish the effects of catecholamine release in patients with hypoglycemic reactions to insulin. Propranolol, corticosteroids, or anxiolytic agents may lead to depression in patients with a known predisposition to depression. Some effects of these interactions of one drug with other drugs and of drugs on other illnesses are well known; others are not. It is probably wise for physicians to familiarize themselves in detail with medicines that they frequently prescribe, and we believe, to limit the number of drugs that they use often. If you are not fully familiar with a drug that you consider using, or the patient is using other unfamiliar drugs or has another important disease, you should seek assistance before prescribing the new drug. The *Physician's Desk Reference* (PDR), the medicine package information

insert (if available), standard reference books on pharmacology and drug treatment, and pharmacology experts who are now often available in many medical centers can be helpful. When in doubt, discuss the new drug with the patient's internist or the physician who is treating the patient's other condition(s). Some computer programs are available and others are being written that warn physicians about potentially adverse conditions or interactions that might effect prescription and dosage of pharmacological agents.

When we were in training the neurologic pharmacopoeia was sufficiently limited that one could easily master it. We now witness an ever-expanding pool of potential agents that we must choose from as well as the explosion in drugs used for other diseases that have potential for neurologic side effects. The growing enthusiasm for alternative therapies may result in interactions of herbals and other nonstandard remedies with prescribed drugs. The patient may be reluctant to tell the physician of self-medication with herbals and the potential interactions may not be known to the physician. Try not to start more than one agent at a time. Osler admonished doctors "Remember how much you do not know. Do not pour strange medicines into your patients."[10]

4. *Failure to monitor for side effects of treatment.* Some potential side effects of prescribed drugs are well known. Leukopenia with carbamazepine, muscle and liver dysfunction with statins, thrombotic thrombocytopenic purpura and leukopenia with ticlopidine, and liver dysfunction with phenytoin, valproate, and isonicotinic acid hydrazide are examples of problems detectable by laboratory monitoring. Other potential effects, for example, postural hypotension with L-dopa or propranolol, or nystagmus and ataxia related to phenytoin and barbiturates, are detected by physical examination. Some side effects, such as depression, drowsiness, and difficulty concentrating, are discovered by taking a history from the patient. Patients should be told of common potential side effects, and monitoring measures should be planned. The frequency of phone call surveillance, follow-up examinations, and laboratory testing will depend on the frequency and severity of potential complications.

5. *Failure to warn about potentially serious side effects.* Sometimes, seemingly innocent side effects can lead by a chain of events to a serious outcome that can precipitate legal redress. A patient given antihistamines or anxiolytic agents that can cause sedation may fall asleep while driving or operating machinery and so develop or cause serious injury. Warn patients about possible sedative effects and about driving or any activity that might be hazardous under those circumstances. Warn them about taking alcohol, sleeping pills, or other potential sedatives. Record the fact that you have warned the

patient in the chart. Start the pills at a low dose and at bedtime if possible, only gradually escalating the dose.

6. *Failure to obtain informed consent.* This is especially important if complications are frequent and potentially serious. Courts have varied in their determinations of how much need be told to patients. Physicians have argued, occasionally successfully, that full disclosure might have unduly disturbed or adversely affected the treatment. Disclosure in these cases is omitted "for the good of the patient." Substantial risk of harm by disclosure might consist of severe emotional distress or probable refusal of a diagnostic procedure or therapy that is likely to be very effective. Courts are increasingly skeptical about the argument that possible adverse emotional impact on the patient justifies nondisclosure. Some courts decide on the extent of informed consent in relationship to the accustomed practice in the community or nationally. There are no firm guidelines or rules on this subject. We believe it is wise to tell the patient or the family the common and important risks. If there are cogent reasons for omitting some disclosures, note these circumstances in your records or the hospital chart. It is also best to make a note of your discussion with the patient and/or the family and what you have told them.

7. *Failure to stop treatment when side effects or complications have occurred.* This point is an extension of failure to monitor. When side effects do occur, the risk/benefit ratio of continuing or stopping the treatment must be discussed with the patient and noted in your records.

Patients and families sometimes sue because they feel that the doctor's fees and outstanding bills are unreasonable. Especially when the outcome is bad, suits may be instituted at least partially to protest excessive fees. Some persons would like nothing better than to get back at "rich doctors." In poor outcome cases, physicians may want to review their outstanding charges to assess their reasonableness under the circumstances. You may also want to soften your customary bill collection procedures and speak with other colleagues in the case, such as neurosurgeons and radiologists, to advise them not to aggressively pursue payment at risk of suit.

Our advice for prevention of these causes for litigation can be summarized briefly. Befriend and be considerate of the patient; communicate often, openly, and honestly. Use tests liberally, especially those with little or no risk, and consult often. Bill fairly, and keep as complete records as possible.

THE NEUROLOGIST AS A CONSULTANT TO LAWYERS IN CASES OF POSSIBLE MALPRACTICE AND AS AN EXPERT WITNESS IN COURT

Retaining your own ethical principles is important and must be the first consideration. Neurologists who feel morally compromised when dealing with lawyers and the courts should avoid the system as much as possible. Yet neurologic, medical, and surgical colleagues are frequently sued for bad outcomes unrelated to any negligence on their parts. They badly need our help. No one wants to see patients who are legitimately injured by negligence not be compensated fairly. For these reasons, I think it is important that capable medical experts testify for their colleagues and for patients when they believe the cause is just.

Physicians should not testify when they are not expert in the issues being considered. Clearly, they should not testify to untruths. Yet unqualified experts and physician "hired guns" who testify for either side for money are at least partially responsible for the problems in the medicolegal system.

What Are the Legal Issues?

In order to testify or to even review cases for possible malpractice, you must know something about the relevant law, legal procedures, and legal lingo. There are five essential conditions that must be met to establish malpractice, and the plaintiffs must prove them all.

1. The doctor had a duty to the patient, that is, a doctor-patient relationship or contract existed. If the doctor did establish a doctor-patient relationship, he or she has an obligation to practice up to the standard of other physicians in that specialty.
2. The standard of care was in fact breached, and the physician practiced below the standard. Since few standards are written in detail, this nearly always involves testimony by other physicians as to what is the standard of care and how the physician departed from it in the particular case.
3. The plaintiff must have suffered an injury or damages. Negligence alone does not constitute malpractice. There must have been a definite injury to the patient. Though the injury can be physical, emotional, or economic, nearly always there must be at least some physical component.
4. There must be a proximate causal relationship between the breach of the standard and the plaintiff's injury. In some cases, the physician has committed an error that has little to do with the adverse outcome. The breach of the standard of practice must have caused the injury.
5. Plaintiff's damages are actual and quantifiable.

As discussed in the section on civil claims, there are several rules or tests that courts have applied concerning the issue of causality. The negligence must be a proximate and substantial cause of the injury, not a remote or minor factor. But for the defendant's negligent act, the plaintiff would not have sustained an injury. Nonnegligent conduct would have led to a better result.

We know of several recent cases in which, though neurologist defendants did not perform well, the disorder they misdiagnosed was not treatable even had it been correctly diagnosed. One physician missed the diagnosis of aneurysmal subarachnoid hemorrhage that led to death five hours after admission. In this case, even the best therapy would not have reversed the eventual outcome. In other cases, the correct diagnosis of subarachnoid hemorrhage or cryptococcal meningitis was made only after some delay. The plaintiffs had the burden of showing that the delay led to an adverse outcome. Missing the diagnosis of glioma, motor neuron disease, or multiple sclerosis can lead to lawsuits, but it is very difficult to show that the patient has been injured since very effective treatment for these disorders is not available even if the diagnosis had been recognized quickly and accurately. When doctors render an opinion about the above cited failings, the courts do not insist on absolute certainty and also do not request or demand that physicians back up their assertions with documentation from literature citations. Physicians must couch their opinions, using the term "with reasonable medical certainty." This term is not easily defined or quantitated. "Almost surely," "more likely than not," "probably," and "in the vast majority of instances" are some interpretations.

What Are the Different Activities Requested of Neurologist Experts?

Probably the most common request made of doctors by lawyers is to review the facts of a particular case to determine if, in their opinion, malpractice did occur, and whether they would be willing to render an opinion or testify in the case on behalf of the lawyer's client. There are lawyers who support plaintiffs in suits against doctors, and there are other lawyers who defend physicians against malpractice allegations. Most firms confine their activity to be either strictly defense or plaintiff advocates. Most lawyers ask that the reviewing physician look over the available materials and call the lawyer with verbal comments before submitting a written report. Written reports are admissible in court and can be used by the opposing lawyers if the opinion is unfavorable to the case of the requesting lawyer.

Be sure you know what side of the case the law firm is on. Do they represent the plaintiff or are they acting in defense of a physician or hospital? Are they defending all the parties in the case or just one of the doctors? If not all parties, which physician do they represent? Before rendering an opinion, be certain that you have seen all the available documents, including relevant laboratory studies and imaging tests. You should also discuss with the requesting lawyer, up front, your fees and limitations on your services in the case, such as rendering an opinion only or testifying in court or by deposition.

L.R.C. sometimes refuses to render an oral opinion. When there has been no physician negligence, L.R.C. has on occasion sent a firm statement to that effect to the requesting plaintiff's lawyer and to the lawyer defending the physicians in the case. This is meant to deter lawyers who "shop around," requesting opinions of multiple physicians until they finally find one who will support their cause. The naysayers never get mentioned to the court, only the doctor who agrees.

After reviewing the materials, if your opinion seems favorable to the requesting lawyer, you may or may not be asked to write a report stating your opinion. Reports are most helpful in attempting to settle the case out of court. The lawyer will use knowledge of your involvement in the case to push for a settlement or surrender before a trial proceeding is begun. Most legal cases are settled after considerable jockeying by the respective parties in the case. If the case will definitely come to court, lawyers may not want to "tip their hand" as to what tactics or arguments their side will follow. Your report, discoverable to the opponents, may yield clues that the lawyer would rather not disclose before trial. If a report is written, it should generally conform to that outlined in the beginning of the chapter. First, state the documents reviewed in formulating your opinion. Then, outline the facts of the case. State if there has or has not been a breach of the standard of care and why or why not. Has there been an injury and, if so, what and how was it related to the supposed deviation from the standard of care? Suggestions for the written format and content of medicolegal reports are available.[11]

Discovery and Deposition

Lawsuits are initiated when a claimant's lawyer files a complaint that outlines the names of the defendants and states the general grounds for the suit. After the complaint is filed, the defendant files an answer that denies all the allegations or admits some statements, while denying others. The defendant could admit errors but deny responsibility for harm or cite contributory problems or wrongdoing on the part of the claimant. After the complaint and answers, the court hears preliminary motions from either side and may dismiss the case. In some states, the case is then heard by a screening panel of lawyers, doctors, and citizens who render an opinion of whether the suit has sufficient grounds to warrant a trial.

After the initial filings, each side in the case is entitled to discovery. This means that opposing parties are given access to relevant evidence on each side so that they can better prepare a defense or might be so impressed by the weight of the evidence that they will settle or dismiss the case. As part of the discovery process, lawyers from either side can ask for a discovery deposition, during which they can examine the opposition's experts to determine what those individuals will testify to in court. The deposition is available to all parties in the suit.

Ordinarily, the deposition occurs in the lawyer's or doctor's office. Present are the testifying physician, the opposing lawyers or their designated assistants, and a clerk who records the proceedings. Testimony is taken under oath. The questioning lawyer (the plaintiff's lawyer if the expert is hired by the defense or the defense lawyer if the expert is testifying for the plaintiff) spars with the expert, usually trying to determine (1) the expert's background and credentials, (2) the expert's previous court experience (Will the lawyer be able to impeach the expert as a frequent testifier in court, as a "money grabber," or as a partisan always testifying for one side?), (3) the witness's character (Is the witness firm and forthright or wavering and wishy-washy? How shakable are the statements? How well articulated? Is the jury likely to be sympathetic with the expert?), and (4) the substance of the testimony (What are the major points of argument that will be testified to in court?). Good lawyers often use the discovery deposition as an opportunity to educate themselves about the medical and neurologic aspects and nuances of the case so that they can better understand the arguments for and against their position and can better search for literature that will support their contentions.

During the discovery deposition, opposing lawyers can object to the line of questioning or the form of specific questions, but, since no judge is present, the objections are simply recorded by the clerk. Under some circumstances, the deposition may be stopped and a judge could be asked for a ruling before a question is allowed. Cross-examination can be performed, but usually the lawyer hiring the expert does not want to give away strategy and will remain relatively quiet. If there are multiple parties in the case, lawyers for other defendants or claimants may question the expert to determine his or her position in relation to their clients.

Most clerks are not very familiar with medical terminology. Speak slowly and clearly and spell or write out any complex medical terms for the recording clerk. Your statements during depositions and your written report can later be used to discredit your trial testimony if there are discrepancies between what you say at trial and what you have said during the deposition. Consider your answers carefully. After the testimony is typed out, experts can ask to review their depositions, correct errors, and sign as to their accuracy, or can "waive signature." It is always best to "reserve signature" until you review the document.

If other witnesses have been deposed before you, the lawyers requesting your services usually make these depositions available to you before your testimony. The lawyer should be charged for time spent in reviewing charts, depositions, and other materials, writing a report, and preparing testimony.

Testifying in Court

For the novice, a court appearance can be a very difficult and memorable experience. In the passage cited at the beginning of this chapter, Hamilton describes her consternation at the process of testimony in court.

In most instances, the lawyer who has retained your services will meet with you before your discovery deposition and before your court appearance to review the questions and material to be covered. Pretrial meetings or discussions between the lawyer and testifying physician are very important. You need to know what questions the lawyer is likely to ask. The lawyer will want to know, in general, what the answers to these questions are likely to be. You can help the lawyer prepare the best legal defense by educating the lawyer about the medical facts, issues, and literature relevant to the case. As in preparing for a formal debate, if you are able to anticipate the strong and weak points on each side, a better defense and offense can be planned. Yet some lawyers, usually those who are less skillful, seem willing to skip or hold only perfunctory pre-trial meetings and so find themselves unprepared to deal with problematic testimony that could have been anticipated and handled by better advance preparation.

The first rule for the expert witness is to be well prepared even before appearing at the courtroom. You will be asked about your background, including your education, training, and experience, so provide the lawyer with an up-to-date curriculum vitae and bring one with you to court. If you cared for or examined the patient yourself, make yourself very familiar with your office and hospital notes and reports. If you simply reviewed materials and did not see the patient, refamiliarize yourself with the materials. During your testimony, you are free to ask to refer to your prior notes and reports and any documents entered in evidence. You may be asked about whether you have testified before and if so for plaintiffs, defendants, or both. You may also be asked about your fees or other remuneration for testifying. You are entitled to a fee for your time and expertise. Prepare yourself for the answers to these questions and those that you have been told will be covered during direct examination by the lawyer who has retained your services.

You must, of course, prepare yourself not only for the friendly questioning of the lawyer you are assisting, but also for parrying questions that might be posed to you by the not-so-friendly opposing lawyer during cross-examination. Act as if you were preparing for a formal debate. What arguments are the opposition likely to espouse and pursue? If you were on their side, how would you try to tear down the testimony you propose to give? How can you respond to these counterarguments? By adopting the opposition's view, you can be better armed for queries or attacks during vigorous cross-examination. Reading the depositions on each side and discussion with the lawyer who has retained you will give clues as to the tactics of the opposing case that will help you prepare to testify.

When you appear in court, dress neatly but not too formally, pretentiously, or ostentatiously. This is a very serious business, and testimony should be considered, careful, and earnest. Do not appear angry or hostile about testifying. The jury would also rather be elsewhere. Speak slowly, audibly, and clearly, and direct your gaze to the questioning attorney and to the jury. Answers should be short, concise, and directly responsive to the question asked. Avoid complex medical terms. If they must be used, define them simply as a way of explanation. Remember that you are testifying to a lay jury and to a judge who may have little detailed medical knowledge. Excessive and unnecessary medical jargon will obscure your testimony and may give the jury the impression that you are arrogant and superior and so create an adverse feeling toward your testimony. We find simple diagrams and analogies useful and use examples such as those cited in Chapter 7 on physician-patient communications. Use a chalkboard, large writing tablet, or prepared illustrations to help get your points across. If you anticipate using any of this equipment, ask the lawyer to make sure it is available in the courtroom.

During direct examination, the lawyer will gradually build up your testimony by sequential questions and answers. For example, you will be asked if you have an opinion about a particular finding. You reply yes, you do or no, you do not have an opinion (but you have not been asked yet what that opinion is). You may then be asked if you can state an opinion with a reasonable degree of medical certainty. Again, you are expected to answer only yes or no. Only then will you be asked what that opinion is. Usually, the direct examination by the lawyer who has engaged your services goes smoothly. You have already prepared yourself for the questions. The lawyer wants to place your testimony in the best light and will be very gentle with you. Avoid giving the impression of being overly partisan. Despite the fact that one side has retained you and the case is decided by which side has the best advocacy, we believe that expert witnesses should take the position that they are there to testify for truth and equity. Although you might, in general, support one side, the issues are sometimes gray, not black or white. Admit errors or oversights on either side. Your testimony, if fair and balanced, will appear more believable to the jury than if you take an obviously militant partisan stand.

Cross-examination is more difficult and more anxiety producing. The opposing lawyer will try to discredit you and your testimony. He or she will try to make you angry and nervous. Remain cool and dispassionate. Pay careful attention to the questions. If you do not fully understand a question, ask for clarification before responding. Particularly difficult are hypothetical questions in which the lawyer may lay out a very complex multifactual tortuous set of conditions and series of events ("I will ask you to assume . . . and further to assume that . . . and that, etc."). When the question is too complex and contains too many clauses, it is best to say that you cannot answer the question as posed but would be glad to answer single propositions from it. You may be directed to answer questions using only yes or no replies. There are questions that are not answerable by yes or no, or by true or false. Many answers require qualifications and "ifs" and "ands" and "buts" to place the answer in perspective. You might tell the judge that you cannot answer the question by yes or no without further qualifications.

At times, the opposing lawyer will cross-examine you by asking questions that are off the topic and irrelevant to the argument or merely partially true. In a case in which L.R.C. testified for a defendant physician accused of negligently missing the diagnosis of cryptococcal meningitis, L.R.C. was asked, "Did the patient have a headache? Did the patient have a stroke?" The answer to both questions was definitely yes. Next, he was asked, "Does cryptococcal meningitis cause headache? Does it cause stroke?" The answers were also yes, but anyone with any medical experience knows that an extremely tiny minority of patients with either headache or stroke have cryptococcal meningitis. The questions as posed do not put the issue in perspective. As expert witness, you should as calmly as possible merely answer the questions as asked. Rely on the lawyer who has retained you to, on redirect examination, ask questions that will clarify the frequency and perspective and expose for the jury the fact that your answers were correct, but constituted only half-truths. The pretrial discussions should have prepared the lawyer to be able to accomplish this. You may ask the judge if you can be allowed to qualify or comment on your answers in order to clarify your testimony for the jurors. The cross-examining lawyer may object and the judge may deny your request, but in doing so, the message is conveyed to the jury that you have not been fully heard on the subject and your answers represent only a part of the story. The lawyer who engaged you is alerted to pursue the topic further on redirect questioning.

After having been involved in a number of court cases, the medical expert witness can serve as a valuable aid and consultant to lawyers by clarifying the issues, raising cogent arguments on either side of the case, identifying experts knowledgeable on these issues, and citing references from the literature that would help educate lawyers on the medical concepts. We believe that defending innocent physician colleagues is a noble undertaking, and any help that can be given to defendant lawyers is useful. Keep in mind, however, that medical peers are not deciding the case. The case is being played on a turf foreign to you; the court procedure and evidence are legal, not predominantly medical or scientific. Legal tactics are chosen to convince the judge and jury. These strategies are quite different from those that would convince our medical colleagues. Give advice, but don't try to run the case.

THE NEUROLOGIST AS A DEFENDANT IN A MALPRACTICE ALLEGATION

Being a defendant in a malpractice proceeding is almost always a disaster for the physician accused of wrongdoing. Readers are urged to read a book by Charles and Kennedy about being a defendant in a malpractice suit.[3] Physicians seek to help patients: Primum non nocere (do no harm), the medical student is taught. It is very difficult for physicians to think that they might have caused harm or injury to the very patient that they have sworn to heal. Soul searching is a natural response when there is even the perception of a kernel of merit to the accusation. When the physician finds absolutely no merit in the accusations, the usual response is anger. Sued doctors get angry with the claimant, the involved lawyers, the medicolegal system, the insurance carriers, and virtually anyone else in sight. Especially heinous to some physicians is the prospect of financial settlement in a case in which the physician feels that no injustice or negligence occurred. Frustration, despair, loss of confidence, and depression are common sequelae of lawsuits, even those that are successfully defended. Lawsuits clearly cause alterations in physician behavior, some positive and some negative and undesirable. In one study, more than half of sued physicians developed depression or stress-induced symptoms.[12] Litigation generated great internal turmoil and was identified by 23 percent of those sued as being the single most stressful period of their lives.[12] Practice afterward was nearly always altered; more defensive strategies were used, and less satisfaction and more stress accompanied physician-patient interactions.[13]

If one of your patients has had an adverse outcome and you suspect that a possible suit might ensue, take immediate action. Meeting with the patient and family to express your concern probably helps. Make sure that outstanding bills are not vigorously pursued or sent out for collection. Let the insurance company that handles your malpractice insurance know of the possibility of litigation. Most hospitals now have risk management or similarly titled personnel who can help with prevention of a suit. If a suit cannot be prevented, these people can help prepare a defense while the information and events are recent and fresh in memory. When a legal complaint is pursued, begin the process of self-psychology, psyching yourself. Especially if you feel that you have done no wrong, you must not and cannot let the suit destroy you and your family.

There is a wonderful story that we find relevant. A psychiatrist was walking down a street with another psychiatrist. All of a sudden, he felt pain in his right arm. He looked about but saw no one except the other psychiatrist to his right. He continued to walk but soon felt another sharp blow to his right arm. He looked askance at his companion and then walked on. After the next blow, he asked his friend to stop hitting him. After several more minutes, he received the most severe blow of all to his right arm. He became incensed, took off his coat and put up his fists to fight. He then paused for a moment, thought, and said, "Hey, wait a minute. Why am I getting so upset? It's your problem!" Similarly, if you have done no wrong, the problem is the patient's, or the lawyers', or the law, or the legal system, but not yours. Get yourself the best legal advice available. There are many distinguished and able expert physicians who will be glad to help and testify for you. Keep up your daily activities, help prepare your defense, and go forward with your life. The crisis will pass.

Many of today's physicians are discouraged by the external pressures they perceive and real threats to their autonomy. We have avoided a doomsday philosophy and have tried to keep this book as upbeat as possible considering the changes in modern medicine. Advice to physicians has emphasized better patient care. Physicians will win public confidence and support only if they are viewed as strong patient and public health advocates. In this chapter about lawyers and medicolegal issues, it has clearly been difficult to maintain our optimism and positive approach. There is little good that can be said about the medical malpractice problem and, admittedly, we have little confidence in the fairness and equity of the legal process or in some lawyers. A standard joke among lawyers is, "When the decision is rendered and justice is done, protest immediately and seek a retrial."

The best protection physicians have against allegations of malpractice is to take superb and humane care of their patients and to keep impeccable and detailed records of their care. Knowledge of the laws and legal processes relevant to medical care is also advisable.

REFERENCES

1. Hamilton A. *Exploring the Dangerous Trades*. Boston: Little, Brown, 1943.
2. Wilbur R. Council of Medical Specialty Societies Executive Report. Vol. 21, Number 5, 1988.
3. Charles SA, Kennedy E. *Defendant: A Psychiatrist on Trial for Medical Malpractice*. New York: Vintage Books, 1986;171.
4. U.S. Dept. of Health, Education, and Welfare. *Report of the Secretary's Commission on Medical Malpractice*, 1973.
5. Beresford HR. *Legal Aspects of Neurologic Practice*. Philadelphia: F.A. Davis, 1998.
6. Rapp JA, Rapp RT (eds). *Illinois Medical Malpractice: A Guide for the Health Sciences*. St. Louis: Mosby, 1988.
7. *Guides to the Evaluation of Permanent Impairment*. Chicago: American Medical Assocation, 1995.
8. Webster J. Medical "experts" in litigation. *Ann Int Med* 1988;108:637–638.
9. Biller J. *Iatrogenic Neurology*. Boston: Butterworth–Heinemann, 1998.
10. Bean RB, Bean WB. *Sir William Osler: Aphorisms from His Bedside Teachings and Writings*. Springfield, IL: Charles C Thomas, 1961.
11. Fox RM. *The Medicolegal Report*. Boston: Little, Brown, 1969.
12. Charles SC, Wilbert JR, Franke K. Sued and nonsued physicians' self-reported reactions to malpractice litigation. *Am J Psych* 1985;142:437–440.
13. Charles SC, Wernicke R, Wilbert J, Lichtenberg R, Dejesus C. Sued and nonsued physicians, satisfactions, dissatisfactions, and sources of stress. *Psychosomatics* 1987;29:462–488.

15

Tying Things Together and Last Words

We have repeatedly emphasized in the chapters of this book the need to look ahead (planning) and to look back (reviewing and revising). Following this advice, we will in this section briefly try to tie up loose ends, add things that did not fit well into the individual chapters, emphasize key points, and attempt to unite the various sections of the book more closely.

THE PROBLEM FACING PHYSICIANS

Undoubtedly, these are difficult times for organized medicine, and physicians in particular. Part of the reason for doctors' troubles is their own success. People are living longer and when they age medical problems grow dramatically, especially if terminal illnesses are long. Most elderly patients develop problems that affect their nervous systems. Care of the elderly accounts for a disproportionate amount of medical expenses. Most expenditures on health care occur in the last years of life. Intensive care units often care for patients with little hope for survival at great expense. Research and technology have grown and have improved the potential for accurate diagnoses and more effective treatment, but these modern improvements are costly. Governments and big businesses are exerting major pressures to curb costs. Physicians are generally seen as the ones who determine costs by controlling care. The public's expectations for high-quality care are also higher, and often quite unrealistic. Governments, the public, big businesses, and lawyers stand ready to exact their individual wills and the dictates of their purses on doctors—those smug, arrogant, fellows who drive around in big Cadillacs and are always playing golf while getting fat on the system.

THE SOLUTION

In our opinion, there are three ways that individual physicians can respond. First, become active in local and national physician groups and specialty societies. Make your thoughts, ideas, and feelings known. Together physicians may be able to influence the ongoing changes in health care. Second, improve your clinical capabilities and activities so that patient care is optimized and personalized. Physician self-images must be improved. The essence of professionalism is the individual's sense of accomplishment, control, and responsibility. Most physicians enter medicine to be good doctors and to improve health. The advertisements on television enticing youngsters into the armed forces say, "Be all that you can be." Isn't that what pride and self-respect are about? The physician's goal is to use science and scientific advances to improve the health and well-being of patients. This book is aimed at this aspect of professionalism—how to use the science of medicine in the art of the care of the patient. Third, reaffirm the concept that physicians exist to care for patients and to keep people from becoming ill. Physicians must work to improve the lot of patients. This means getting to understand them and their problems, their environments, and their stresses. This book has attempted to familiarize physicians with the patient's perspective regarding hospitals, ambulatory care, tests, treatments, and consultations. We have emphasized the importance of the socioeconomic milieu. Physicians must become patient advocates in the best and fullest sense of that term, both in their political activities and their every interaction with their own patients. Though the book is aimed at and for clinical physicians, in many ways, the heroes are the patients.

PROFESSIONALISM—WHAT THE CLINICIAN DOES!

Science

Science is key. Art is wasted if the doctor has little understanding of the scientific basis of the problem. The difference between medicine and other helping professions such as the clergy is medical science. The bedrock of training is an intimate knowledge of anatomy, pathology, and physiology. The neurologist must have intimate knowledge of the basic sciences and the central and peripheral nervous systems to practice clinical neurology well. All else can be learned later. The foundation cannot be added after the building had been constructed. Medical curricula and training programs must continue to emphasize these subjects. The technical execution of procedures such as the neurologic examination, history taking, lumbar puncture, and electromyography must be supervised during training and learned well. We emphasized in the first part of this book the need to practice systematically and logically—in a word, scientifically. For some reason, physicians often behave in a schizophrenic way in reference to their laboratory research and practice. In the lab, they espouse hypotheses, systematic observations, quantification, sequential testing, and analysis, yet in the clinic their approach is more casual and haphazard. We argue herein for an identical approach in the lab and clinic. All aspects of the care of the patient are based on careful observation and generation of hypotheses. Systematic, sequential data gathering and hypothesis testing are crucial. Quantification helps convey the data to others and to the same physician seeing the patient at a later time. Record keeping in the laboratory should be precise and complete. So should it be in the hospital and ambulatory facilities.

The first part of the book emphasizes the technique and style of the physician. The history, examination, laboratory evaluation, information transmittal, and treatment are handled sequentially. Each step depends on the preceding steps. Each should be logical and thorough.

Art

Art is much more difficult to define than science. By *art* we mean skills and style as well as the broad cultural background that falls under the general heading of "liberal arts" in college curricula. Art is all that is not science that relates to a physician's activities and scope. The breadth of the physician's and patient's environment is vast. We have tried to emphasize the many different aspects of the art of clinical care.

Communication

We have included a full chapter (Chapter 7) on information transmittal in Part II, but in reality, success of the physician in the entire breadth of activities depends on facility of communication. We communicate not only with patients, but also with colleagues, other personnel, and with the public. Some of the communication is informal and spontaneous, and some formal and prepared. Most communication is verbal and face-to-face or by phone, but much is written.

Because communication skills are so key, medical schools require college English as a prerequisite for admission. Physicians must keep improving and maintaining their language skills and become self-conscious about their own skills and styles of communication. An excellent way to maintain skills is to continue to read and write. Osler urged students and physicians to read each night, but not medical material. Sherlock Holmes or a good novel are excellent ways of ending the day and relaxing. Write! Physicians should review their notes and hospital charts, office records, and reports to see if they are clear and convey what was intended. Do they reflect the observations accurately? Could someone unfamiliar with the patient be able to visualize the person and findings described? Physicians should maintain and improve their writing skills by writing medical papers and case reports and reviews. Try also writing nonmedical materials.

Most physicians are called on to discuss a clinical case at a morbidity and mortality conference, grand rounds, or a resident conference. It is important to realize that careful preparation for such sessions is most helpful to the presenter and offers the ability to deepen one's understanding of the situation being discussed. Each patient offers something new and an opportunity to read and enhance skills. Robert Loeb used to tell his medical students that they would remember information when it was tied to a patient. Each patient will present multiple issues. It is best to select a specific aspect of the case to study in depth, rather than trying to gather a smattering of multiple areas.

ASSISTANCE

Nothing substitutes for experience. Although trainees and young practitioners may be familiar with a disease or a phenomenon through instruction during medical school or formal training, there are almost always issues and nuances in the care of patients with that disease or problems that have not been covered and need to be learned. Even experienced clinicians frequently encounter situations or problems that are relatively unfamiliar to them. Learn to seek help often. Assistance can sometimes be gained from consultation with other physicians who are available and knowledgeable. Sometimes sharing the case informally with associates or colleagues suffices to answer specific conundrums. The literature is also usually helpful. Personal filing systems containing articles from journals and reprints prove very helpful when files are kept up to date. Computers now offer ready access to specific points in question. Perhaps more important is access to individuals we like to call oracles, individuals with experience and wisdom. Medicine and neurology are now so complex that physicians should cultivate and use a stable of individuals who are knowledgeable in different subspecialty areas such as stroke, epilepsy, cognition and behavior, neuro-ophthalmology, and different disciplines such as neuroimaging, electromyography, and neuropharmacology. Call often. Taking care of sick patients is a lifelong education. The "oracles" called usually do not mind and often also learn from the encounters. The oracles who are called often enjoy and learn from sharing these cases and problems. Learn as much as possible from each experience. There are physicians who have seen many patients, but have learned little. Use all of the resources available. The effective clinician is a lifelong student.

Systems

The problems and responsibility of each individual physician are too large and diverse to be handled casually. The human brain is a very remarkable organ, but even it cannot store and parcel all of the data and tasks required regularly. Physicians must rely on other people to help. Much of Chapter 11, on ambulatory care, discusses secretaries, triage personnel, billing staff, and the physician's understanding the roles and capabilities and limitations of these individuals to optimize their use. Similarly, systematic interactions with hospital personnel such as nurses, technicians, and trainees can be of great help to physicians. Rules, techniques, filing systems, protocols, and routines also help ensure that responsibilities will not be neglected and that patients and data will not slip through the cracks. Computers can now help greatly with these functions if they are properly harnessed and used. Computers can certainly aid physicians in quickly accessing their patient files and the medical literature.

PHYSICIANS' AWARENESS OF THEMSELVES, THEIR ROLES, AND THEIR ENVIRONMENT

Much in this book, especially Part III, centers on the environment in which the physician works. The more physicians understand their roles and environmental stresses, the better position they will be in to do their best. The clinician should be most concerned about the patient—that is why we have devoted the entire Part II to the physician-patient interaction in all of its phases. Part III discusses the broader physician environment, which includes an array of key individuals. Physicians interact with many other doctors, especially in the hospital, and in relation to consultations and laboratory, radiographic, imaging, and physiologic testing. In the hospital, interfaces with nurses, clerks, technicians, medical students, and trainees dramatically affect the physician's activities and capabilities. In the ambulatory facility, secretaries, billing staff, and other office personnel contribute to success or failure in optimizing patient care. Lawyers and the legal system more and more encroach on physician roles and we have devoted Chapter 14 to that subject. The doctor is influenced not only by people, but also by institutions—hospitals, clinics, doctor's offices, universities, insurance systems, legal and governmental institutions. Academia is very important to many and we have included a chapter (Chapter 13) on this subject. Any in-depth discussion of research and patient involvement in research has been omitted because the complexity of the subject puts it beyond the scope of this book.

The physician and his or her environment have been the subject of a number of books. For example, *The Citadel*, by A.J. Cronin; *Middlemarch*, by George Eliot; *Arrowsmith*, by Sinclair Lewis; *Of Human Bondage*, by W. Somerset Maugham; and *The Physician*, by Noah Gordon. Maugham and Cronin were themselves physicians. These books are excellent reading for prospective doctors and for all physicians. Self-awareness of the physician's role and of the physician's own style and procedures has to be helpful in maintaining and improving effectiveness.

PATIENTS AND THEIR ENVIRONMENT

We end the book with brief comments about patients, for their care is the focus of this work. They are the raison d'être of medicine. Physicians are granted unique access into the pain, triumphs, and souls of their patients. William Carlos Williams, a great American writer and poet as well as a physician, used his observations as a physician to write about his patients and their lives. In order to understand patients, physicians must know them, their families, and their environments in the broadest sense. The patient is not a disease, but an individual whose life experience and personality are entwined with and determinative of the expression of their illness. Physicians work in and influence patients' environments as they relate to their sicknesses. Hospitals, clinics, offices, laboratories, academia, research personnel and research studies, lawyers, other physicians, consultants, and the media impact patients greatly, just as they impact physicians. But the impacts and influences are different. The physician should mentally put himself or herself in the role of the patient. In Part III we have tried to note the influence of the various sites of care, personnel, and institutions on patients as well as doctors. To be effective the clinician must understand the patient, in the very broadest sense, as well as the disease that the patient has.

16

The Ten Commandments of Doctoring

1. Always ask yourself: What would I want were I or one of my loved ones the patient?
2. Care about the patient and show it.
3. Listen to each patient. They want to tell you about their disease and about themselves.
4. Be thorough. Check and double check.
5. Be honest and straightforward.
6. Give the patient and the problem enough time.
7. Always deliver to all patients:
   Kindness
   Interest
   Thoughtfulness
   Concern
   Attention
   Respect
   Empathy
8. Learn as much about the patient as about the disease the patient has.
9. Find out what is wrong with each patient with as much detail and precision as possible.
10. Be a teacher. Doctors need to teach patients and their families about their disease and its likely course and management, and about their health and their risks of illness.

Index

Note: Page references followed by "f" denote figures; page references followed by "t" denote tables.